Total care of the stroke patient

Total care of the stroke patient

Mary T. O'Brien, R.N., M.S.

Neurological Nurse Clinician, Peter Bent Brigham Hospital, Division of the Affiliated Hospitals Center, Inc., Boston

Phyllis J. Pallett, R.N., M.P.H.

Lecturer, Institution for Social and Policy Studies, and Department of Epidemiology and Public Health, Yale University School of Medicine, New Haven. Formerly Director, Department of Patient Care Studies, Yale—New Haven Hospital

Little, Brown and Company, Boston

To the many patients and their families who have shared with us the difficulties they encountered and the triumphs they achieved in coping with stroke

Preface

According to national mortality statistics, death due to stroke appears to be decreasing continuously in many countries. It is still unclear whether this downward trend can be attributed to a reduction in the incidence of stroke, to an improvement in the survival rates for stroke victims, or simply to changes in the practice of coding the cause of death. In spite of the decline in the number of deaths from stroke, it still ranks as the third most common cause of death in the United States and many other countries.

In 1975, the mortality rate for stroke in the United States was 91.8 per 100,000. During any one year approximately half-a-million persons in our country will suffer a stroke; less than half of these people will survive beyond a month. Of these, only 10% will recover fully, 40% will be left with a mild disability, another 40% will be left severely disabled, and the remaining 10% will require care in an institution for the remainder of their lives. At any one time, roughly 2.5 million people in the United States are living with the disabilities common to stroke: hemiplegia, aphasia, and sensory and perceptual impairments, many also suffering from the complications of these disorders. Stroke is no respecter of age. While it is commonly thought of as a disease of the aged, it can and does occur in infancy, childhood, adolescence, and young adulthood. No single health problem places so heavy a demand on our nation's health care resources.

While stroke is a critical public health problem, its impact on the individual patient and his family cannot be expressed merely in epidemiologic terms. This devastating illness can render its victim totally helpless and incapable of communicating even the most basic needs.

Proper management of the patient with stroke depends on knowledge of the pathological process involved. Unfortunately, the complexity of the pathological processes involved in the stroke syndrome and the principles of care for them are poorly understood by many health care professionals. The purpose of this book is to familiarize health care practitioners with these pathological manifestations and their physiological basis and to provide standards for care. Since survival immediately following stroke and the quality of that survival beyond the acute phase depend in large part on meticulous nursing, these standards are for nursing care. This book grew out of a study of the effectiveness of certain nursing measures in the prevention and control of complications frequently occurring in the acute stage of stroke which inhibit effective rehabilitation. Complications of stroke involve all of the major body systems. Many can be prevented by nursing measures. This study, carried out at the Peter Bent Brigham Hospital, Boston, Massachusetts, showed that such complications could be prevented when patient care was organized according to a protocol designed to assist the nursing staff in patient assessment and the initiation of specific preventive and therapeutic measures.

Total Care of the Stroke Patient is directed primarily to the hospital nurse whose responsibilities in caring for patients with stroke run the gamut from acute lifesaving measures (such as providing respiratory support) to helping the family accommodate their home to the patient's sensory and motor deficits.

Our major goal is to help the nurse become aware of the variety and complexity of neurological dysfunctions that can occur in different patients depending upon the cause of the stroke and the area of the brain that is involved. We hope the nurse will be inspired to accept the responsibility for coordinating the various services the stroke patient requires from the initial stages of illness through the rehabilitative phase.

The text should also be helpful to nurses in the community and long-term care facilities and to therapists, physicians, social workers, and dieticians who care for patients with stroke in the hospital, long-term care facilities, and the community,

We wish to express our special thanks to our editors Christopher Campbell and Julie Stillman of Little, Brown for their continued support and advice, to Michele L'Heureux for her illustrations, to Gladys Caterinicchio and Kenneth Noyes for their diligence in typing the manuscript, and to our families for their patience and encouragement throughout the writing of this book. We also acknowledge with appreciation those people who read sections of the manuscript and offered helpful comments and suggestions, in particular: H. Richard Tyler, M.D., David Dawson, M.D., H. Harris Funkenstein, M.D., Joseph Alpert, M.D., Michael Moskowitz, M.D., Howard Zubick, Ph.D., Thomas McCourt, D.D.S., and Anne Burns, R.N.

M. T. O.
P. J. P.

Contents

Total care of the stroke patient

1. Introduction

DEFINITION

The term *stroke* or *cerebral vascular accident* (CVA) refers to an impairment of the cerebral circulation due to a pathological process in one or more of the blood vessels supplying the brain. Changes in cerebral tissue resulting from the impairment are due to ischemia, infarction, or hemorrhage. Brain tissue that is deprived of an adequate supply of blood and oxygen undergoes ischemic changes that can result in necrosis or infarction. When hemorrhage occurs in the brain, increased intracranial pressure exerted by the extravasated blood can also lead to infarction. Infarction of brain tissue is irreversible. The three pathological processes involved are (1) thrombus, (2) embolus, and (3) hemorrhage. It should be noted, however, that cerebral infarction may be present without definitive identification of any of these processes. The typical sequence of events is a relatively sudden development of a neurological deficit followed by a fairly rapid evolution of it. The neurological deficit reflects the size and location of the ischemic area, infarction, or hemorrhage. Usually the onset is a matter of seconds, minutes, or hours; however, the condition may develop over a period of several days. A *completed stroke* is the unchanging state after the maximum neurological deficit has been produced [1, 3].

The classic sign of cerebrovascular disease is *hemiplegia*. It occurs with lesions of either of the cerebral hemispheres and also may occur with lesions of the brainstem. Hemiplegia is a spastic or flaccid paralysis of one side of the body, including the extremities. Hemiparesis, a weakness of one side of the body, may also be seen. Sensation may remain intact on the affected side but frequently is impaired or absent. The paralysis or paresis is manifested on the opposite side of the body to the cerebral hemisphere in which the occlusion or rupture of the artery occurs. Other deficits accompanying hemiplegia or hemiparesis are homonymous hemianopsia and other visual defects, impairment of speech, impairment of cognitive functions, and perceptual deficits. Specific focal neurological signs of stroke, such as hemiparesis, quadriparesis, aphasia, homonymous hemianopsia, and ataxia, reflect the location of the lesion in the brain. When the initial insult does not terminate in death, partial or even complete recovery may take place in a relatively short period of time. For some patients, however, the process of recovery may extend to weeks or months. Evidence of ongoing restitution may continue to be seen for many months [1, 3].

In contrast to the sudden manifestation of an acute neurological impairment, there is often a slower process, referred to as a *progressing stroke* or "thrombus in evolution." Impairment develops gradually over hours or days [3]. During this time one particular sign or symptom may worsen, and new neurological defects may develop. Usually this slower evolution of stroke is caused by an increasing stenosis of the involved artery by a mural thrombus, with extension of the thrombus along the artery, blocking its branches and thereby interfering with collateral circulation. The thrombus may extend the entire length of the artery [1, 3].

TYPES OF STROKE

Cerebral thrombosis

The most common cause of cerebral infarction is atherosclerotic thrombosis. Atherosclerotic plaques usually form at the branching of blood vessels. Thrombosis will develop most readily wherever these atheromatous plaques have caused a narrowing of the vessels. The sites most frequently affected are (1) the internal carotid artery at the carotid sinus, (2) the bifurcation of the middle cerebral artery, (3) the junction of the vertebral and basilar arteries, (4) the posterior cerebral artery as it winds around the cerebral peduncle, and (5) the anterior cerebral artery as it curves over the corpus callosum [1, 3].

The process by which the thrombus builds up over the atherosclerotic area is not well understood. It is known, however, that development of atherosclerosis in the smaller cerebral vessels is influenced by hypertension. Hypertension and diabetes mellitus are the two major predisposing factors to atherosclerosis in the vascular system. During the evolution of a thrombotic stroke, prodromal transient ischemic attacks are seen which are thought to be the result of a partial occlusion of the affected artery. The state of the atherosclerotic vessels and the progression of signs and symptoms will vary from patient to patient. However, as the thrombus continues to develop, the neurological deficit may progress until a fully established stroke is manifested [1, 3].

CLINICAL PICTURE

In approximately eighty percent of the cases of stroke which are due to thrombosis there is a history of one or many transient ischemic attacks. These prodromal episodes signal the developing lesion or occlusion in a specific artery or its branches. Disease of the carotid and its branches will result in transitory hemiparasthesias, hemiplegia, monoplegia, confusion, blindness in one eye, or speech disturbance. When the vertebral and basilar arteries are affected, the attacks will consist of dizziness, diplopia, numbness, impaired vision, headaches, or dysarthria. Such warning attacks may start anywhere from months to hours before a full-blown stroke actually occurs [1, 3].

The main stroke resulting from thrombotic occlusion of a cerebral vessel can develop in any one of the following ways:

1. as a single attack completed within a period of several hours
2. intermittently progressing over a period of hours or days
3. as a partial stroke followed by a period of improvement and then by further neurological impairment
4. as several brief episodes of impairment followed by a longer attack and then by complete and permanent paralysis [3]

The signs of neurological impairment in patients with stroke vary depending on the collateral circulation available and on the location and size of the ischemic area or infarction resulting from the arterial occlusion. When the carotid system is involved, signs are usually unilateral: hemiplegia, hemianopsia, aphasia, and agnosia.

Bilateral motor and sensory signs along with disturbances of the cranial nerves, cerebellum, or brainstem will be found most commonly with occlusion of the basilar arterial system. A more detailed description of the differences in clinical picture according to the vessel involved is presented in a subsequent section.

LABORATORY FINDINGS
On lumbar puncture no blood will be found in the cerebrospinal fluid, and the pressure will be normal unless there is severe swelling due to an unusually large infarct. The skull film will also be normal, and the pineal will not be shifted from the midline unless there is severe cerebral edema. Electroencephalogram readings will often show a slower frequency and a lower voltage than normal. Computerized axial tomography (CAT scanning) can usually demonstrate small infarctions early. Arteriography demonstrates the occluded vessel and provides information about collateral blood flow [1, 3].

COURSE AND PROGNOSIS
The course of illness and immediate prognosis following cerebral thrombosis is difficult to foretell. Unfortunately, most often the clinical course is one of progression of the neurological deficit. This may involve a temporary worsening of the patient's condition for a day or so or a progression to total paralysis and coma. This progression is most likely related to increasing stenosis of the involved artery or to extension of the thrombus into adjacent vessels. With cerebral infarction, swelling of the necrotic tissue can result in increased intracranial pressure and even herniation of the brain [1, 3].

If the patient survives the initial insult, he usually improves eventually. This improvement can run the gamut from total recovery beginning in a few days, if the infarct is small, to little significant recovery after months of intensive therapy, when there has been a large infarct with severe neurological deficits. It appears that the longer the period before spontaneous movement of the affected limbs is seen, the poorer the prognosis for recovery of motor activity and speech. Hemianopsia persisting beyond a few weeks or any paralysis remaining five to six months following the stroke is usually permanent [1, 3]. Aphasia, dysarthria, and cerebellar ataxia, however, can continue to ameliorate for a year or longer, and sensory improvement has been known to continue for up to two years [1, 3, 5].

With paralysis resulting from stroke, the affected muscles are initially flaccid. Then spasticity develops, giving the patient the characteristic posture of a flexed, adducted arm and an extended, adducted leg. It is important to keep in mind that early development of spasticity is usually a positive indication for functional recovery, while slow development of this condition means that the patient is less likely to regain function [1, 3].

If infarction of the cerebral cortex has occurred, the patient may become subject to epileptic seizures. Patients with hypertension remain in danger of extension of the stroke or development of thrombosis in another area in the future [3].

TREATMENT
Treatment of a completed stroke due to cerebral thrombosis requires critical measures for management of the acute manifestations and also prompt initiation of

physical therapy and rehabilitation. Treatment of a thrombus still in evolution is directed toward halting progression of the stroke and restoring cerebral circulation. Prevention of factors predisposing to stroke is essential, whether a stroke has already been completed or not. Measures usually employed to improve cerebral circulation include bed rest in a horizontal position for 7 to 10 days, maintenance of systemic blood pressure, correction of anemia if it exists, and avoidance of over-sedation, rapid diuresis, and procedures which might interfere with cerebral blood flow and oxygen supply or precipitate a hypotensive episode [3].

Anticoagulant therapy may be prescribed as a preventive measure for patients with transient ischemic attacks or a thrombus in evolution. It is not used if there is even a remote possibility of hemorrhage.

Surgical procedures may be employed as a preventive measure if the location of a lesion causing transient ischemic attacks due to stenosis or early manifestations of a thrombus in evolution make endarterectomy and bypass grafts feasible [3]. New techniques of microsurgery may allow surgical repair in a larger number of cases than was once thought possible.

Transient ischemic attacks

CLINICAL PICTURE
The term *transient ischemic attack* (TIA) refers to brief, recurrent episodes of a neurological deficit that clears completely. These episodes usually happen prior to a thrombo-occlusive stroke and neuropathologic studies link them almost exclusively to atherosclerotic thrombosis [3, 8].

At the onset of such an attack the patient suddenly becomes aware of a functional loss. Depending upon whether the carotid or vertebral basilar circulation is involved, the loss of power takes place in the hand or foot and progresses rapidly to the entire extremity or side of the body. The patient may experience numbness, partial or complete loss of vision in one or both eyes, diplopia, dysarthria, vertigo, deafness, or "drop attacks" in which he or she has a sudden loss of awareness and falls to the ground. The attack rarely exceeds 30 minutes (but may in some cases last as long as 12 hours) with full recovery within 24 hours. Many very brief attacks lasting only seconds may occur in one day or there may be fewer than one per month. In all cases the findings on neurological examination are negative between attacks [1, 3, 5].

TREATMENT
Treatment may include anticoagulation or surgical endarterectomy, as already discussed under treatment of cerebral thrombosis.

COURSE AND PROGNOSIS
Approximately one third of the patients who suffer from transient ischemic attacks will later have cerebral infarction due to a thrombotic stroke. Another third will continue having these transient episodes without ever developing any permanent disability, while for an equal fraction the attacks will cease spontaneously [5].

Cerebral embolism

Embolism is the second most common pathological process of stroke. In most cases the embolic material has broken away from a thrombus within the heart and lodged within the cerebral hemispheres. Since three times more blood flows through the carotid artery (more than 300 ml/min) than through the vertebral (less than 100 ml/min), the majority of intracranial embolisms occur in the cerebral hemispheres, which are supplied by branches of the carotid. The middle cerebral artery is a direct continuation of the internal carotid artery, and nearly 80% of the blood which are supplied by branches of the carotid. The middle cerebral artery is a direct continuation of the internal carotid artery, and nearly 80% of the blood have a direct route into the middle cerebral artery and can lodge in any one of its branches. This is the area most frequently involved in ischemic infarction due to cerebral embolism.

Embolic material that enters the vertebral artery can cause an occlusion just below its junction with the basilar artery. However, the clot usually continues on through the basilar artery, which is larger, and may then become lodged at the point where the basilar artery bifurcates, causing deep coma and total paralysis. Most often it continues further to enter one or both of the posterior cerebral arteries, resulting in damage to the visual cortex and development of a unilateral or bilateral homonymous hemianopsia. While large masses of embolic material will occlude the larger vessels, the embolus frequently breaks up into such tiny particles that the resultant area of infarction goes undetected [1, 3, 5].

ETIOLOGY
Cerebral embolism is primarily a manifestation of heart and carotid artery disease. In young adults it usually occurs subsequent to rheumatic valvular disease, while in the older age groups it is most often the result of atherosclerosis. In either case it arises from blood clots forming in the heart which grow large enough to be forced into the circulatory system by the continued movement of the beating heart. Atrial fibrillation, therefore, will increase greatly the possibility of this occurring and is the commonest direct cause of cerebral embolism. Heart conditions that can lead to cerebral embolism are

1. active rheumatic endocarditis
2. postrheumatic valvular disease
3. bacterial endocarditis
4. myocardial infarction with mural thrombus
5. congenital heart disease
6. atrial fibrillation and other arrhythmias with arteriosclerotic, hypertensive, rheumatic, or congenital heart disease [3, 5].

Emboli composed of cholesterol crystals from atheromatous plaques lining the carotid, basilar, and vertebral arteries can also lodge in the cerebral vessels to cause infarction. Trauma to any portion of the vasculature can allow air or solid foreign particles to enter the blood and move to the brain, causing occlusion of a vessel. Fat embolism, although rare, can result either from particles of fat dislodged by trauma or by introduction of an oily substance for diagnostic or therapeutic purposes. Fat embolism is most often a complication of fracture of the long bones [1, 3, 5].

PATHOLOGICAL PHYSIOLOGY

The initial obstruction resulting from cerebral embolism usually occurs where the vessel bifurcates, since the lumen of the branches is smaller than that of the main vessel. It may cause an occlusion of one or both branches, resulting in hypoxia to the tissue normally perfused by the branches. If the embolus moves on to the more distal branches before irreversible damage occurs, neuron function will be restored. Often a large embolus will produce a severe but temporary neurological deficit that clears as the clot breaks up in its passage through the artery. It then passes in many small pieces into a small vessel that supplies a less vital portion of the brain [1, 5].

Quite unlike thrombosis, embolism develops very rapidly. There is therefore little opportunity for establishment of collateral circulation to supply the area distal to the occlusion [3].

CLINICAL FEATURES

Stroke due to cerebral embolism is characterized by a sudden loss of function with no warning signs. Embolism may strike at any time — whether the person is asleep or involved in strenuous physical activity — but it is more likely to occur when he or she is active. Usually the patient suffers an abrupt onset of hemiplegia or impairment of vision with no loss of consciousness. Aphasia will be present if the embolism occurs in the dominant hemisphere, but ordinarily the patient is alert and able to comprehend explanations. He may experience headache on the affected side. Unless a large embolism occludes a major vessel or there are multiple emboli with brainstem involvement, there will be no impairment of vital functions. Delirium, stupor, or coma will occur, however, with a brainstem infarct or secondary to increased intracranial pressure from cerebral edema. The precise neurological deficit manifested will reflect that area of the brain supplied by the occluded vessel. The most significant factors in identifying a stroke due to cerebral embolism are usually the acute onset of the neurological deficit and a history of a source of emboli. Evidence of peripheral emboli and presence of atrial fibrillation and/or valvular disease further reinforces the likelihood of embolism [1, 3, 5].

LABORATORY FINDINGS

No laboratory tests provide definitive proof that cerebral embolism has occurred. In the initial phase of the stroke the findings on analysis of cerebrospinal fluid, skull films, and scans ordinarily are within normal limits. An electroencephalogram may help to localize the lesion. Although arteriography may demonstrate the area of obstruction, it is usually not recommended when an intracranial embolism is suspected. A chest x-ray and urinalysis may provide supportive evidence by suggesting rheumatic heart disease or renal emboli, and the electrocardiogram will reveal cardiac arrhythmias or the presence of a silent myocardial infarction (MI), which may have led to the embolism [5].

As the clinical course progresses, test results change. Infarction of the tissue surrounding the embolism can become hemorrhagic, in which case an increased protein level and red blood cells will be found in the cerebrospinal fluid. The area of infarction will show up on a scan, and secondary edema resulting in displacement of the pineal body will be seen on the skull film [3, 5].

PROGNOSIS AND COURSE

The course of illness and immediate prognosis following cerebral embolism is as difficult to predict as it is for cerebral thrombosis. Massive brainstem infarction following embolic occlusion of the basilar artery is nearly always fatal. Most patients recover from cerebral embolism, some with no neurological deficits. When a patient dies, it is usually due to the secondary effects of cerebral edema. There may be a remarkable return of neurological functioning, with observable improvement just hours after the attack. This may be due to disappearance of arterial spasm or to the progression of the embolic material into smaller distal branches of the artery. The long-term prognosis depends largely on the severity of the underlying disease responsible for producing the embolism and the likelihood of subsequent embolization. Improvement in the resulting neurological deficits is identical to that described for cerebral thrombosis [3, 5].

TREATMENT

The treatment of patients who have suffered a cerebral embolism is directed toward (1) management of the acute manifestations of the arterial occlusion, (2) institution of therapeutic measures for the underlying systemic disease process in order to prevent any recurrent emboli, and (3) prompt initiation of rehabilitation procedures just as for patients with thrombosis [3, 5].

In the case of extracranial embolism, located either in the carotid, brachiocephalic, or subclavian arteries, the clot may be surgically removed. Newer techniques of microsurgery allow surgical intervention for intracranial arterial obstruction in some cases.

If the heart has been identified as the source of the embolism, bed rest will be prescribed during the initial phase to keep the heart rate down and discourage further distribution of embolic material.

Anticoagulants have proved effective in prevention of embolism associated with atrial fibrillation, myocardial infarction, and prosthetic heart valves. Since cerebral infarction secondary to embolism may become hemorrhagic, administration of anticoagulants during the acute phase of embolic stroke is not without risk. However, clinical evidence suggests that anticoagulant therapy does not increase the degree of hemorrhage within a hemorrhagic infarct. Therefore, unless there is gross hemorrhage, as demonstrated on lumbar puncture, and CAT scan is normal, anticoagulant therapy is usually instituted.

Intracranial hemorrhage

The third most common cause of stroke is intracranial hemorrhage. In most cases hemorrhage is due to hypertension or to rupture of a saccular aneurysm. Hypertension results in hemorrhage within the brain tissue, whereas a ruptured saccular aneurysm bleeds into the subarachnoid space. These two causes of intracranial hemorrhage will be discussed separately.

HYPERTENSIVE INTRACRANIAL HEMORRHAGE
It is not known precisely what vascular lesion leads to the rupture of the vessel in hypertensive intracerebral hemorrhage. The rupture usually occurs in the arteries that penetrate the brain itself rather than in the circle of Willis [3, 5].

Extravasation of blood from an intracerebral hemorrhage due to hypertension will create a mass that compresses and displaces adjacent brain tissue. As bleeding continues, the mass increases in size. In the case of a large hemorrhage, the vital centers will be compromised. Coma and death may ensue. Extravasated blood from a large hemorrhage may seep into the ventricles, causing the spinal fluid to be bloody on lumbar puncture. If the hemorrhage is small and occurs away from the ventricles, the spinal fluid may never become bloody [1, 3, 5].

The most common sites of hemorrhage, according to Mohr, Fisher, and Adams [3], due to hypertension are, in order of frequency

1. the putamen and adjacent internal capsule (50% of all cases)
2. various parts of the central white matter
3. the thalamus
4. the cerebellar hemisphere
5. the pons

Clinical picture. With intracerebral hemorrhage, stroke occurs abruptly, most often without warning and while the patient is up and active. It evolves steadily and usually rapidly, although its duration can be from minutes to days, depending upon the rate of bleeding. Severe headache is a common symptom, and vomiting may also occur at the onset. Hypertension will be noted. Although the patient may be alert initially, coma ensues if the bleeding is massive. Some patients have focal seizures [3].

With intracerebral hemorrhage due to hypertension there is usually only one episode of bleeding, without recurrence. Resorption of the extravasated blood will take place slowly, over a period of weeks or months [1, 3, 5].

The particular neurological signs and symptoms seen will depend on the site of bleeding and the size of the hemorrhage. With *putaminal hemorrhage,* which affects the internal capsule, the patient has a gradual loss of power in the facial muscles, arm, and leg, with slurred speech or aphasia and deviation of the eyes away from the paralyzed limbs. As the stroke evolves, the hemiplegia may worsen, and the patient may become stuporous. A large hemorrhage will cause compression of the upper brainstem, resulting in coma, irregular breathing, fixed dilated pupils, and occasionally decerebrate posturing [3, 8].

Thalamic hemorrhage can also affect the internal capsule, causing hemiplegia, usually with a greater sensory than motor loss. Bleeding into the subthalamic area will cause a variety of ocular disturbances, including deviation of eyes downward and pupils unreactive to light. If bleeding occurs in the dominant hemisphere, the patient may become dysphasic.

Cerebellar hemorrhage causes repeated vomiting. The patient will also complain of an occipital headache and inability to walk. Dysphagia and dysarthria are usually symptoms, and there will be oculomotor disturbances, including deviation of the eyes laterally. The patient will remain conscious unless bleeding is extensive and causes brainstem compression [1, 3, 8].

Usually *pontine hemorrhage* is fatal within a very short time. In the early stage contralateral hemiplegia and homolateral facial paralysis are present, but complete paralysis, coma, and decerebrate rigidity ensue rapidly. The eyeballs are fixed, with tiny reactive pupils, and are permanently deviated away from the side of the lesion. Deepening coma, rapid rise in temperature, and extension of paralysis to both sides of the body are all ominous signs since they indicate extension of bleeding into the ventricles [8].

Laboratory findings. The CAT scan has revolutionized the diagnosis of intracerebral hemorrhage and is particularly helpful in identifying small hemorrhages that were previously unrecognized clinically. In the absence of CAT scan equipment, examination of cerebrospinal fluid is extremely important in establishing whether an intracerebral hemorrhage has occurred. Spinal fluid is most often bloody and under pressure. Lumbar puncture is not without risk in patients with cerebral hemorrhage, since the procedure may lead to increased herniation. In contrast to cerebral thrombosis, in which skull x-ray is usually normal, a shift of the calcified pineal gland from the midline away from the side of the hemorrhage may be noted on the skull film [3, 5].

Course and prognosis. The prognosis in cases of massive cerebral hemorrhage is extremely grim. Putaminal, thalamic, cerebellar, and pontine hemorrhage are all usually large, and approximately seventy percent of patients afflicted with this type of stroke die as a result of brainstem compression within a very short time. When the hemorrhage is small, prognosis for complete recovery, once the extravasated blood is absorbed, is good, since rebleed is not likely and there may have been no destruction of brain tissue. (The hemorrhage may push the brain tissue aside rather than destroy it.) However, 75% of all patients with intracerebral hemorrhage die because bleeding extends into the ventricles or causes midbrain compression and possibly herniation [3, 8].

Treatment. Very little can be done to control the hemorrhage or restore damaged tissue. Treatment is supportive, directed to decreasing intracranial pressure and managing the acute manifestations of the stroke. In *cerebellar hemorrhage* surgical intervention with evacuation of the clot may be necessary as a lifesaving measure to prevent herniation. Surgical procedure in other areas has not been successful [3, 5].

RUPTURED SACCULAR ANEURYSM

Saccular aneurysms are small, thin-walled outpouchings which develop on the arteries that form the circle of Willis and on their major branches. Frequently these sac-like formations are referred to as "berry" aneurysms. They are usually found at the bifurcations of the vessels. They range from 2 mm to as large as 3 cm in diameter, with an average diameter of approximately 8 to 10 mm. They vary in shape as well as size. Some are blister-like protrusions from the artery, some appear as round sacs attached to the vessel by a slender stalk, while others develop a narrow cylindrical shape [1, 3, 8].

It is thought that saccular aneurysms result from developmental defects of the arterial wall, developing over years in parallel with the evolution of the arterial defect. The aneurysms themselves are not congenital anomalies. Protrusion of the artery at the site of the defect will occur and enlarge gradually over time. Eventually the arterial wall at the dome of the aneurysm may rupture. These aneurysms are rare in children and are seen most frequently in patients between the ages of 35 and 65 years [3].

The majority of saccular aneurysms according to Mohr, Fisher, and Adams [3] (90–95%) are found on one of the following sites of the anterior portion of the circle of Willis:

1. in the anterior communicating artery
2. where the posterior communicating artery arises from the internal carotid artery
3. at the first bifurcation of the middle cerebral artery
4. where the internal carotid artery bifurcates to form the middle cerebral artery and the anterior cerebral artery [3].

Clinical picture. In most cases saccular aneurysms cause no symptoms and therefore go undetected unless rupture occurs. Occasionally, very large aneurysms cause symptoms by compression of adjacent nerves prior to rupture. Minor leakage may precede rupture and may cause a warning headache. Rupture of saccular aneurysms occurs most often when the patient is active and often is precipitated by sexual intercourse or other physical exertion. With rupture there will be hemorrhage under pressure into the subarachnoid space, and one of the three following patterns will be noted:

1. sudden occurrence of excruciating headache followed immediately by loss of consciousness
2. sudden excruciating headache without loss of consciousness
3. sudden loss of consciousness with no other symptom [1, 3]

With massive hemorrhage, death may ensue within minutes or following several days of deep coma due to intracerebral dissection into the ventricles. If the hemorrhage is small, there may be no loss of consciousness or it may be regained within minutes. The patient will remain confused for as long as ten days and experience severe headache and stiff neck. There will be no lateralizing neurological signs if bleeding is confined to the subarachnoid space. However, if there is intracerebral clot formation or cerebral infarction in the area surrounding the site of rupture, the patient will become comatose, and lateralizing signs such as hemiplegia or aphasia will be seen [3].

Mohr, Fisher, and Adams have outlined specific neurological manifestations that can help to identify the location of the hemorrhage [3]. *Third nerve palsy* is indicative of rupture of an aneurysm at the junction of the posterior communicating artery and the internal carotid artery. The patient will have ptosis of the eyelid, diplopia, mydriasis, and oculomotor paralysis. A brief initial episode of *lower limb paralysis* (in one or both legs) can indicate hemorrhage from an aneurysm of the anterior communicating artery which caused ischemia of the motor areas. *Hemiparesis* or *aphasia* suggests impaired circulation due to rupture of an aneurysm at the bifurcation of the middle cerebral artery. A unilateral blindness usually denotes rupture of an aneurysm which lies anteromedially in the circle of Willis. *Akinetic mutism* with no loss of consciousness is indicative of rupture of the anterior communicating artery which has caused ischemia or hemorrhage into the frontal lobes, hypothalamus, or corpus callosum [3, 8].

Laboratory findings. The cerebrospinal fluid is usually grossly bloody following rupture of a saccular aneurysm and is under extremely high pressure. Leukocytosis is commonly seen. Skull films are generally normal. However, if a subdural or intracerebral clot has formed, the pineal gland may be shifted from the midline. CAT scanning will show a localized clot adjacent to the ruptured aneurysm but carotid and vertebral angiography is the only certain means of showing the aneurysm. The electroencephalogram has little to offer but may corroborate clinical findings when there is a neurological deficit [1, 3].

Course and prognosis. Unfortunately hemorrhage due to rupture of a saccular aneurysm tends to recur. The first major hemorrhage is fatal for approximately fifty percent of patients. A significant proportion of those who survive will die as a result of a subsequent hemorrhage occurring within 6–12 months following the first attack. The prognosis for this condition is grave, especially when rebleeding occurs shortly after the first attack [1, 3].

Treatment. Treatment is directed toward (1) decreasing arterial blood pressure in order to stop the bleeding and prevent a recurrence and (2) management of the acute manifestations of the stroke. The patient is kept at absolute bed rest for 4–8 weeks. Care of the patient is planned around avoiding any form of exertion including coughing, vomiting, straining at stool, and seizure activity. The patient should always be fed by the nurse. Medications may be prescribed to control seizures, nausea and vomiting, and blood pressure. According to Mohr, Fisher, and Adams [3], a systemic antifibrolysin (Amicar) which is administered intravenously to prevent lysis of the clot at the site of the ruptured aneurysm, seems to reduce the recurrence of hemorrhage significantly. Intravenous therapy is instituted cautiously to prevent increased intracerebral pressure.

Surgical intervention may be required for evacuation of an intracerebral clot. Ligation of the common carotid artery or intracranial resection of the aneurysm itself may also be carried out to prevent recurrence of hemorrhage. Since communicating hydrocephalus can occur following rupture of an aneurysm, ventricular shunting may also be required [1, 3].

Table 1-1 contrasts some of the clinical manifestations of the early stage of strokes caused by thrombus, embolism, hemorrhage, and rupture of saccular aneurysms.

Table 1-1
Clinical manifestations found in the early stage of stroke

Clinical Manifestation	Type of Stroke			
	Thrombosis	Embolism	Hypertensive Hemorrhage	Ruptured Aneurysm
Prodromal warning	Often	No	No	Infrequently
Development	Intermittent	Sudden	Gradual	Sudden
Quick reversal	Possible	Possible	Never	Possible
Bloody CSF	No	Uncommon	Nearly always	Always
Headache	Not infre-quently	Not infre-quently	Often, not always	Often
Coma	Not usually	Not usually	Often	Often
Hypertension	Often	Not neces-sarily	Nearly always	Often
Nucchal rigidity	No	No	Yes	Yes
Signs of carotid occlusion	Often	No	No	No
Onset during sleep	Often	Rarely	Almost never	Almost never

CLINICAL PICTURE ACCORDING TO VESSELS INVOLVED

The syndromes produced by stroke depend upon the site of the vascular occlusion, infarction, or hemorrhage. A description of the syndromes accompanying involvement of the major vessels and their branches follows.

Middle cerebral artery

The middle cerebral artery is one of the two terminal branches of the internal carotid artery. The middle cerebral artery and its branches are more frequently affected by stroke than any of the other cerebral vessels. Usually the infarction is due to embolic occlusion. This artery provides 80% of the blood supply to the cerebral hemispheres [3].

The branches of the middle cerebral artery supply (1) the putamen and caudate nucleus except for the frontal portion, (2) the lateral section of the globus pallidus, and (3) those sections of the anterior limb, genu, and posterior limb adjacent to the putamen. When the middle cerebral artery is occluded at the origin, the blood flow to the penetrating vessels as well as to the superficial vessels will be blocked, resulting in superficial as well as deep middle cerebral infarction. This will appear as the classic picture of (1) contralateral hemiplegia including paralysis of the face, arm, and leg, (2) hemianesthesia, and (3) homonymous hemianopsia. If the lesion occurs in the dominant hemisphere, the patient will also have aphasia. If the nondominant hemisphere is involved, his speech will remain intact, but he will have apractagnosia: He may neglect half the space surrounding him and half his body. There will be distortion of visual coordinates and inaccurate localization in half his field of vision. Consequently, his ability to judge distances will be impaired, with visual-spatial disorientation and disturbance in body image. There may be visual illusions with upside-down reading and loss of topographic memory. If sufficient collateral circulation is established, the resulting ischemia will be limited, thereby reducing the number of these signs and symptoms [3, 4].

Occlusion of any branch of the middle cerebral artery will result in a corresponding partial deficit. If the superior division of the middle cerebral artery region is involved, there will be sensorimotor disturbances. With dominant hemisphere lesions this will be accompanied by aphasia. Wernicke's aphasia is associated with occlusion of the lower division [3].

The individual penetrating branches of the middle cerebral artery which supply the internal capsule and putamen may also become occluded. Involvement of the internal capsule will result in a motor hemiplegia; when the thalamus is affected, there will be a hemisensory defect. Occlusion in the area of the midbrain will produce the syndrome of hemiparesis with cerebellar ataxia on the same side. In the area of the pons, occlusion will result in dysarthria, with a clumsy hand or hemiplegia [3, 8].

Anterior cerebral artery

The anterior cerebral artery arises from the internal carotid artery. It supplies (1) the cortex of the motor area of the lower limb and the motor pathways to the head and arm in the internal capsule; (2) the septal area located on the medial surface between the two hemispheres, which influences consciousness, and (3) the corpus callosum with pathways from the dominant hemisphere to the motor area of the nondominant hemisphere, interruption of which can result in apraxia [4].

The syndrome accompanying stroke in the territory of the anterior cerebral artery is not yet well defined. The outcome of stroke in this area depends on the size of infarction and can vary from patient to patient according to differences in the anatomical structure of the circle of Willis. It is known, however, that occlusion of this artery or its branches results in contralateral hemiplegia with cortical sensory loss over the leg. The arm may also be affected, but to a much lesser degree. Urinary incontinence, lack of spontaneity, and gait apraxia may also result. When occlusion of a common anterior cerebral stem causes bilateral infarction, there will be paraplegia with profound mental symptoms. When only one of these arteries is occluded, collateral circulation is usually supplied by the other [3, 8].

Internal carotid artery

The entire brain receives its blood supply from two sets of arteries: the internal carotids and the vertebral arteries. The vertebral arteries will be discussed subsequently.

As is true of stroke in the area of the anterior cerebral artery, occlusion of the internal carotid by a thrombus or embolism can produce widely differing manifestations, from a completely asymptomatic stroke to a massive fatal infarction. This is so because of (1) anatomical differences in patients' cerebrovascular systems, (2) the possibility of a previous asymptomatic occlusion of the opposite internal carotid, (3) and the many structures and major vessels supplied by the internal carotids. The middle cerebral arteries, anterior cerebral arteries, and anterior choroidal arteries all derive directly from the internal carotids. The internal carotid artery also supplies the optic nerve and retina [3, 4].

In most cases occlusion of the internal carotid results in stroke in the territory of the middle cerebral artery. The syndrome produced is the same as that of middle cerebral artery occlusion (already discussed), usually with contralateral hemiplegia and aphasia, if there is a lesion of the dominant hemisphere. If, however, the anterior communicating artery, which joins the two anterior cerebral arteries, is small, the anterior cerebral territory will also be affected. If both anterior cerebral arteries derive from a common stem, infarction of the anterior cerebral territory may occur bilaterally. In some people the posterior cerebral artery arises from the internal carotid rather than from the basilar artery. Such a person with occlusion of the internal carotid artery may experience contralateral or bilateral homonymous hemianopia, apraxia of ocular movements, verbal dyslexia, memory defect, topographic disorientation, and possibly visual hallucinations. Patients whose stroke involves the combined territories of several major arteries are always considerably less responsive than those with more limited involvement. The area supplied by the anterior choroidal artery can also become infarcted by occlusion of the internal carotid artery [3, 8].

It is important to note that when one internal carotid artery is occluded and collateral flow is restricted, the most distal portions of the anterior cerebral and middle cerebral territories will be affected. In such a case, paresthesias and weakness of the upper extremity and possibly of the face and tongue will be seen [3].

Since the internal carotid supplies the optic nerve and retina, progressive occlusion of the internal carotid may produce transient warning attacks of blindness in one eye. This happens to approximately twenty-five percent of the patients who eventually suffer major strokes due to occlusion of the internal carotid artery [3].

Vertebral—basilar—posterior cerebral system

POSTERIOR CEREBRAL ARTERY
The posterior cerebral artery arises from the bifurcation of the basilar artery. It and its branches supply (1) most of the diencephalon, (2) the midbrain, (3) the medial and lateral portions of the thalamus, (4) the visual cortex, (5) the lateral and lower surface of the occipital lobe, (6) the choroid plexus of the lateral and third ventricles, (7) the hippocampus, and (8) portions of the tegmentum [4].

The signs and symptoms arising from occlusion of the posterior cerebral artery will vary with the exact location and size of the resultant infarct and with the extent of collateral circulation available to prevent ischemia. The sign most often associated with stroke in the posterior cerebral artery area is homonymous hemianopsia due to damage of the calcarine cortex. Bilateral homonymous hemianopsia and cortical blindness can also occur with bilateral occipital lobe involvement. Frequently some portion of the visual field remains intact. The patient may be unaware of his visual defect. He may also be unable to perceive certain movements or objects not centrally located. He may run into objects or be unable to enumerate them. Some lesions produce extreme visual distortion [3, 8].

When the obstruction is located close to the basilar artery, where the posterior cerebral artery has its origin, evidence of damage to the thalamus, cerebral peduncle, and midbrain will be seen. The *thalamic syndrome* occurs when the sensory region of the thalamus becomes infarcted. This results in a sensory loss or diminution on the opposite side of the body. This loss may be manifested in a number of ways. Usually both deep and superficial sensation are affected including pain, temperature, touch, and proprioception or position sense. On occasion only one or two of these sensory modalities will be involved, e.g., pain and temperature. Position sense is the most frequently affected. The patient may suffer disabling intractable pain, which he will describe as "torturing" or "agonizing," in response to any stimulus in the affected parts. Various manifestations of motor disability may arise, such as hemiballismus, choreoathetosis, incoordination, intention tremor, asynergy, and muscle spasms [3, 7].

Occlusion of branches supplying the red nucleus will produce a gross ataxia on the opposite side of the body. Third nerve palsy may also be seen. Infarction of the posterior commissure area will be evidenced by a paralysis of the conjugate verticle gaze. Intracerebral hemorrhage in the peduncle as well as infarction due to occlusion of branches of the posterior cerebral artery supplying that area can result in hallucinations. With infarction of the midbrain, deep coma and decerebrate posturing will be present.

VERTEBRAL ARTERY
The vertebral arteries arise from the subclavian artery, follow the anterolateral surfaces of the medulla, and join to form the basilar artery at the caudal border of the pons. With the internal carotid arteries they are the source of blood supply to the entire brain. The vertebral arteries supply (1) the medulla, (2) the lower section of the pyramid, (3) the medial lemniscus, (4) the lateral medullary region, (5) the restiform body, and (6) the posteroinferior part of the cerebellar hemisphere [2, 3].

The outcome of infarction due to occlusion of the vertebral arteries will vary. Occlusion of one artery may be asymptomatic if collateral circulation from the circle of Willis is able to provide an adequate blood supply. It is well known, however, that there is considerable size difference between the two vertebrals. In a few cases only one of the two is large enough to provide a blood supply to the brain. Blockage of this artery would in effect result in bilateral infarction, which is identical to the basilar artery syndrome (described next).

The clinical picture most often seen with occlusion of the vertebral artery is referred to as the *lateral medullary syndrome*. It is due to infarction of a small section of the medulla when one or more of the five vertebral branches supplying the medulla become occluded. The patient may experience pain, numbness, or impaired sensation over the face. He may develop ataxia and falling to the affected side. Vertigo, nausea, and vomiting as well as nystagmus and diplopia may occur if the vestibular nucleus is involved. Dysphagia, hoarseness along with paralysis of the palate and vocal cord, and impaired gag reflex will result when the ninth and tenth nerve fibers are affected. When the spinothalamic tracts are affected, the patient will have diminished pain and thermal sense on the side of the body opposite to the lesion [3, 8].

BASILAR ARTERY
As has already been described, the basilar artery is formed by the junction of the two vertebral arteries at the lower border of the pons. It then subdivides to form the two posterior cerebral arteries. The basilar artery supplies (1) the pons, (2) the upper part of the cerebellum, and often (3) the posterior cerebral areas as well [4].

Thrombosis in the basilar system is most likely to occur in one of the branches of the basilar artery. These are (1) the paramedian branches that supply portions of the pons, (2) the short circumferential branches that supply the lateral sections of the pons and the middle and superior cerebellar peduncles, and (3) the long circumferential branches that supply the cerebellar hemispheres [3].

Basilar occlusion due to thrombosis may be due to an atherosclerotic plaque in the artery itself, occlusion of both vertebral arteries, or occlusion of one when the lumen of the other is unusually narrow. Embolism usually occurs where the basilar artery bifurcates to form the posterior cerebral arteries or within one of these two arteries. Occlusion of the basilar artery will produce a combination of various brainstem syndromes as well as those syndromes associated with occlusion in the area of the posterior cerebral artery. These include bilateral motor and sensory impairment with cerebellar and cranial nerve abnormalities [1, 3].

The most common signs of occlusion in the branches of the basilar artery are (1) cerebellar ataxia on the side of the lesion; (2) nausea and vomiting; (3) slurred speech; (4) loss of sensation of pain and temperature over the face, trunk, and extremities of the opposite side; (5) Horner's syndrome, dizziness, nystagmus, tinnitus, or deafness and disorders of ocular movements; and (6) hemiplegia [3].

Before a major stroke due to total occlusion of the basilar artery by thrombosis, symptoms of basilar insufficiency due to gradual stenosis of the artery usually have been present for some time. The syndrome associated with complete basilar artery occlusion includes (1) paralysis of all extremities; (2) diplopia, paralysis of conjugate lateral and/or vertical gaze, and horizontal and/or vertical nystagmus; (3) blindness, impaired vision, or various visual field defects; (4) bilateral cerebellar ataxia; and (5) coma [1, 3]. With a brainstem lesion there will be bilateral motor and sensory signs because the tracts for both sides of the body run in close proximity.

REFERENCES

1. Alpers, B. J., and Mancoll, E. L. *Clinical Neurology*. Philadelphia: Davis, 1971. Pp. 189–250.
2. Carpenter, M. B. *Core Text of Neuroanatomy*. Baltimore: Williams & Wilkins, 1974. Pp. 1832–1868.
3. Mohr, J. P., Fisher, C. M., and Adams, R. D. Cerebrovascular Disease. In G. W. Thorn et al. (eds.), *Harrison's Principles of Internal Medicine* (8th ed.). New York: McGraw-Hill, 1977. Pp. 1832–1868.
4. Smith, C. G. *Basic Neuroanatomy* (2nd ed.). Toronto: University of Toronto Press, 1971. Pp. 222–246.
5. Toole, J. R., and Patel, A. N. *Cerebrovascular Disorders*. New York: McGraw-Hill, 1974. Pp. 187–197; 215–225; 332–343.
6. Tyler, H. R., and Funkenstein, H. The diagnosis and treatment of stroke. *Primary Cardiology* 2:4, April, 1976.
7. Victor, M., and Adams, R. D. Disorders of Sensation. In G. W. Thorn et al. (eds.), *Harrison's Principles of Internal Medicine* (8th ed.). New York: McGraw-Hill, 1977. Pp. 109–114.
8. Walton, J. *Brain's Diseases of the Nervous System* (8th ed.). New York: Oxford, 1977. Pp. 311–374.

2. Anatomy and physiology of the brain

The brain consists of three major sections — the cerebrum, the cerebellum, and the brainstem — which rest within the cranial cavity of the skull. The foramen magnum, a large opening at the base of the cranial vault, allows for communication of the cranial cavity with the vertebral canal. It is through this foramen that the medulla, which is the distal portion of the brainstem, connects with the spinal cord. Because of its soft gelatinous consistency, the brain would be particularly vulnerable to trauma without adequate protection. Therefore, it is encased within the rigid structure of the skull, which is lined by three sets of membranes, the meninges. The meninges surround the brain and provide support and protection for it. The meninges are called the dura mater, the arachnoid mater, and the pia mater [2, 5, 13] (Fig. 2-1).

The outermost meningeal layer, the *dura mater,* consists of relatively inelastic dense connective tissue. This dural layer gives rise to several deep folds or septa, which separate the cranial cavity into compartments. The largest of these septa is the *falx cerebri,* which divides the cranium into the two compartments that house the cerebral hemispheres. The second septum, the *tentorium cerebelli,* provides a separation between the section that houses the cerebral hemispheres and that of the cerebellum. A third septum, the *falx cerebelli,* serves to divide the compartments in which the two lobes of the cerebellum rest. The dura receives its major blood supply from the middle meningeal artery, a branch of the maxillary artery which enters the skull through the foramen spinosum [5].

The middle meningeal layer, the *arachnoid mater,* is a very delicate, web-like, nonvascular membrane. It is separated from the dura mater by a potential space known as the *subdural space,* and from the pia or innermost meningeal layer by the *subarachnoid space,* which is filled with cerebrospinal fluid. The arachnoid passes over the sulci without dipping into them. Except in the depths of the sulci the sub-arachnoid space is quite narrow over the convexity of the cerebral hemispheres. At the base of the brain and surrounding the brainstem there are wide separations between the arachnoid and pia layers. These are referred to as *subarachnoid cisterna.* The largest is the cerebromedullary, or *cisterna magna,* between the medulla and cerebellum, through which cerebrospinal fluid flows from the fourth ventricle [5].

The innermost meningeal layer, the *pia mater,* is a vascular membrane which is closely adherent to the surface of the brain, following the convolutions and dipping into the sulci. The cortical distribution of the cerebral arteries and veins lies upon the surface of the pia, within the subarachnoid space. The blood vessels that are integral parts of the choroid plexuses are carried by the pia mater into the ventricles where cerebrospinal fluid is formed. The outer surface of the brain wall in the area of the ventricles adheres firmly to the pia to provide anchorage of the choroid plexuses within the ventricles [2, 5, 14].

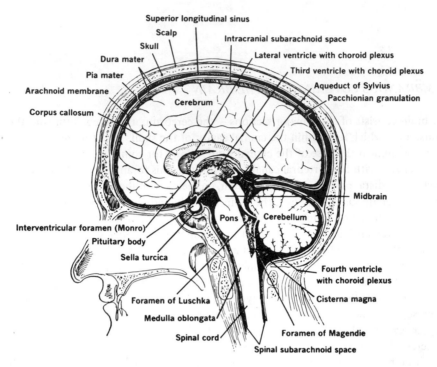

Superior longitudinal sinus
Scalp
Skull
Intracranial subarachnoid space
Dura mater
Lateral ventricle with choroid plexus
Pia mater
Third ventricle with choroid plexus
Arachnoid membrane
Aqueduct of Sylvius
Pacchionian granulation
Corpus callosum
Cerebrum
Midbrain
Interventricular foramen (Monro)
Pons
Cerebellum
Pituitary body
Sella turcica
Fourth ventricle
with choroid plexus
Cisterna magna
Foramen of Luschka
Medulla oblongata
Spinal cord
Foramen of Magendie
Spinal subarachnoid space

Figure 2-1
Lateral view of the head showing the brain and meninges in relation to the skull.
(From Esta Carini and Guy Owens. Neurological and Neurosurgical Nursing *[6th*
ed.]. St. Louis: The C. V. Mosby Co., 1974.)

CEREBROSPINAL FLUID AND VENTRICULAR SYSTEM

VENTRICLES

The ventricular system consists of four interconnected cavities, called ventricles,
located within the brain and the brainstem. They are identified as the two lateral,
the third, and the fourth ventricles. Each of the two *lateral ventricles* is located in
one of the cerebral hemispheres. Each lateral ventricle is divided into an anterior
horn, located within the frontal lobe; a body, located in the parietal lobe; a posterior horn, in the occipital lobe; and an inferior horn, in the temporal lobe. Both
lateral ventricles communicate with the centrally located *third ventricle* via the
foramen of Monro, which is also referred to as the *interventricular foramen.*
The third ventricle communicates with the *fourth ventricle* through the *aqueduct*
or foramen of Sylvius. The floor of the fourth ventricle is formed by the pons
and medulla, and the cerebellum forms its roof. There are three openings in
the fourth ventricle that serve to connect it with the subarachnoid space. These
are the two lateral *foramina of Luschka* and the *foramen of Magendie* [14],
(Fig. 2-1).

CEREBROSPINAL FLUID

Cerebrospinal fluid (CSF) is formed in the choroid plexus, which consists of tufts of dilated capillaries that project into the walls of the ventricles. Two large strips of choroid plexus are located in the floor of the lateral ventricles, and smaller ones are located in the roofs of the third and fourth ventricles. Cerebrospinal fluid flows from the lateral ventricles through the foramen of Monro to the third ventricle, then on through the aqueduct of Sylvius to the fourth ventricle, and through the apertures of the fourth ventricle to circulate through the subarachnoid space surrounding the brain and spinal cord. Most of the fluid is returned to the venous system by the *arachnoid villi.* These are tufted prolongations of the cerebral pia and arachnoid meninges which protrude into the venous sinuses. It is estimated that approximately 45–130 milliliters of cerebrospinal fluid are produced daily. The system normally contains about 125 milliliters. Under normal conditions cerebrospinal fluid is clear and colorless with a specific gravity of 1.004 to 1.007. It is composed of small amounts of glucose, protein, and potassium and relatively large amounts of sodium chloride [5, 6].

Cerebrospinal fluid serves to cushion the delicate structures of the central nervous system against trauma. It also provides a pathway for chemical substances to reach the intercellular spaces of the brain. Since the brain is confined within a rigid bony structure, the combined volume of cerebrospinal fluid, intracranial blood, and brain tissue must be kept fairly constant to prevent injury of the brain tissue resulting from pressure against the cranium. Any increase in volume of any one of these three components will be at the expense of one or both of the other two [5].

CEREBRAL HEMISPHERES

Structure

The cerebrum, the largest part of the brain, is divided into two hemispheres, the right and the left. The surface of the cerebrum is composed of highly convoluted layers of gray cortex. The ridges of the convolutions are called *gyri* and the furrows between them, *sulci.* These surface markings are useful in identifying the position of functional areas of the brain. The two hemispheres are partially separated from each other by the *longitudinal fissure,* into which a dural septum, the falx cerebri, fits. The longitudinal fissure completely separates the frontal and occipital regions of the two cerebral hemispheres. In the central section of the cerebrum, however, the fissure extends only to the level of the corpus callosum, a broad band of fibers that connects the two hemispheres and that plays an important role in interhemispheric transfers of learned discriminations, sensory experience, and memory [5, 14].

The *lateral surfaces* of the two hemispheres as shown in Figure 2-2 are highly irregular due to the many sulci created by infolding of the cerebral cortex. This arrangement allows for an increase in the cortical area without an actual increase of the surface area of the two hemispheres. The lateral sulcus (*sylvian fissure*) separates the frontal and temporal lobes. The central sulcus or *sulcus of Rolando* separates the frontal lobe from the parietal [5].

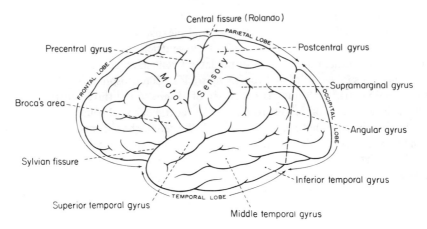

Figure 2-2
Lateral view of the left cerebral hemisphere. (From John F. Simpson and Kenneth R.
Magee. Clinical Evaluation of the Nervous System. *Boston: Little, Brown and*
Company, 1973.)

The medial surface of the cerebral hemispheres can only be exposed by dissection
of the brain along the midsagittal plane, as shown in Figure 2-3. Here the cortical
convolutions are flatter than those on the outer convexity. The interhemispheric
commissure, the *corpus callosum,* which serves to connect the two cerebral hemispheres, is the most prominent structure on the medial surface. It is composed of myelinated fibers and forms the floor of the longitudinal fissure and part of the roof of the
lateral ventricle. The callosal sulcus separates it from the gyrus that lies above it [5].

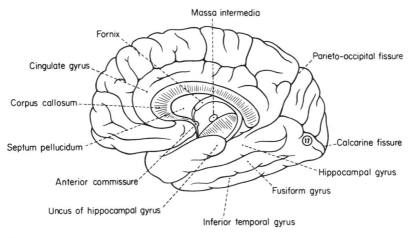

Figure 2-3
Medial view of the right cerebral hemisphere. (From John F. Simpson and
Kenneth R. Magee. Clinical Evaluation of the Nervous System. *Boston: Little,*
Brown and Company, 1973.)

The *inferior surface of the cerebrum* is divided by the base of the lateral sulcus into two parts. The posterior or tentorial part, which consists of the inferior surface of the temporal and occipital lobe, rests on the tentorium cerebelli and the middle cranial fossa. The anterior or orbital part consists of the orbital surface of the frontal lobe, which is divided by the olfactory sulcus. The olfactory bulb and tract lie within this sulcus [5, 13] (Fig. 2-4).

Topography of the cerebral hemispheres

The cerebral hemispheres each consist of five lobes, divided by fissures and sulci (Figs. 2-2, 2-3, and 2-4). These lobes are somewhat arbitrarily defined according to the bones of the skull that lie above them: (1) frontal, (2) parietal, (3) temporal, (4) occipital, and (5) central or insular. The cingulate gyrus, hippocampus, and adjacent cortex are often considered collectively as a sixth lobe, the limbic [5, 14].

FRONTAL LOBE

The frontal lobe is the largest and accounts for about one third of the hemispheric surface. It extends back to the central sulcus (fissure of Rolando), which separates it from the parietal lobe. The lateral sulcus (sylvian fissure) defines its inferior boundary and separates it from the temporal lobe. The precentral gyrus, which lies in front of the central sulcus, contains the higher centers for motor control of

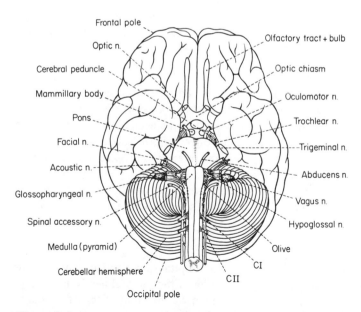

Figure 2-4
View of the inferior surface of the brain, showing the lobes and brainstem. (From John F. Simpson and Kenneth R. Magee. Clinical Evaluation of the Nervous System. *Boston: Little, Brown and Company, 1973.)*

movements of the opposite side of the body. The frontal lobe consists of three convolutions, the superior, middle, and inferior gyri, which are delineated by the superior and inferior frontal sulci running from the precentral sulcus. The inferior gyrus is further subdivided into the orbital, triangular, and opercular portions. In the dominant hemisphere, which is usually the left in right-handed persons, the triangular and opercular portions are known as *Broca's area,* the cortical center for motor formulation of speech [5, 14].

PARIETAL LOBE

The boundaries of the parietal lobe are not as easily demarcated as those of the frontal lobe. Anteriorly the parietal is separated from the frontal lobe by the central sulcus (fissure of Rolando). Posteriorly it is separated from the occipital lobe by an arbitrary vertical line drawn from the upper end of the parieto-occipital sulcus to the preoccipital notch, which is a shallow depression about four centimeters from the occipital pole. The sylvian fissure or lateral sulcus separates the parietal lobe from the temporal lobe below. The configuration of this lobe varies greatly. However, there are two major sulci, the postcentral, which runs parallel to the central sulcus, and the intraparietal, which runs back to the occipital lobe. The *postcentral gyrus,* which lies just behind the central sulcus, represents the *cortical sensory area.* Lesions in the postcentral gyrus cause a person to lose the ability to localize a painful stimulus or measure the intensity of pain. The *intraparietal sulcus* separates the superior and inferior parietal lobules or gyri. The inferior parietal lobule consists of two gyri, the supramarginal and angular. Lesions in the angular gyrus of the dominant hemisphere characteristically produce an inability to understand the written word. Lesions of the inferior parietal gyrus produce astereognosis, or inability to correlate and interpret a variety of sensory impressions [5, 14].

TEMPORAL LOBE

The anterior boundary of the temporal lobe is the lateral sulcus (sylvian fissure), which separates it from the frontal and parietal lobes. An arbitrary line drawn from the posterior end of the lateral sulcus to the front of the occipital lobe serves as the posterior boundary. This lobe is composed of three gyri, the superior, middle, and inferior, which are separated by the superior and inferior sulci. The superior sulcus runs parallel to the lateral sulcus (sylvian fissure). Its ascending terminal portion is surrounded by the *angular gyrus.* The superior gyrus contains the auditory projection area of the cortex. Lesions in this area are associated with inability to understand the spoken word [5, 14].

OCCIPITAL LOBE

The occipital lobe is marked off by the parieto-occipital sulcus and an arbitrary line drawn from this fissure to the inferolateral border of the cerebral hemisphere. The outer surface is quite variable and much less extensive than that of the other lobes. The lateral surface is divided by the lateral occipital sulcus into an inferior and superior group of irregular gyri. The medial aspect is divided by the *calcarine sulcus,* which joins the parieto-occipital sulcus. The *visual cortex* is located on both sides of the calcarine sulcus [5, 14].

CENTRAL LOBE

The insula or central lobe lies within the lateral sulcus. It is overlapped by a section of the temporal, frontal, and parietal cortex known as the opercula and is separated from these three lobes by a circular sulcus. It can be seen only when the temporal and frontal lobes are separated. The insula is a triangular cortical area with its apex directed forward and down into the floor of the lateral fossa. The opening leading to it in the floor of the lateral fossa is called the limen [5, 14].

CEREBRAL CORTEX

The cerebral cortex is the mantle of gray matter that covers the convoluted surface of the cerebral hemispheres. It makes up about forty percent of the brain and covers an area of approximately 2,200 square centimeters (2.5 square feet). One third of this covers the outer surface of the convolutions, while the remaining two thirds lie in the depths of the sulci. The cerebral cortex is composed of nerve fibers, neuroglia, blood vessels, and about fourteen billion neurons. A neuron, or nerve cell, is the functional and anatomical unit of the nervous system. Each neuron consists of a cell body and one to many processes, called nerve fibers, which serve to receive and conduct impulses. *Afferent fibers* conduct impulses toward the neuron, and *efferent fibers* conduct impulses away from the cell body. Within the central nervous system information is transmitted through a succession of neurons. The transmission of impulses from one neuron to the next may be blocked, changed, or integrated with impulses from other neurons to create highly intricate patterns. These functions are referred to as *synaptic* functions [11]. The juncture from one neuron to the next over which impulses are transmitted is called a synapse. Each neuron is composed of a soma or cell body, a single axon (conducts impulses away from the cell body), and many dendrites (conducts impulses to the cell body). Numerous small knobs called synaptic knobs lie on the surface of the soma and dendrites. They are terminal ends of nerve fibers originating in other neurons. Some are excitatory and others inhibitory. These knobs are separated from the neuronal soma by a space referred to as the synaptic cleft.

Neurons throughout the central nervous system differ in size of cell body, length and size of axon, and the number of synaptic knobs. Chemical compounds involved in impulse transmission, called *neurotransmitters,* are secreted by the synaptic knobs (presynaptic terminals), cross the synaptic cleft, and — depending on the type of transmitter substance secreted — either inhibit or excite action potentials in the postsynaptic neuron. Impulses are conducted in only one direction, from the presynaptic region that receives the stimulation to the postsynaptic region. The major neurotransmitters that have been identified with some certainty are acetylcholine, norepinephrine, and dopamine, all of which are excitatory transmitters. Acetylcholine is active in the parasympathetic system at the neuromuscular junction and at the ganglionic junctions. Norepinephrine, by its action at most postganglionic sympathetic terminals, maintains sympathetic tone and circulatory homeostasis. Dopamine, a precursor to norepinephrine, functions in the brain to effect motor coordination [3, 6, 7, 11]. Gamma-aminobutyric acid (GABA), identified as an inhibitory transmitter, has been found in many brain nerve terminals.

Within the gray matter of the cerebral cortex neurons are aggregated and arranged in extensive layered sheets. There are three types of neurons, classified according to the nature of their connections: projection, association, and commissural. *Projection neurons* conduct impulses to subcortical areas such as the corpus striatum, thalamus, and brainstem. *Association neurons* interrelate with other more superficially located cortical nerve cells in the same hemisphere. *Commissural neurons* connect with cortical areas in the opposite hemisphere. Most of these commissural fibers are found in the corpus callosum, which joins the two cerebral hemispheres. The connections between the fibers within the cortex allow for conduction of the nerve impulses [1].

The nerve cells and fibers of the cerebral cortex are arranged in layers. Ninety percent of the cerebral cortex in man is *neocortex,* which is mainly association cortex and has six layers. Starting from the surface, these are the I. molecular, II. external granular, III. external pyramidal, IV. internal granular, V. internal pyramidal, and VI. multiform. In addition to this horizontal layering, the cells are also loosely arranged into vertical columns [5]. The pattern of distribution of cortical cells varies in different parts of the brain. Any direct evidence we have concerning the functions of the cerebral cortex in man is derived from the study of localized destructive lesions, from sensations and responses of conscious patients who have underdone electrical stimulation of specific points on the cortical surface, and from patterns of response in epileptic seizures arising from lesions of the cortex [6]. Several cytoarchitectural maps have been drawn that show the specialized functions of areas of the cortex. Brodmann's 52 anatomical areas are often used for descriptive purposes (Fig. 2-5). It is important to note, however, that no one cortical area is exclusively concerned with one function.

Functions of the specific cortical areas

The three main areas of the cerebral cortex are (1) the sensory areas, which are involved in general sensation, vision, and hearing; (2) the motor areas; and (3) areas of association, which are related to primary sensory areas and the functions of the higher mental processes. The cortex of the parietal, occipital, and temporal lobes is concerned with reception and conceptual elaboration of sensory data, while the cortex of the frontal lobe is concerned mainly with motor responses, foresight, mood, and judgment [1].

SENSORY AREAS

The primary sensory areas are regions on the cerebral cortex to which impulses concerned with specific sensory modalities are projected. These areas are concerned with integration of sensory experience and discrimination of the quality of sensation. Three primary sensory areas have been established: (1) the somesthetic area, (2) the visual area, and (3) the auditory area. There is some evidence that secondary sensory areas exist outside the principal area of projection but adjacent to the primary areas. Sensory impulses reach the cortex from the ascending pathways of the spinal cord via the projection fibers of the thalamus. Cortical projections relay specific sensory

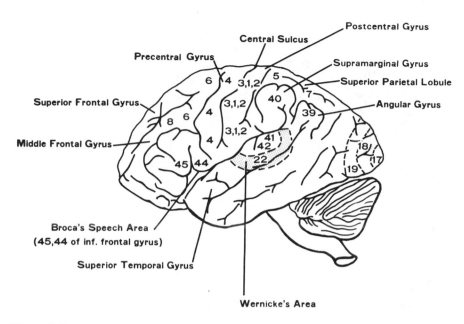

Figure 2-5
Lateral view of the brain, showing the most significant areas of Brodmann. (From
R. G. Clark [6]).

impulses to the appropriate sensory areas of the parietal, occipital, and temporal
lobes [5].

Somesthetic.   The *primary somesthetic* or general sensory area occupies areas 1, 2,
and 3 on the Brodmann cytoarchitectural map (Fig. 2-5). Projection fibers from the
thalamus convey data for the various modalities of sensation (touch, pain, temperature) to the general sensory area. Fibers related to cutaneous sensibility end in the
anterior portion of this cortical area, while fibers for deep sensibility end in the
posterior part. Figure 2-6 illustrates the proportionate representation, in the primary
somesthetic area, of sensations in the various regions of the body. It shows dramat-
ically the functional importance given to sensitivity in certain parts of the body,
such as the mouth and fingers [1, 5].

Awareness of crude sensory modalities such as pain, thermal sense, and contact
occurs at the level of the thalamus. The somesthetic area of the cortex is necessary
for the more discriminative sensations of fine touch, recognition of spatial relationships, response to stimuli of varying intensity, and appreciation of differences or
similarity in external objects coming into contact with the body. Therefore, with
lesions occurring in the primary somesthetic areas, there may be a loss of discriminative touch, ability to differentiate various intensities of stimuli, and appreciation of
position sense; only a crude awareness of pain, temperature, touch, and pressure will
remain [1].

The *secondary somesthetic* area lies along the superior bank of the lateral sulcus

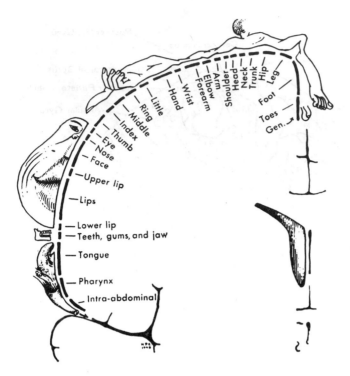

Figure 2-6
Sensory homunculus. A figure showing the disproportionate cortical representation of the body's sensory functions. (From Wilder Penfield and Lamar Roberts. Cerebral Cortex of Man: A Clinical Study of Localization of Function *[Reproduction of 1950 ed.]. New York: Hafner Press, 1968.)*

(sylvian fissure) and extends posteriorly into the parietal lobe. Representation of the various regions of the body is in reverse sequence to that found in the primary somesthetic area which were shown in Figure 2-6. Lesions occurring in this area do not cause detectable sensory defects. Its function is not completely understood but seems to be related to sensation of pain [5].

Visual.   The primary visual area — sometimes called the striate area — is located in the walls of the calcarine sulcus, which divides the medial aspect of the occipital lobe (area 17 of the Brodmann cytoarchitectural map, Fig. 2-5). The complex process of vision is initiated when images fall upon the retina of the eye. The process by which these images are transformed into perceived images takes place partly in the retina but primarily in the brain. The eyes are fixed in such a way that the retinal image of any object will be focused on the macula lutea, which is responsible for central vision. The remainder of the retina is concerned with paracentral and peripheral vision. Retinal nerve impulses travel to the visual cortex via the visual pathway, which passes from the optic nerve through fibers of the optic chiasm, encircles the hypothalamus and continues to the geniculate bodies of the thalamus.

Hence the fibers form the optic radiation or geniculocalcarine tract, which relays the impulses to the primary visual cortex on the two sides of the calcarine sulcus. This area is discussed further in relation to the thalamic radiations. Visual defects resulting from injury to the visual cortex or any part of the visual pathway vary according to the location and extent of the damage. *Homonymous* defects are those restricted to a single field of vision, either the right or the left; *heteronymous* defects involve both right and left fields of vision [1]. A lesion which results in unilateral destruction of the entire visual cortex will produce a contralateral homonymous hemianopsia — that is, blindness in the nasal field on the side of the lesion and blindness on the temporal field of the opposite side. When only a portion of the visual cortex is destroyed, the result will be homonymous quadranopsia, in which blindness will occur in either the superior (when the lesion is in the temporal lobe) or the inferior (when the lesion is in the parietal lobe) half of the contralateral visual field. When a lesion occurs in the area of the optic chiasm, where the fibers cross, the result is usually a bitemporal hemianopsia and occasionally a binasal hemianopsia [1, 5, 6]. Central vision may be unaffected by lesions of the visual cortex following occlusion of the posterior cerebral artery. This is referred to as "macular sparing" and is thought to be due to collateral circulation provided by branches of the middle cerebral artery. One third of the area of the visual cortex is involved with central vision.

There are two *secondary visual areas,* usually classified as II and III. Visual area II is located anterolateral to area I in Brodmann's area 18. Visual area III is located in Brodmann's area 19. Both receive projections from the primary visual area, which is the only visual area to receive projections directly from the lateral geniculate body [5].

Auditory. The *primary auditory (acoustic) area* is located within the lateral sulcus (sylvian fissure) and the two transverse gyri (Heschl's convolutions), which lie on the surface of the superior temporal convolution. This area corresponds to areas 41 and 42 on Brodmann's cytoarchitectural map (Fig. 2-5). The auditory area of the sensory cortex where sound is heard is located in Brodmann's area 41. Recognition of sound takes place in the association area of the cortex, Brodmann's area 42 [1, 5, 6]. The auditory pathway is described in a further section in relation to the thalamic radiations.

The taste, or *gustatory area,* is located in the sylvian fissure adjacent to the parietal operculum represented by Brodmann's area 43. The exact pathway for taste sensation is not known [1].

The precise location of the *vestibular area* in the cerebral cortex has not been definitely established. Recent evidence seems to suggest that it is in the postcentral gyrus of the parietal lobe, but fiber connections from the vestibular nuclei to the thalamus and cerebral cortex have not been demonstrated [1, 6].

MOTOR AREAS
As has just been described, the sensory or somesthetic area occupies the postcentral gyrus on the dorsolateral surface of the cerebral hemisphere and the paracentral lobule on its medial surface. The motor area is very near it, located in the precentral gyrus, and includes the anterior wall of the central sulcus on the dorsolateral surface

of the cerebral hemisphere and the anterior part of the paracentral lobule on its medial surface. These two areas that surround the rolandic fissure have overlapping functions and connections and, although described separately here, are usually considered together as a *sensorimotor strip.* Projection fibers from the motor area convey impulses concerned with motor function, modification of muscle tone, reflex activity, modulation of sensory impulses, and alteration of sense awareness. These fibers originate from the cortical areas and project impulses to brainstem nuclei, the basal ganglia, and the spinal cord [1, 5].

Primary motor area.   The cortical motor area is usually called the primary motor area and corresponds to area 4 of Brodmann's map (Fig. 2-5). The corticospinal tract, which transmits impulses for highly skilled volitional movements arises here, but it is not known precisely which cortical areas contribute fibers to this tract. Charts of motor representation of various parts of the body have been prepared based upon movements elicited by electrical stimulation, under local anesthesia, of various sites on the motor area. The disproportionate parts of the body in Figure 2-7 represent graphically the relative size of the motor area that controls their movement. Lesions in the primary motor area cause flaccid paralysis, on the contralateral

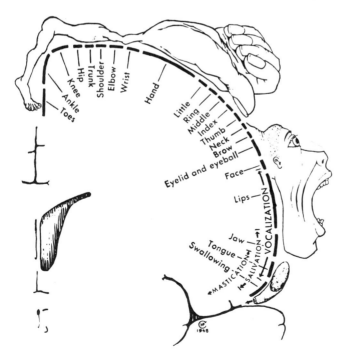

Figure 2-7
Motor homunculus. A figure showing the disproportionate cortical representation of the body's motor functions. (From Wilder Penfield and Lamar Roberts. Cerebral Cortex of Man: A Clinical Study of Localization of Function *[Reproduction of 1950 ed.]. New York: Hafner Press, 1968.)*

side, that part of the body controlled by the damaged area of the motor cortex. When the lesion extends beyond the motor area to interrupt the motor projection fibers, a spastic paralysis results. When there is partial recovery, the residual paralysis is usually in the distal portion of the extremities, where loss of movement is always greatest [1, 5].

Premotor area.   The premotor area (Brodmann's area 6) is situated in front of the primary motor area along the lateral aspect of the frontal lobe. It has both commissural and association fibers and receives fibers from subcortical connections with the thalamus, corpus striatum, and cerebellum. It is thought that the premotor area may be concerned with complex learned motor activity, as *apraxia,* an impairment in performance of a learned motor activity in the absence of a motor paralysis, is known to result from lesions in this area. There is a section located in the lower part of Brodmann's area 8, on the lateral surface of the hemisphere in the caudal aspect of the middle frontal gyrus, that represents the *frontal eye fields* and that may be included in the premotor cortex [1, 5, 6]. Stimulation of this area produces conjugate deviation of the eyes to the opposite side. It is felt that this area controls voluntary scanning movements of the eyes.

Supplementary motor area.   A supplementary motor area has been identified on the medial surface of the superior frontal gyrus and is believed to be concerned primarily with the mechanisms of posture and movement. Stimulation of the area is known to produce raising of the opposite arm, turning of the head and eyes, and bilateral synergistic contractions of trunk and leg muscles [1, 5, 6].

ASSOCIATION AREAS
A large cortical area known as the *prefrontal cortex* lies anterior to the premotor area, has connections with the dorsomedial nucleus of the thalamus, and receives many association fibers from other areas of the brain. It is believed that complex memory patterns formed in the parietal, temporal, and occipital lobes may be transmitted to the prefrontal cortex for synthesis into memory constellations that form the basis of abstract thinking [1, 5, 6, 15]. This area is also believed to control affect or mood of thought.

Somesthetic.   The somesthetic association cortex is situated in Brodmann's areas 5 and 7 of the superior parietal lobule (Fig. 2-5). Here data from the various senses are integrated. Lesions that occur in this area will result in agnosia and astereognosis. *Agnosia* is a defect in understanding the significance of sensory information. *Astereognosia* involves a loss of awareness of the body image or relationship of body parts and may cause the patient to ignore or fail to recognize parts of his body [1].

Visual.   The visual association cortex surrounds the primary visual area and includes such complex aspects of vision as relating what is being seen to what has been seen in the past; it allows visual recognition. Lesions in this area cause a *visual agnosia.* Although the patient sees, he is unable to recognize what is in his opposite field of vision [1].

Auditory.   The auditory association cortex *(Wernicke's area)* is located in Brodmann's area 22, adjacent to the primary auditory sensory area. Fibers from the auditory association cortex connect with the primary sensory area and with cortical areas of the parietal, occipital, and insular lobes. Lesions of this area in the dominant hemisphere cause "word deafness" or sensory aphasia. Although the patient can hear, he is unable to interpret the meaning of sounds, especially speech [1, 5].

Additional areas.   In addition to those related to specific sensory functions, there are additional areas of association cortex in the inferior parietal lobule and the posterior portion of the temporal lobe. In these areas, data that arrive at the primary sensory areas of the cerebral cortex and are analyzed in the adjacent association cortex are correlated to allow for assessment of the immediate environment. Memory traces, or *engrams*, which are laid down over the years, form the basis of learning at an intellectual level. The neuron connections within the cerebral cortex allow these engrams to be used in the formation of ideas and abstract thinking. Connections between the sensory association areas, the prefrontal association cortex, and the motor cortex allow for formation and overt expression of complex behavior patterns based upon experience [1].

The use of language relies heavily on certain mechanisms within the association areas of the cerebral cortex. Because disorders arising in this area are so commonly manifested in stroke, the anatomy and physiology of these areas have been presented in detail in Chapter 5, which deals with aphasia.

CORTICOFUGAL SPINAL SYSTEM

Efferent fibers arising from specific regions of the cerebral cortex form a massive *corticofugal fiber system* in which each fiber follows a definite course and terminates in a particular area of the nervous system. Most of these fibers can be grouped into three systems, the corticospinal, the nonpyramidal corticofugal, and the corticopontocerebellar system. The overall functioning of the central nervous system depends on the integration of the activities of all three systems. The *corticospinal system* is concerned primarily with fine, discrete, skilled movements of the distal extremities. It is often referred to as the *pyramidal system* because corticospinal tracts pass through medullary tracts which are pyramid shaped [6]. The *nonpyramidal corticofugal system* is concerned with integration of all somatic, visceral, and sensory functions of the nervous system. The *corticopontocerebellar system* relates the cortical areas and the cerebellum [5, 6].

CEREBRAL DOMINANCE

Motor and sensory impulses on both sides of the body project contralaterally but almost equally to corresponding cortical areas. Information received by a cortical area in one hemisphere can be transferred to the other via commissural neurons. There are, however, many functions which are not represented equally in the cortex of both hemispheres. Since one hemisphere appears to take the lead for certain higher cortical functions, such as language, that hemisphere is usually termed the *dominant*. Disturbances related to language due to lesions arising in the dominant hemisphere are discussed in Chapter 5. A number of cortical areas affect only the contralateral side of the body. When a lesion occurs in such an area, the resulting disturbance of function is seen only contralaterally regardless of which side is the dominant. This is the case with lesions of the primary motor and sensory areas and those of the parietal lobes that result in astereognosis. In other syndromes of the parietal lobe the deficits are more likely to occur in the nondominant hemisphere, as with disorders of body image and awareness [5]. These disturbances are discussed in detail in Chapter 6.

WHITE MATTER

The substance that constitutes the *medullary center* of the cerebrum is usually referred to as *white matter*. Each cerebral hemisphere includes a large core of white matter that accommodates the many nerve fibers running to and from the cerebral cortex. The medullary center is bounded by the cortex, lateral ventricle, and corpus striatum (Fig. 2-8). The nerve fibers in the medullary center are classified by the nature of their connection. *Association fibers* connect one cortical area with another within the same hemisphere. *Projection fibers* establish connections between the cortex and subcortical levels of the nervous system. *Commissural fibers* serve to connect similar cortical areas between the two hemispheres [1, 5].

   Association fibers are the most numerous and are divided into long and short groups. The *short association fibers* connect adjacent convolutions by traversing the long axis of the sulci. *Long association* fibers connect cortical areas in different lobes within the same hemisphere and form three main fiber bundles — the uncinate fasciculus, the arcuate fasciculus, and the cingulum. The *uncinate fasciculus* connects the orbital frontal gyri and inferior and middle frontal gyri with the anterior portion of the temporal lobe. The *arcuate fasciculus* connects the superior and middle frontal gyri with parts of the temporal lobe. It provides an important communication between the sensory and motor language areas. The *cingulum* connects regions of the frontal and parietal lobes with parahippocampal and temporal cortical regions [1, 5].

   Projection fibers, which convey impulses to and from the cerebral cortex, are arranged in a radiating mass *(corona radiata)* that converges toward the brainstem. At the upper part of the brain the fibers form a compact band called the *internal capsule*. The internal capsule consists of (1) an anterior limb, which separates the caudate nucleus and the putamen and includes the anterior thalamic radiation fibers; (2) a posterior limb, which contains the optic radiation fibers; and (3) the genu, which connects the anterior and posterior limbs. Afferent fibers, or *thalamocortical radiations*, in the internal capsule arise primarily from the thalamus and project to nearly every cortical area. The efferent fibers arise from various cortical areas and project to masses of nerve cells in the brain and spinal cord. These are classified as *corticothalamic, corticospinal, corticopontine*, and *corticobulbar fibers* [1, 5].

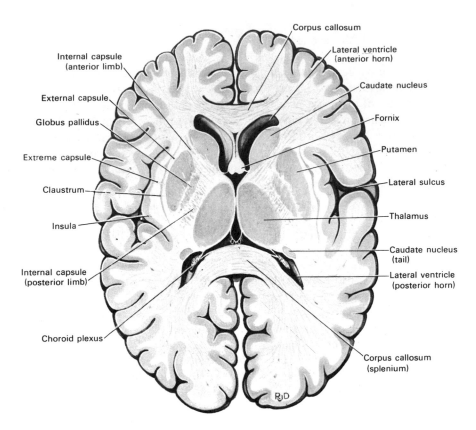

Figure 2-8
Horizontal section of the brain, showing the cerebral cortex, white matter, basal ganglia, thalamus, and ventricles. (From M. B. Carpenter [5]).

Commissural fibers interconnect corresponding areas of the two hemispheres. The two commissures are the corpus callosum and the anterior commissure. The *corpus callosum* is a broad plate of myelinated fibers that traverses the floor of the hemispheric fissure and fans out to connect regions of the cortex in all lobes with corresponding regions in the opposite hemisphere. The *anterior commissure* is a small bundle of fibers that provides additional communication between the two temporal lobes [1, 5].

BASAL GANGLIA

The basal ganglia include several masses of gray matter embedded within the white matter of each cerebral hemisphere: the corpus striatum, the subthalamic nucleus, and the substantia nigra, which are motor nuclei. Lesions affecting these structures will result in involuntary, uncontrollable, purposeless movements and other motor signs (Fig. 2-8) [1].

Corpus striatum

The corpus striatum is a major center of the complex extrapyramidal motor system. It consists of two sections, the lenticular nucleus and the caudate nucleus, which are separated partially by the internal capsule. The *lenticular nucleus* is subdivided into the putamen and the globus pallidus. The *putamen* is the largest and most lateral section of the basal ganglia. It is connected to the head of the caudate nucleus by numerous gray strands, which extend across the internal capsule. Cells of the *globus pallidus* form the principal efferent fiber system of the corpus striatum. The *caudate nucleus* is an elongated, arched structure in the form of an anterior head tapering into a slender tail. The head of the caudate nucleus protrudes into the anterior horn of the lateral ventricle, and the tail lies along the dorsolateral border of the thalamus, then forward along the inferior roof of the ventricle and terminates at the amygdaloid nucleus [1, 5].

Neural connections of the basal ganglia

The corpus striatum participates in three main neuronal pathways: (1) from the thalamus to the neostriatum (this term refers to the putamen and caudate nucleus); (2) from the globus pallidus to the red nucleus and reticular formation for relay to lower motor neurons; and (3) from the cerebral cortex through the neostriatum, paleostriatum (globus pallidus), and ventral thalamic nuclei to motor and premotor areas of the frontal lobe. The cerebral cortex and basal ganglia are connected through corticostriate fibers. Other pathways connect the globus pallidus to lower motor neurons via brainstem centers [1].

Nerve fibers that connect with the corpus striatum from the cerebral cortex, thalamic nuclei, and substantia nigra are referred to as *striatal afferent fibers* and are classified as corticostriate, thalamostriate, and nigrostriate. *Corticostriate fibers* originate in various parts of the cerebral cortex, mainly in the frontal and parietal areas, to connect with the caudate nucleus and putamen. Fibers that project contralaterally cross from one hemisphere to the other via the corpus callosum, which joins the two cerebral hemispheres. Corticostriate fibers arising in areas other than the sensorimotor cortex, however, have only an ipsilateral projection. The *thalamostriate fibers* are one of the most important groups of afferent fibers passing to the caudate nucleus and putamen from the thalamus. *Nigrostriate fibers* from the substantia nigra project to the putamen of the corpus striatum by traversing the internal capsule and globus pallidus [1, 5].

Subthalamic region

The *subthalamic fasciculus* is a connection that consists of fibers passing in both directions across the internal capsule from the subthalamic nucleus to the globus pallidus. The subthalamic nucleus is one of the extrapyramidal motor nuclei. Lesions occurring in this area, usually due to hemorrhage, will result in a motor disturbance known as *hemiballismus* and characterized by involuntary, forceful, purposeless, flailing movements of the extremities. These movements involve the proximal musculature of the upper and lower extremities and occur on the side opposite to the lesion [1, 5, 6].

Additional nuclei in the subthalamic region are the zona incerta and those of the tegmental fields of Forel. Fiber bundles, the pallidofugal fiber system (ansa lenticularis, lenticular fasciculus, thalamic fasciculus), which represents the principal efferent system of the corpus striatum, and the subthalamic fasciculus pass through the subthalamic region [5].

Functions of the basal ganglia

The contribution of the corpus striatum to motor function is poorly understood, but it is felt that the caudate nucleus and putamen function together to initiate and control gross intentional body movements. Two neuronal pathways are thought to transmit impulses for performance of this function:

1. a route into the globus pallidus by way of the thalamus to the cerebral cortex, then down to the spinal cord via the corticospinal and extracorticospinal pathways
2. a route through the globus pallidus and substantia nigra via short pathways into the reticular formation, and into the spinal cord via reticular tracts

While the caudate nucleus and putamen help to regulate gross intentional movements, normally performed unconsciously, this control involves the cortical motor areas with which both the caudate nucleus and putamen are connected closely [1, 10].

Evidence suggests that the principal function of the globus pallidus is to provide background muscle tone for intended movements, whether they are initiated by cortical impulses or impulses from the caudate nucleus and putamen. It is believed that the globus pallidus provides this function through two pathways:

1. by way of feedback circuits to the thalamus and cerebral cortex and on to the spinal cord via the corticospinal and extracorticospinal tracts, and
2. by way of short pathways to the reticular formation of the brainstem and on to the spinal cord by way of the reticulospinal tracts [10]

The basal ganglia are concerned with control of automatic associated movements of the body such as the arm swing that occurs in alternation to the legs when a person walks. To regulate such movements the basal ganglia function in coordination with the cerebellum, thalamus, and cerebral cortex and have many neural connections with the reticular formation of the midbrain [2].

DISTURBANCES ASSOCIATED WITH EXTRA-PYRAMIDAL DISEASE

Since the basal ganglia are subcortical nuclei, neurologists have used the term *extra-pyramidal* to group basal ganglia with brainstem nuclei that are related to somatic motor functions. As has already been stated, the pyramidal system includes cortico-spinal tracts involved with discrete skilled movements and is so called because the corticospinal tracts occupy pyramid-shaped tracts on the medulla. The extrapyramidal motor system includes (1) the basal ganglia, (2) the subthalamic nucleus, (3) the substantia nigra, (4) the red nucleus, and (5) the brainstem reticular formation.

Clinically two basic types of disturbances are associated with disease of the extrapyramidal system, dyskinesias, or abnormal involuntary movements, and disturbances of muscle tone. Dyskinesias can take one of the following forms:

Tremor   A rhythmical, alternating, involuntary activity with a relatively regular frequency and amplitude, occurring at rest or upon voluntary movements.

Athetosis   Slow, writhing, involuntary movements, especially of the extremities, although the face and neck may be included. The axial musculature is primarily involved, and there is severe torsion of the neck, shoulder girdle, and pelvic girdle.

Chorea   A brisk, graceful series of successive involuntary movements of considerable complexity. These movements involve primarily the distal portions of the extremities, muscles of facial expression, the tongue, and deglutitional musculature.

Ballism   Violent, forceful, flinging movement involving primarily the proximal appendicular musculature and the muscles about the shoulder and pelvic girdles.

An increase in muscle tone is present to a nearly equal degree in antagonistic muscle groups (both flexor and extensor muscles). Although it is increased during athetoid movements and persists after their completion, tone may gradually diminish thereafter. Variable degrees of hypotonus are usually associated with chorea and ballism [1, 5].

DIENCEPHALON

The diencephalon lies between the cerebral hemispheres and the midbrain and is almost completely surrounded by the hemispheres. It consists of four parts, each of which is represented bilaterally: the thalamus, subthalamus, epithalamus, and hypothalamus [5].

Thalamus

The *thalamus* is the largest portion. It is a large nuclear mass of gray matter that lies between the interventricular foramen and the posterior commissure and extends from the third ventricle to the medial border of the posterior limb of the internal capsule (see Figure 2-8). The thalamus serves as a station from which impulses of all types are relayed to the cerebral cortex.

THALAMIC NUCLEI
The major thalamic nuclei can be classified as specific relay nuclei or as association nuclei. *Relay nuclei* project to and receive fibers from well-defined cortical areas

that are related to specific functions, such as the temporal gyrus of Heschl for hearing and the calcarine sulcus for vision. The *association nuclei* do not receive direct fibers from ascending systems. They do, however, have many connections with other nuclei of the diencephalon, and they project to cortical association areas of the frontal and parietal lobes and to a lesser extent to those of the occipital and temporal lobes. Other thalamic nuclei have predominantly subcortical connections, such as the hypothalamus and corpus striatum, through which the thalamus can influence visceral and somatic effectors [2, 5].

The thalamic nuclei can also be classified into the four following groups according to their function and connections with other parts of the brain.

Reticular nucleus.   The thalamic portion of the reticular formation of the brainstem, the reticular nucleus receives data from the reticular formation of the brainstem, which extends into the subthalamus and is continuous with the thalamus. Fibers project from this nucleus to widespread areas of the cortex, and it is through this nucleus that the reticular formation participates in the ascending activating system.

Midline and intralaminar nuclei.   These nuclei receive afferent fibers from the reticular formation of the brainstem and project to other parts of the diencephalon. The *midline nucleus* consists of clusters of nerve cells adjacent to the third ventricle. The principal source of afferent impulses is the reticular formation of the brainstem, especially for data of visceral origin. This nucleus is also involved in autonomic responses at the diencephalon level and has connections with the medial thalamic nucleus, which has a role in affective reactions. The *intralaminar nuclei* receive afferent impulses from the reticular formation of the brainstem, through which most sensory data are relayed. They project to surrounding parts of the thalamus, which then project to various cortical areas. They constitute the key generator of synchronized cortical activity. The reticular formation of the brainstem is the anatomical basis of consciousness and alertness. Lesions affecting this area will cause lethargy, somnolence, and a diminished response to sensory stimulation.

Specific nuclei projecting to motor and sensory cortical areas.   The medial geniculate nucleus is concerned with hearing, the lateral geniculate nucleus with vision, and the ventral posterior nucleus with general sensation and taste. The ventral lateral and ventral anterior nucleus receive data from the cerebellum, corpus striatum, and substantia nigra and project to cortical motor areas of the frontal lobe [1].

The *medial geniculate nucleus* forms a swelling on the posterior surface of the thalamus. It is part of the auditory pathway and receives auditory stimulation from both ears but mainly from the opposite side. Efferent fibers from the medial geniculate nucleus form the auditory radiation which terminates in the auditory area of the temporal lobe (the transverse gyrus of Heschl) [1].

The *lateral geniculate nucleus* is the terminus of almost all the fibers of the optic tract. Each nucleus receives data originating in the retina and related to the opposite field of vision. There is a point-to-point projection of the retina on the lateral geniculate nucleus. The nucleus projects efferent fibers that terminate in the visual area of the occipital lobe, the site of awareness and discriminative analysis of visual stimuli [1].

The *ventral posterior nucleus* is the thalamic center for general senses and taste. The lateral and ventral spinothalamic tracts, the medial lemniscus, and the trigemino-thalamic tract, as well as fibers from the gustatory nucleus of the brainstem, all terminate here. There is a detailed topographical projection of the opposite half of the body on this nucleus. This projection, together with that on the somesthetic area of the cortex, is the basis for precise recognition of the source of stimuli. Nerve fibers from the ventral posterior nucleus end in the general sensory area of the parietal lobe and also project to other thalamic nuclei. There is an awareness of general sensory stimulation at the thalamic level, but cortical participation is necessary for refinement of sensation, awareness of discriminative touch, and proprioception [1].

The *ventral lateral nucleus* receives input from the cerebellum, substantia nigra and globus pallidus and sends fibers to the motor and premotor areas of the frontal lobe. These projections influence voluntary motor activity. Lesions occurring in this area may result in dyskinesias. The connections of the *ventral anterior nucleus* are not well identified. There is some overlapping with the functions of the ventral lateral nucleus, and it is thought that this nucleus is involved in evoking cortical responses related to the alerting system of the brain [1].

Nonspecific thalamic nuclei.   The nonspecific thalamic nuclei have reciprocal connections with association areas of the cortex. They include the medial and anterior nuclei, the pulvinar, the lateral posterior nucleus, and the lateral dorsal nucleus [1].

The *medial thalamic nucleus* has several subnuclei, the most important being the dorsomedial. Its connections with other parts of the thalamus and the association cortex of the frontal lobe are many and varied. It constitutes part of a system that contributes to mood and feeling tone and appears to play a part in memory. Projections to the corpus striatum allow for motor responses to mood change. Projections to the medial thalamic nucleus and hypothalamus influence visceral reactions to mood change [1].

The *anterior thalamic nucleus* is included in the limbic system of the brain and appears to have an important function with regard to memory and preservation of both the individual and the species [1].

The *dorsal tier of lateral nuclei* includes the pulvinar, the lateral posterior nucleus, and the lateral dorsal nucleus, all of which have similar connections and functions. They all receive projections from other thalamic nuclei. In view of their reciprocal connections with cortical association areas, it is believed that the activity of the cortex with respect to analysis of sensory input and development of intellect is reinforced by these nuclei [1].

THALAMIC RADIATIONS
Fibers that form reciprocal connections between the thalamus and the cerebral cortex constitute the thalamic radiations [5]. These thalamocortical and cortico-thalamic fibers form a continuous fanlike projection that emerges along the entire

lateral extent of the caudate nucleus. Fiber bundles radiate forward, backward, upward, and downward to form large portions of the internal capsule. The radiations connect with almost all parts of the cortex. The most abundant projections are to the frontal granular cortex, the precentral and postcentral gyri, the calcarine area, and the gyrus of Heschl. The posterior parietal and adjacent areas of the temporal lobes also have many thalamic connections. These radiations are grouped into four subdivisions, referred to as thalamic peduncles. The *anterior* or *frontal peduncle* connects the frontal lobe with the medial and anterior thalamic nuclei. The *superior* or *centroparietal* peduncle connects the rolandic area and adjacent portions of the frontal and parietal lobes with the ventral thalamic nuclei. The *posterior* or *occipital* peduncle connects the occipital and posterior parietal convolutions with the caudal portions of the thalamus. This includes the optic radiation from the lateral geniculate body to the calcarine cortex. The *inferior* or *temporal* peduncle includes scanty connections between the temporal lobe and the insula, among them the auditory radiation from the medial geniculate body to the transverse temporal gyrus of Heschl [5] .

A large portion of the *internal capsule,* a broad, compact band composed of all the afferent and efferent fibers going to and from the cerebral cortex, is composed of thalamic radiations. The rest of the capsule is composed of efferent cortical fiber systems that descend to the lower portions of the brainstem and spinal cord [5] .

Visual pathway. The visual pathway from the retina of the eye to the visual cortex of the occipital lobe, relies heavily on the thalamic relay nuclei. There is a point-to-point projection from the retina to the lateral geniculate nucleus in the thalamus and from the lateral geniculate nucleus to the visual cortex of the occipital lobe. This allows the cortex to receive a spatial pattern that corresponds to the image of the visual field the retina has received. The visual pathway begins at the *retina;* images of objects in the right field of vision are projected on the right nasal and left temporal half of the retina. Impulses from the rods and cones of the retina are conveyed to each *optic nerve.* The optic, or second cranial nerve, enters the cranial cavity, and the right and left optic nerves unite to form the optic chiasm. At the *optic chiasm,* nerve fibers coming from the nasal half of each retina cross to the opposite side, while nerve fibers coming from the temporal half of both retinas remain uncrossed. This partial crossing of optic nerve fibers is the basis for binocular vision. In the optic chiasm, fibers from the nasal half of each retina join the uncrossed fibers from the temporal half of the retina to form the optic tract. Impulses conducted to the right hemisphere by the right optic tract represent the left field of vision, and those conducted to the left hemisphere by the left optic tract represent the right field of vision. Each optic tract encircles the hypothalamus, and most of the fibers terminate in the *lateral geniculate body.* From there the geniculocalcarine tract becomes the last relay on the visual pathway. Fibers of the *geniculocalcarine tract* traverse the internal capsule to form the optic radiation and terminate in the *visual cortex* on both sides of the calcarine sulcus [1, 5] .

Visual defects will occur whenever there is an interruption of the visual pathway. The nature of the defect will depend on the location and extent of the lesion. The *left visual field* is represented in the right geniculate nucleus and the visual cortex of the right hemisphere. Visual defects restricted to a single visual field, right or left, are *homonymous*; those in which parts of both fields are involved are *heteronymous*. Homonymous defects are caused by a unilateral lesion beyond the optic chiasm in the optic tract, lateral geniculate body, optic radiation, or visual cortex. A complete destruction of any one of these will result in a loss of the entire field of vision for the side opposite to the lesion. This is referred to as *homonymous hemianopsia*. A lesion resulting in a partial destruction of any of these structures can result in less extensive visual defects, sometimes referred to as *quadrantic homonymous* defects. When the optic nerve is damaged, there will be blindness in the corresponding eye with loss of the direct pupillary reflex. The consensual reflex will be retained. A lesion of the optic chiasm will cause a bitemporal hemianopsia, however. Pressure on the lateral edge of the chiasm from a carotid aneurysm can cause a nasal hemianopsia in one eye [1, 5].

Auditory pathway.   The auditory pathway, from the cochlear nerve in the ear to the auditory cortex of the temporal lobe, relies on several synaptic relays between the cochlear nuclei of the ear and the medial geniculate nucleus of the thalamus. This is a complicated pathway. Projections from the ventral *cochlear nucleus* proceed to the ipsilateral olivary nucleus of the pons and on to the lateral lemniscus. Fibers projecting from the dorsal cochlear nucleus pass over the inferior cerebellar peduncle to the contralateral olivary nucleus and on to the *lateral lemniscus,* which is the principal auditory pathway in the brainstem. Impulses are carried from the lateral lemniscus to the inferior colliculus and end in the *medial geniculate nucleus* of the thalamus. From the medial geniculate nucleus the impulses pass through the *auditory radiation* of the internal capsule to the auditory cortex of the *temporal lobe*. Parallel with neurons conducting information to the auditory cortex are descending and efferent neurons conducting impulses in the opposite direction for feedback circuits. These connect the auditory and adjacent cortex with the medial geniculate nucleus and inferior colliculus, then proceed to the cochlear nuclei and olivary nucleus, which are in turn joined to the cochlear nerve. All along this pathway there is a processing of auditory data depending on pitch, timbre, and volume of sound perception [1].

Destruction of the cochlea, cochlear nerve, or cochlear nuclei will of course result in complete deafness on the affected side. Lesions of the lateral lemniscus will cause a partial deafness on both sides but greatest on the opposite side, since the fibers in this section of the pathway are both crossed and uncrossed. Each lateral lemniscus conducts stimuli from both ears. With a unilateral lesion of the auditory cortex there will be only a slight diminution of hearing in both ears, more pronounced on the side opposite the lesion. Complete destruction of the cortex of one hemisphere will produce difficulty in judging the direction and distance of the source of sound [1, 5].

THALAMIC FUNCTIONS
The thalamus is played upon by two sources of efferent fibers, the peripheral and the cortical. With the exception of the olfactory, all sensory impulses concerning the individual's internal and external environment terminate in the thalamus. From

the thalamus these impulses are projected to specific cortical areas via the thalamic radiations. In addition, the thalamus has subcortical efferent connections with the hypothalamus and corpus striatum by which it influences visceral and somatic effectors.

It is felt that the complex structure and organization of the thalamus indicate a more elaborate function than that of a simple relay station. There is evidence that it plays a major role in regulation of the state of consciousness, alertness, and attention through its functional influence on cortical areas. It seems certain that it is the chief sensory integrating mechanism of the cortical nervous system. Since certain thalamic nuclei receive principal efferent projections from the cerebellum and basal ganglia, it appears that the thalamus may also serve as an integrative center for motor function. Simple impulses from peripheral receptors do not pass through the thalamus without some modification. Many impulses are synthesized and integrated at the thalamic level before projection to specific areas of the cortex [5].

There are two aspects to sensation, the discriminative and the affective. By *discrimination,* stimuli are compared with respect to intensity, locality, and relative position in space and time. Sensory impulses are integrated into perceptions of form, size, and texture; and movements are judged as to direction, amplitude, and sequence. The *affective* character of sensation is concerned with agreeableness or disagreeableness, pleasure and pain. Pain is a highly subjective sensation with an affective character that is difficult to describe and nearly impossible to measure. Temperature and most other tactile sensations also have a marked affective tone [5].

Lesions of the thalamus or the thalamocortical connections will cause complete contralateral anesthesia with sense impairment, or loss of tactile localization, two-point discrimination, position sense, and movement. With certain lesions, after a brief period, there will be some return of crude touch, pain, and thermal sense, but the sensations recovered will be poorly localized and accompanied by an increased "feeling tone," usually of an unpleasant nature. With lesions of the thalamus, the threshold of excitability will be raised on the affected side, and tactile and thermal stimuli that were not previously experienced as unpleasant will evoke disagreeable sensations.

The thalamus is a sensory center for the brain and an integral part of the neural mechanism for emotional response to sensory experience. The *thalamic syndrome* is a disturbance of this aspect of thalamic function. This syndrome results most often from vascular lesions that affect the thalamus or its connections. The symptoms vary in intensity and location with the extent and location of the lesion, but basically, when the threshold of sensation has been reached, the sensation becomes exaggerated, perverted, and extremely disagreeable. Spontaneous, intractable pain may occur. The syndrome may also include emotional instability with spontaneous or forced laughter and crying [1, 5].

Subthalamus

The subthalamus is a complex area between the thalamus and internal capsule. It includes the subthalamic nucleus, which is a motor nucleus, sensory fiber tracts that terminate in the thalamus, and bundles of fibers from the cerebellum and corpus striatum. Lesions of the subthalamic nucleus will result in hemiballism on the opposite side of the body [1, 5].

Epithalamus

The epithalamus includes the pineal gland and the habenular nuclei with their connections. The *pineal gland* is a small cone-shaped body that is attached to the diencephalon by a stalk into which a recess of the third ventricle extends. The pineal contains no nerve cells. The site of action of the pineal hormone and the physiological importance of the gland are still being assessed. Since radiopaque granules of calcium and magnesium salts appear in the pineal after the age of 16, this structure can be useful as a landmark in skull films. The *habenular trigone* contains several nuclei that are concerned with the olfactory and limbic systems of the brain and constitute part of a pathway that is related to basic emotional drives and the sense of smell [1, 5].

Hypothalamus

The hypothalamus is the part of the diencephalon most concerned with visceral, endocrine, and autonomic functions. It is bounded by the wall of the third ventricle and extends from the region of the optic chiasm to the caudal border of the mammillary bodies. The hypothalamus is divided into a medial and a lateral zone. The lateral contains fewer nerve cells. The *medial zone* is further subdivided into three regions. These are the anterior, also called supraoptic or suprachiasmatic, the tuberal, and the mammillary.

The *anterior region* of the medial zone lies above the optic chiasm. This area secretes the antidiuretic hormone (ADH) in response to overly concentrated body fluids, thereby regulating renal excretion of water. ADH is stored in the posterior pituitary gland and when released into the blood causes a resorption of water by acting on the collecting ducts of the kidneys, thus causing a decrease in loss of water into the urine. Stimulation of the paraventricular nuclei causes the secretion of the hormone oxytocin which regulates uterine contractibility and milk ejection by the breasts [10]. The *tuberal region* is where the hypothalamus reaches its widest extent. This region possesses three sets of nuclei, in which most of the efferent hypothalamic fibers to caudal portions of the brainstem originate. Each nucleus consists of small nerve cells. The *mammillary region* includes the mammillary bodies, which are made up of small neurons, and the posterior hypothalamic nucleus, which consists of large neurons and small nerve cells [1, 5].

Although the hypothalamus is very small, it has extensive and complex fiber connections with the cerebrum, brainstem, and spinal cord. Intrahypothalamic fibers also exist. The hypothalamus receives information from many sources and serves as the main integrator of the autonomic nervous system. While some fiber tracts of the hypothalamus are organized into definite conspicuous bundles, others are extremely difficult to trace. *Afferent* connections arise from the basal olfactory regions, periamygdaloid region, olfactory bulb, hippocampal formation, and various portions of the frontal lobe, orbital cortex, and thalamus. Tegmental nuclei of the midbrain project mainly to the lateral mammillary nucleus. These afferent connections convey data of visceral origin, among them the sense of taste. Somatic sensory information, especially from the erotogenic zones, is also conveyed to the hypothalamus. Some afferent fibers are related to basic emotional drives and the sense of smell. The hypothalamus is an integral part of the limbic system and essential to the relationship between emotional drives and visceral function [1, 5, 6].

Efferent fibers project from the hypothalamus to thalamic nuclei, the frontal cortex, the midbrain, brainstem, and spinal cord. Impulses of hypothalamic origin reach the parasympathetic salivatory and lacrimal nuclei as well as the dorsal motor nucleus of the vagus nerve. Lower motor neurons, including the trigeminal and facial nerves and the hypoglossal nucleus, receive hypothalamic impulses in connection with eating and drinking. The hypothalamus also influences the motor neurons of the spinal cord to regulate temperature through shivering. Hypothalamic activity, which is conveyed to the thalamus and cerebral cortex, influences affective states [1, 5, 6].

The hypothalamus is intimately concerned with the hormonal activity of the entire endocrine system and in particular with that of the anterior lobe of the pituitary gland (adenohypophysis), which causes secretion of gonadotropic (LH and FSH), adrenocorticotropic (ACTH), thyrotropic (TSH), growth (GH), and melanocyte stimulating (MSH) hormones [1, 5]. Regulation of anterior pituitary hormone secretion depends entirely upon release of hypothalamic regulatory hormones from neurosecretory cell bodies in the basal hypothalamus. It is postulated that each anterior pituitary hormone is controlled by a specific hypothalamic hormone. To date three have been identified: thyrotropin-releasing hormone (TRH), luteinizing hormone—releasing hormone (LHRH), and somatostatin, the growth hormone release—inhibiting hormone [12].

The hypothalamus regulates body water through control of intake and output by creating the sensation of thirst and controlling excretion of water in urine. When electrolytes within the neurons of the thirst center located in the lateral hypothalamus become too concentrated, the sensation of thirst develops; when body fluids become too concentrated, neurons in the superoptic nuclei are stimulated, causing secretion of the antidiuretic hormone (ADH), or vasopressin, which is stored in the posterior portion of the pituitary gland. When this substance is released into the blood, it acts on the collecting ducts of the kidneys, causing massive resorption of water. ADH acts to conserve water and concentrate urine by helping to maintain the constancy of the osmolality and volume of body fluids. High concentrations of ADH can result from severe hypotension through activation of carotid and aortic baroreceptors, which stimulate release of the hormone. Decreases in plasma volume, particularly when the left atrium and pulmonary circulation are affected, stimulate release of ADH through neural impulses from the left atrium via the vagus nerve to the supraoptic nuclei of the hypothalamus. Administration of water lowers the plasma osmolality and expands blood volume, thereby inhibiting ADH secretion [16]. Interference with this mechanism as a result of stroke is discussed in Chapter 9 in relation to disorders of fluid balance.

The hypothalamus is the chief subcortical center for regulating sympathetic and parasympathetic activities. Diverse disturbances of autonomic functions, such as water balance, sugar and fat metabolism, and temperature regulation, can all result from lesions in the hypothalamic area [1, 5].

THE OLFACTORY PATHWAYS, AMYGDALA, AND HIPPOCAMPAL FORMATION

OLFACTORY SYSTEM

The olfactory system consists of the olfactory mucosa, bulbs, and tracts, together with that portion of the cerebral cortex having olfactory functions and its projections. The olfactory cortex extends from the uncus of the temporal lobe across the anterior perforated substance of the midbrain to the medial surface of the frontal lobe beneath the genu of the corpus callosum.

The pathway begins with the *olfactory mucosa,* which covers a small area in the upper part of each nasal cavity. Olfactory cells in this area are the functional unit of the olfactory system. These cells are neurons and serve as both sensory receptors and conducting neurons. Axons from the olfactory cells converge to form the olfactory or first cranial nerve. These nerve tracts pass through the cribriform plate of the ethmoid bone. They become attached to the brain in front of the anterior perforated substance, where they divide to form the lateral and medial striae, which are bands of nerve fibers. The *olfactory bulb,* which is the terminal nucleus of the olfactory nerve, appears as an expansion of the olfactory tract just above the cribriform plate. The lateral striae of the olfactory tract pass along the lateral margin of the anterior perforated substance of the midbrain to the prepyriform region. Impulses from the olfactory bulb are thereby conveyed via the olfactory tract to olfactory areas of the cerebral cortex in order to establish awareness of odors and make connection with other areas of the brain for emotional and autonomic response to the olfactory stimuli. The prepyriform cortex and the periamygdaloid area, which receive fibers from the olfactory striae, constitute the primary olfactory cortex. The prepyriform area, which is often referred to as the lateral olfactory gyrus, extends along the lateral olfactory striae to the amygdaloid region [1, 5].

Olfaction is a complex sense which conjures up memories and emotions and contributes to the pleasures of eating. Loss of this sense cannot be compared to the disability of blindness or deafness, however, nor is it a primary sign of significant neurological dysfunction.

AMYGDALA

The amygdaloid nucleus (amygdala), which is part of the limbic system, is a mass of gray matter situated in the temporal lobe between the top of the inferior horn of the lateral ventricle and the lenticular nucleus. Nearly all parts of the amygdaloid nucleus receive direct or indirect afferent olfactory connections. The most prominent efferent pathway terminates in the hypothalamic nuclei [2, 5].

HIPPOCAMPAL FORMATION

The hippocampal formation consists of the hippocampus, that portion of the para-hippocampal gyrus that is directly continuous with it, and the dentate gyrus. It is a curved structure located in the floor of the inferior horn of the lateral ventricle. It is a submerged gyrus that forms the largest part of the olfactory cerebral cortex; and it is included together with the limbic lobe and parts of the amygdaloid nucleus, thalamus, and hypothalamus in what is referred to by some researchers as the limbic system of the brain. The structure and functional aspects of this system are exceedingly complex, but recent research indicates that they are associated with the emotional aspects of behavior, visceral responses to emotion, and brain mechanisms for memory. When an infarction in the hippocampal area due to arterial occlusion is followed at a later time by infarction of the hippocampal area in the opposite hemisphere, recent memory will be impaired. Patients so affected will be unable to commit any new information to memory, although they will retain memories of earlier events. This has definite implications with regard to teaching such patients to cope with their illness [1, 5].

The *fornix* is a band of white fibers that constitute the main efferent fiber system of the hippocampal formation. Both direct and indirect pathways connect the hippocampal formation with thalamic nuclei, the hypothalamus, and the reticular formation of the midbrain. It is theorized that the fornix provides one of the main pathways by which impulses related to subjective emotional experience from the cerebral cortex reach the hypothalamus, where they are integrated to allow emotional expression [1, 5].

The *limbic lobe* is a large convolution on the medial surface of the cerebral hemisphere, which surrounds the head of the brainstem and the interhemispheric commissures. It is formed by the cingulate gyrus, the parahippocampal gyrus, the subcallosal gyrus, the hippocampal formation, and the dentate gyrus. The extent to which these cortical areas function together as a unit has not been well established [5].

THE CEREBELLUM

The cerebellum is situated in the posterior cranial fossa and separated from the overlying occipital lobes of the cerebrum by the tentorium cerebelli, a transverse fold of the dura mater (Figs. 2-1 and 2-9). It consists of (1) an outer layer of gray matter, the cerebellar cortex, (2) an inner medullary core of white matter, and (3) four pairs of central nuclei. The cerebellum is attached to the brainstem by three pairs of peduncles, which contain afferent and efferent fibers. The superior peduncle connects with the midbrain, the middle peduncle connects with the pons, and the inferior peduncle (or restiform body) connects with the medulla. The cerebellar surface is divided into a middle section, called the vermis, and two lateral lobes, the cerebellar hemispheres. A deep cleft between the two hemispheres, called the posterior cerebellar notch, is occupied by the falx cerebelli, a fold of the dura mater. The cerebellar cortex has an irregular surface composed of numerous transverse ridges and folds called folia. Five transverse fissures divide the cerebellum into three lobes:

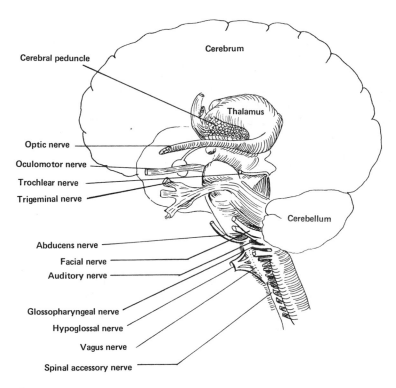

Cerebral peduncle

Cerebrum

Thalamus

Optic nerve

Oculomotor nerve

Trochlear nerve

Trigeminal nerve

Cerebellum

Abducens nerve

Facial nerve

Auditory nerve

Glossopharyngeal nerve

Hypoglossal nerve

Vagus nerve

Spinal accessory nerve

Figure 2-9
Lateral view of the brain, showing brainstem and cranial nerves (except olfactory).
(From Esta Carini and Guy Owens. Neurological and Neurosurgical Nursing *[6th ed.]. St. Louis: The C. V. Mosby Co., 1974.)*

the flocculonodular, anterior, and posterior. The flocculonodular lobe consists of small appendages (flocculi) in the inferior part of the vermis. The anterior lobe is the part of the superior surface that lies anterior to the primary fissure. The posterior lobe is located between the other two and contains the major portion of the two hemispheres [1, 5, 6, 9].

The *cerebellar cortex* is composed of three layers, the molecular layer, the Purkinje cells, and the granular layer. The intricate relationships between the various neurons in the various cortical areas are extremely complex. Afferent fibers to the cerebellum are conveyed primarily to the cerebellar cortex, entering mainly through the inferior and middle cerebellar peduncles. These fiber tracts include the spinocerebellar, cuneocerebellar, olivocerebellar, vestibulocerebellar, and pontocerebellar [5, 6].

Four pairs of *cerebellar nuclei* are embedded in the medullary center of the white matter, the fastigial, globose, emboliform, and dentate. The dentate is the largest. All parts of the cerebellar cortex project fibers to these nuclei. In addition, these nuclei receive input from motor areas of the cerebrum via the cerebro-olivocerebellar and cerebroreticulocerebellar systems [5, 6].

The cerebellum is essentially a motor part of the brain, its function is to maintain coordination of muscle action and equilibrium. It is responsible in particular for synchronization of the actions of muscles that comprise a functional group, so that movements may be performed smoothly and accurately. To carry out this function the cerebellum receives large numbers of *afferent fibers* from the cerebral cortex, muscles through the spinocerebellar tracts and all the sensory modalities. These fibers convey information to the cerebellum concerning motor activity. The vermis receives input from the spinal cord, the flocculonodular lobe receives input from the vestibular system, and the two cerebellar hemispheres receive input from the cerebral cortex.

These afferent signals are evaluated by the cerebellum, and appropriate nerve impulses are conveyed via *efferent fibers* to modify muscular movements. There are two distinct efferent systems. The first and larger involves fibers from the dentate, emboliform, and globus nuclei. The second involves fibers from the fastigial nuclei. These complex cerebellar efferent systems are organized into three longitudinal zones: (1) The vermal zone, which connects with vestibular nuclei, is predominantly concerned with mechanisms that influence extensor muscle tone. (2) The paravermal zone, which exerts only ipsilateral influence, connects with the red nucleus in the midbrain and is concerned with mechanisms that influence flexor muscle tone. (3) The lateral hemispheric zone is concerned with coordination of somatic motor activity. It has connections with the ventral lateral nucleus of the thalamus on the opposite side and indirectly affects the motor cortex.

In order to assure muscle synergy throughout the body, the cerebellum has three feedback circuits that allow nerve impulses to be returned to the same region from which they originated: (1) The vermal region receives input from the spinal cord. Information is returned to the cord indirectly by the fastigial nucleus via the reticulospinal and vestibulospinal tracts. (2) The flocculonodular lobe receives data from the vestibular system. Information is returned through the fastigiobulbar and fastigioreticulovestibulobulbar pathways. (3) The lateral hemispheric region receives information from the cerebral cortex. Information is returned to the cortex via the dentatothalamocortical path and through the red nucleus (rubrospinal tract) to the spinal cord [1, 5, 6].

Functions of the cerebellum

The cerebellum is chiefly concerned with maintenance of equilibrium, coordination of motor activity, and regulation of muscle tone. Its influence is particularly important for voluntary movements, although it does not initiate them. Impulses from a wide variety of sensory receptors are conveyed to the cerebellum for organization and integration. The major afferent input is from the stretch receptors, whose function is unconscious. Impulses from the stretch receptors trigger the neural mechanism that effects gradual alterations of muscle tension for posture and equilibrium and assures a smooth and orderly sequence of muscular contractions for skilled voluntary movements. The cerebellar system provides the complex reciprocal control of muscle tone and movement that assures an automatic synergistic motor activity. It accomplishes this by transmitting impulses to brainstem nuclei that in turn project to spinal levels and to thalamic relay nuclei, which modify the activity of cortical neurons directly concerned with motor function [5].

When lesions occur in the cerebellum, disturbances of motor function involving voluntary movement without paralysis result. Lesions occurring in the vestibular portion of the cerebellum cause the *archicerebellar syndrome.* Signs of this syndrome are limited to a disturbance of equilibrium. The patient will be unsteady on his feet, walk with a wide base, and sway from side to side. Lesions in the corpus cerebelli or the major afferent and efferent pathways cause the *neocerebellar syndrome,* in which skilled voluntary and associated movements – that is, movements related to the corticospinal system – are affected primarily [4].

The following signs will be noted in varying degrees of severity with the neocerebellar syndrome. Unilateral lesions will result in motor dysfunction on the same side of the body as the lesion due to double crossing of cerebellar-cortical tracts. Some lesions may produce bilateral disturbances.

Ataxia This disturbance is evident during walking. It is characterized by intermittent muscle contractions that are highly irregular in force, amplitude, and direction. Frequently the patient is unsteady when standing, especially if his feet are close together. The patient lurches, reels, and stumbles and has a broad-based gait [4].

Dysmetria When reaching out with a finger to point or to grasp an object, the patient overshoots the mark or deviates from it [4].

Adiadochokinesia Adiadochokinesia is a clumsiness in performing rapid alternating movements such as flexion and extension of the fingers [1].

Asynergy This is a mechanical or puppetlike sequence of movements that would normally flow in a smooth sequence.

Hypotonia With hypotonia the muscles lack tone and tire easily.

Intention tremor This type of tremor occurs primarily during voluntary and associated movements and is characteristically noted at the end of a particular movement [1].

Nystagmus This consists of an involuntary oscillation of the eyes which is seen especially with lesions of the vermis due to involvement of projections to the oculomotor, trochlear, and abducens nuclei. It is most pronounced when the patient deviates the eyes laterally toward the side of the lesion [1, 5].

Asynergy of speech muscles Involvement of the synergistic action of the speech muscles leads to speech disturbance. Speech may be slow and monotonous with some syllables unnaturally separated. There is slurring, and some words are uttered in an explosive manner.

All of the deficits noted above are due to motor disturbances which are superimposed upon volitional movements which remain basically intact [1, 5].

THE BRAINSTEM

The brainstem is composed of the medulla, pons, and midbrain. It connects the cerebral hemispheres with the spinal cord, which merges with the medulla at the level of the foramen magnum of the skull (see Figures 2-1 and 2-9). Although each of the three structures composing the brainstem has individual features, all three share common nerve fiber tracts and each includes cranial nerve nuclei. The brainstem, like the spinal cord, has long afferent tracts passing upward to conduct sensory impulses and long efferent tracts passing downward to conduct motor signals. The various motor and sensory pathways undergo rearrangements in their passage between the spinal cord and brainstem [8]. Ascending tracts convey impulses concerned with specific sensory modalities that reach consciousness as well as impulses from stretch and tactile receptors to the cerebellum that are not associated with conscious sensory perception. Certain motor, sensory, visceral, and integrative functions also originate in brainstem nuclei [1, 4, 5, 6, 9].

The medulla

The medulla is the caudal part of the brainstem and extends from the level of the foremen magnum to the pons. It is approximately three centimeters in length and widens gradually as it passes upward from the spinal cord. The lower half of the medulla contains a continuation of the central canal of the spinal cord. This canal then flares out into an open portion, which contains part of the fourth ventricle. Sulci and nerve roots divide the surface of each half of the medulla into an anterior, a lateral, and a posterior region [1, 5, 6].

ANTERIOR VIEW OF THE MEDULLA

When viewed *anteriorly,* the medulla is noted to have two longitudinal ridges (called pyramids), which contain the descending pyramidal or *corticospinal tracts.* These are motor fibers that pass from the cerebral cortex to the spinal cord. The majority of fibers cross from one side to the other in the medulla. This is referred to as the *pyramidal decussation* and is the anatomical basis for voluntary motor control of half the body by impulses from the contralateral cerebral cortex. The corticospinal or pyramidal tract is one of the largest and most important in the body. This descending tract originates in the primary motor area of the cerebral cortex and traverses the medullary center and internal capsule to reach the brainstem. The fibers continue as a compact fasciculus (fiber bundles having a similar origin) in the midbrain, break up into smaller bundles in the pons, then reform as a compact fasciculus in the pyramid of the medulla. Fiber bundles then connect with motor nuclei of the various cranial nerves [1, 5, 6].

LATERAL VIEW OF THE MEDULLA

From the *lateral aspect,* the medulla is seen to have two longitudinal grooves. These are the anterolateral sulcus, which contains the rootlets of the twelfth cranial nerve (hypoglossal), and the posterolateral sulcus, to which the nerve roots of the ninth (glossopharyngeal), tenth (vagus), and eleventh (accessory) cranial nerves are attached. Between these two sulci is a small swelling created by the *olivary nucleus complex,* located within the medulla. The olivary nucleus plays an important role in functions related to stereotyped movement of postural change and locomotion, efficiency of voluntary movements, and maintenance of equilibrium. Descending fibers from the cerebral cortex and midbrain connect with the olivary nucleus, and other afferent fibers come to it from the spinal cord. Olivocerebellar fibers project to all parts of the cerebellar cortex and to deep cerebellar nuclei.

The vestibular and cochlear nuclei as well as the *nucleus ambiguus,* which is a motor nucleus for the muscles of the pharynx, larynx, and upper esophagus, are also located in the lateral part of the medulla. The nucleus ambiguus receives sensory stimuli from the alimentary and respiratory passages via the trigeminal spinal tract. These connections establish coughing, gagging, and vomiting reflexes. Fibers from the vestibular nuclei form the *medial longitudinal fasciculus (MLF).* The ascending component goes to the cranial nuclei that innervate the extraocular muscles, while the descending fibers provide for change in the tone of neck muscles required to hold the head in various positions. Connections established with cranial nerves allow for coordination of eye and head movements [1].

DORSAL VIEW OF THE MEDULLA
From the *dorsal view* of the medulla, the obex or opening of the spinal cord into the fourth ventricle is seen. The upper portion of the medulla forms part of the floor of the fourth ventricle. On either side of the obex are the *inferior cerebellar peduncles,* which join the medulla to the cerebellum. These peduncles are formed by many fiber tracts from both the spinal cord and medulla, but crossed fibers from the olivary complex constitute the largest component. Below the fourth ventricle are the cuneate and gracilis tubercles, which are nuclear masses related to ascending systems. Fibers from the nuclei gracilis and cuneatus become the internal *arcuate fibers.* These decussate or cross from one side to the other to form a well-defined ascending bundle, the *medial lemniscus.* This pathway traverses the pons and midbrain to terminate in the thalamic nucleus for general sensation. This decussation of the medial lemniscus is part of the anatomical basis for sensory representation of half the body in the contralateral cerebral cortex. The long dorsal column fibers of these systems transmit impulses for discriminative touch, proprioception, and vibratory sense as an ipsilateral pathway for the leg, lower trunk, upper trunk, arm, and neck [1, 4, 5, 6].

FIBERS, TRACTS, AND NUCLEI OF THE MEDULLA
The *lateral spinothalamic tract* for pain and temperature, the *ventral spinothalamic tract* for light touch and pressure from the opposite side of the body and the *spinotectal tract,* which carries somesthetic information to the midbrain, all traverse the lateral area of the medulla. The combination of these tracts is referred to as the spinal lemniscus in the brainstem. The spinothalamic tracts terminate with the medial lemniscus in the thalamus [1].

The *trigeminal spinal tract* and its nucleus are also located in the medulla. Fibers of the spinal tract transmit data for temperature, pain, light touch, and pressure from the distribution of the trigeminal nerve. Fibers projected from this nucleus form the ventral trigeminothalamic tract, which conducts sensory data from the head to the ventral posterior portion of the thalamus [1].

The central canal of gray matter in the medulla is surrounded by a diffuse network of fibers known as the *reticular formation*. This refers to an area of neurons that are not organized in nuclei or tracts. The reticular formation extends up through the entire brainstem and receives input from all sensory systems, somatic and visceral. It serves an important function in the reticular activating system with regard to levels of consciousness and degree of alertness, contributes to the extrapyramidal motor system, and contributes to the autonomic nervous system through neurons that function as cardiovascular and respiratory centers. The lateral and paramedian reticular nuclei have connections with the cerebellum. Parvicellular nuclei receive afferents from sensory systems and have connections with other segments of the reticular system. The ventral and magnocellular nuclei have many branches which allow for impulse transmission throughout the retricular system [1].

Corticobulbar fibers are fibers that arise from the cerebral cortex and terminate in the lower brainstem. These fibers project to sensory relay nuclei, the reticular formation, and certain cranial nerve nuclei. The sensory relay nuclei include the nuclei gracilis and cuneatus, the trigeminal nuclei, and the nucleus of the solitary fasciculus. Corticoreticular fibers project from the motor, premotor, and somesthetic cortex in association with the corticospinal tract and terminate in the gigantocellular reticular nucleus of the medulla and the reticular nucleus of the pons. Fibers of the corticobulbar tract terminate in the motor nuclei of cranial nerves that innervate striated musculature. The trigeminal (V), facial (VII), glossopharyngeal (IX), vagus (X), accessory (XI), and hypoglossal (XII) cranial nerves are involved. Bilateral lesions involving corticobulbar fibers produce a syndrome referred to as *pseudobulbar palsy*. This syndrome, which may be seen with brainstem stroke, includes a weakness or paralysis of the muscles involved in swallowing, chewing, breathing, and speaking and loss of emotional control with inappropriate laughing and crying [5, 6].

CRANIAL NERVES

Four of the twelve *cranial nerves* are attached to the medulla, the hypoglossal (twelfth), the accessory (eleventh), the vagus (tenth), and the glossopharyngeal (ninth) (Fig. 2-9). The *hypoglossal* or twelfth cranial nerve supplies the intrinsic and extrinsic somatic skeletal muscles of the tongue. Its efferent fibers originate in the hypoglossal nucleus, located in the medulla. The nucleus receives stimuli from buccal and pharyngeal mucosa via the sensory trigeminal nuclei for reflex movements of the tongue in swallowing, chewing, and sucking. Fibers from the hypoglossal (XII) and glossopharyngeal (IX) nerves, carrying data for touch from the posterior part of the tongue and pharynx through a reflex pathway that includes the nucleus ambiguus and the hypoglossal nucleus, are important to the gag reflex [1, 5, 6].

The *spinal accessory* or eleventh cranial nerve has two distinct parts, the cranial and the spinal. The cranial part arises in the nucleus ambiguus of the medulla. The spinal part originates in the cervical cord. Fibers of the cranial part assist the vagus and laryngeal nerves to innervate the intrinsic muscles of the larynx. Fibers of the spinal part (which is not a true cranial nerve) innervate the ipsilateral sternocleido-mastoid muscle and the upper part of the trapezius. A contralateral paresis of these muscles will result from upper motor neuron lesions affecting the spinal accessory nerve [1, 5, 6].

The *vagus* or tenth cranial nerve arises in the groove on the medulla between the inferior cerebellar peduncle and the olivary process and passes through the jugular foramen, where it is joined by the cranial portion of the accessory nerve. It contin-ues down the neck and thorax into the abdomen. Afferent sensory fibers arise in the pharynx, larynx, trachea, and taste buds as well as in the abdominal and thoracic viscera. The vagus also supplies sensory fibers to the external ear, auditory canal, and tympanic membrane. Vagal fibers supply receptors in the aortic arch that moni-tor blood pressure and chemoreceptors in the aortic bodies that monitor blood oxy-gen levels. Efferent motor fibers project to parasympathetic ganglia in the abdominal and thoracic areas and to striated muscles of the pharynx and larynx [1, 5].

The *glossopharyngeal* or ninth cranial nerve is closely related to the vagus nerve and has similar functions and common nuclei located in the medulla. The glosso-pharyngeal nerve includes fibers for general sensations of pain, temperature, and touch in the posterior third of the tongue, the upper part of the pharynx, the eusta-chian tube, and middle ear. Special afferent fibers convey taste sensation from the posterior third of the tongue. Fibers from the glossopharyngeal nerve are important to the gag reflex. The glossopharyngeal nerve also receives impulses from the carotid sinus and carotid body [5]. Increased blood pressure stimulates special barorecep-tors in the wall of the carotid sinus. Impulses are conveyed by collateral fibers, which project to the dorsal motor nucleus of the vagus nerve in a reflex arc that brings about reductions in heart rate and arterial blood pressure via vagal fibers to the sinoatrial and atrioventricular nodes and atrial heart muscle. Simultaneously other reflex connections are made to inhibit the vasomotor center, which produces vasodilation of peripheral blood vessels and further reduces blood pressure [5]. The carotid body contains chemoreceptors that respond to carbon dioxide and oxygen content of the circulating blood. Fibers carry impulses to the respiratory center in the medulla, producing inspiration. Stretch receptors in the lungs send impulses via the vagus nerve back to the respiratory center to inhibit respirations [5]. Lesions affecting the glossopharyngeal nerve will cause loss of the gag reflex, loss of the carotid sinus reflex, and loss of taste in the posterior third of the tongue [1, 5, 6].

The pons

The pons lies between the medulla and midbrain of the brainstem in front of the cerebellum. It consists of two areas, the dorsal, known as the pontine tegmentum, and the ventral or basal portion, referred to as the pons proper. The pons is sepa-rated from the medulla by the inferior pontine sulcus and from the midbrain by the superior pontine sulcus. The basilar sulcus, a groove running along the midline of the anterior surface is occupied by the basilar artery [1, 5].

PONTINE TEGMENTUM

The pontine tegmentum contains ascending and descending tracts as well as nuclei of cranial nerves and is a continuation of the medullary reticular formation. With the medulla it forms part of the floor of the fourth ventricle. The ascending tracts are the same as those found in the medulla. These include the medial lemniscus, the medial longitudinal fasciculus (MLF), and the spinothalamic and the ventral spino-cerebellar tracts that traverse the tegmentum and enter into the cerebellum via the superior peduncle. Descending tracts include the central tegmental tract, which carries fibers from the red nucleus, corpus striatum, and other gray areas and receives projections from the reticular formation; the rubrospinal tract, with fibers from the red nucleus; and the tectospinal tract from the midbrain. The cranial nerve nuclei located in the pontine tegmentum (dorsal pons) are those of the fifth (trigeminal), sixth (abducens), seventh (facial) and eighth (acoustic) cranial nerves. The reticular formation in the pontine tegmentum is more extensive than the medullary. It includes the central tegmental tract, with descending fibers from midbrain reticular nuclei that project to the olivary complex in the medulla and ascending fibers from the medullary reticular formation that project to reticular nuclei in the thalamus [1, 5].

PONS PROPER

The *basal* or *ventral portion* of the pons is a large structure composed of longitudinal fiber bundles, nuclei, and transverse fibers that project to the cerebellum. It functions primarily as a large relay station between the cerebral cortex and its opposite cerebellar hemisphere to assure maximum efficiency of voluntary movements. The longitudinal fiber bundles are the (1) corticospinal, with fibers going to the medullary pyramids; (2) corticopontine, which arise from the frontal, parietal, temporal, and occipital cortex and terminate in the pontine nuclei; and (3) corticobulbar fibers. Pontine nuclei give rise to transverse fiber bundles, which enter the cerebellum through the middle cerebellar peduncle. These nuclei make data from the motor area of the cerebral cortex available to the cerebellar cortex. Impulses from the cerebellar cortex influence cortical areas of the frontal lobe. This circuit assures precision and efficiency of voluntary movements [1, 5].

CRANIAL NERVES

The four cranial nerves that originate in the pons are shown in Figure 2-9. The *vestibulocochlear, acoustic,* or eighth cranial nerve is attached to the brainstem at the junction of the pons, medulla, and cerebellum. It consists of two distinct components, the cochlear and the vestibular. These two separate fiber systems are blended into a single nerve trunk. The cochlear nerve is concerned with hearing, while the vestibular nerve is concerned with equilibrium and orientation in three-dimensional space. These two nerves have separate peripheral receptors and distinct connections with the central nervous system.

   The *cochlear nerve* conducts impulses from the organs of Corti in the bony labyrinths of the ear to the junction of the medulla and pons. Auditory impulses are carried to the spinal ganglia of the cochlea, where fibers of the cochlear nerve originate. Fibers of the cochlear nerve pass to the cochlear nuclei, through the inferior cerebellar peduncle, to the contralateral lemniscus. Some fibers also pass to the ipsilateral lemniscus. From the lateral lemniscus fibers, continue to the medial geniculate body through the auditory radiation of the internal capsule and terminate in the auditory center on the transverse temporal convolutions [1, 5, 6].

The *vestibular nerve* fibers enter the brainstem at the junction of the medulla and pons, where they bifurcate, with some fibers going to the vestibular nucleus complex and the rest entering the cerebellum via the inferior cerebellar peduncle. Receptors of this nerve are located in the semicircular canal of the inner ear. The pathway of the vestibular nerve has important connections with nuclei of the three cranial nerves (III, IV, VI) supplying the extraocular muscles. These are important in regulating movements of the eyes, head, and neck in response to stimulation of the semicircular canals. Fibers from the lateral nucleus go to the spinal cord as the vestibulospinal pathway, which regulates muscle tone and posture [1, 5].

The *facial or seventh* cranial nerve has both sensory and motor components. The sensory division of this nerve, which may be referred to as the intermedius or the intermediate nerve, serves the taste buds and the external ear. The *motor segment,* which is the more clinically significant of the two, supplies the facial muscles of expression as well as the submandibular and sublingual salivary glands and the lacrimal gland. The motor nucleus for this nerve is located in the reticular formation of the lower pons. The motor root of the facial nerve consists solely of fibers from this nucleus. The nucleus receives afferent fibers from several sources, which permit the following important reflex actions: (1) Connection with tectobulbar fibers allows for squinting in response to bright light and closing of the eyelids in response to a sudden visual stimulus. (2) Connection with fibers of sensory trigeminal nuclei permits chewing and sucking responses to foods or liquids placed in the mouth, and the blink reflex in response to corneal stimulation. (3) Connection with fibers of the auditory pathway permits contraction of the stapedius muscle in response to noise. Fibers from parasympathetic salivatory nuclei leave the brainstem via the intermediate nerve and continue via the facial nerve on their way to the sublingual and submandibular glands to stimulate secretion. The salivatory nucleus receives impulses from the hypothalamus through the dorsal longitudinal fasciculus and olfactory system via the reticular formation. The lacrimal nucleus also receives impulses to stimulate the lacrimal gland from the hypothalamus for emotional responses and from the trigeminal nucleus in response to corneal and conjunctival irritation [1, 5].

The *sensory* component of the facial nerve originates in the geniculate ganglion. This is located in the bend of the facial nerve, within the temporal bone. Its fibers are conveyed to taste buds in the anterior two thirds of the tongue. Fibers going to the palatal taste buds follow branches of the trigeminal nerve. Impulses for taste from these areas enter the brainstem via the intermediate or sensory root of the facial nerve, are connected to the nucleus of the solitary cell, and pass on to the hypothalamus, the posterior thalamic nucleus, and the cortex of the parietal lobe. Cutaneous sensations from the external ear, auditory canal, and tympanic membrane also enter the brainstem via the facial nerve and are conveyed to the geniculate ganglion. From there they follow the tract of the trigeminal nerve [1].

The *abducens* or sixth cranial nerve arises in the gray matter anterior to the fourth ventricle in the tegmental pons. This nerve, together with the oculomotor (III) and trochlear (IV), supplies the extraocular muscles with motor fibers. The abducens innervates the lateral rectus muscle, which functions to abduct the eyeball or deviate it laterally. Fibers from the abducens nucleus, situated in the pons, emerges from the brainstem at the caudal portion of the pons. The nerve has a long intracranial course and traverses the cavernous venous sinus located on the side of the sphenoid bone in its route to the rectus muscle [1, 5].

The *trigeminal* or fifth cranial nerve is the largest of the cranial nerves and contains both motor and sensory components. It serves as the motor nerve for the muscles of mastication and as the principal sensory nerve for the head. The *motor* nucleus is located in the reticular formation of the pons. The motor root of the trigeminal nerve emerges from the lateral aspect of the pons. Fibers from the motor root form the mandibular nerve, which supplies the muscles of mastication (masseter, temporal, lateral pterygoid, and medial pterygoid muscles), and the tensor tympani, tensor veli palatine, digastric, and mylohyoid muscles, all of which assist in mastication and deglutition. The corticobulbar tract supplies efferent fibers to the motor nucleus. Afferent fibers for reflex action come mainly from the sensory nuclei of the trigeminal nerve.

The *sensory nuclei* for the trigeminal nerve are in the gasserian, or semilunar, ganglion. The projections from this ganglion are the ophthalmic and maxillary nerves and the sensory component of the mandibular nerve. The *ophthalmic* nerve supplies the skin of the forehead, temple, and scalp, upper eyelid, and anterior and lateral surface of the nose. It also supplies the eyeball, upper conjunctiva, cornea, ciliary body, iris, lining of the frontal, ethmoid, and sphenoid sinuses, and upper nasal cavity. The *maxillary* nerve supplies the skin of the side and posterior half of the nose, lower eyelid, upper cheek, anterior temporal region, and upper lip. It innervates the mucous membrane of the lower conjunctiva, maxillary sinus, lower nose, upper lip, cheek, soft palate, oral hard palate, and nasopharynx. The *mandibular* nerve supplies the skin of the side of the head, posterior cheek, temporal area, anterior pinna, upper and outer external auditory canal, lower lip, chin, and mucous membranes of the lower lip and buccal surface, floor of the mouth, teeth, and temporomandibular joint. Efferent fibers from the sensory trigeminal nuclei connect with motor nuclei of the trigeminal and facial nerves, nucleus ambiguus, and hypoglossal nucleus for reflex responses. These include closing of the eyes when the cornea is touched and sneezing in response to irritation of the nasal mucosa. Brainstem lesions causing interruption of the trigeminal motor fibers will result in paralysis of the muscles of mastication [1, 5].

The midbrain

The midbrain, sometimes referred to as the mesencephalon, is the short segment of the brainstem situated between the pons and the diencephalon. It consists of three parts, the tectum, the basis pedunculi or crus cerebri, and the tegmentum. The entire midbrain, exclusive of the tectum, is referred to as the cerebral peduncle.

TECTUM

The tectum or roof of the midbrain consists of four rounded prominences, the two sets of superior and inferior colliculi (corpora quadrigemina). The *superior colliculi* serve as primary relay stations of the visual system and receive fibers from the visual cortex of the occipital lobe, the retina, and the spinal cord. Connections between the cerebral cortex and the superior colliculus are responsible for reflex movements of the eyes and head in response to objects coming within the visual field (automatic scanning) and are important in accommodation of the eyes to near objects through convergence of the eyes, thickening of the lens, and constriction of the pupils. Fibers coming from the retina allow for a reflex that initiates turning the head toward a sudden visual stimulus, raising the arms for protection, and closing the eyelids [1].

The commissure of the superior colliculus connects the two superior colliculi, which give rise to the tectobulbar and tectospinal tracts. Tectobulbar fibers go to the oculomotor, trochlear, and abducens nuclei for eye movements and to the facial nucleus for protective closure of the eyelids. The superior colliculi are also connected with the reticular formation and substantia nigra [1, 5].

The *pretectal region* is a transitional area between the superior colliculus and the thalamus. Nuclei receive fibers from the retina via the optic tract and project fibers to the Edinger-Westphal nucleus of the oculomotor nerve. This is the principal midbrain center involved in the direct and consensual pupillary light reflex. As intensity of light increases, the pupil constricts [5]. The *inferior colliculus* is in the auditory pathway to the cerebral cortex and serves as a relay station, transmitting auditory impulses to the thalamus via the medial geniculate body and to the cerebral cortex. Commissural fibers between the two inferior colliculi allow for bilateral cortical projection from either ear. Some fibers also go to the superior colliculi and from there reach the cranial nerve nuclei that supply the extraocular muscles and motor neurons in the cervical region, to allow a reflex turning of head and eyes in response to auditory stimuli. The trochlear nerve emerges from the brainstem just beyond the inferior colliculus [1, 5].

BASIS PEDUNCULI

The basis pedunculi, which is a dense band of descending fibers, forms the prominent elevation on either side of the midbrain. It is also called the crus cerebri. Most of the descending tracts are from the pyramidal corticospinal tract. In addition, corticobulbar fibers proceed to various cranial nerve nuclei, and corticopontine fibers arising in the parietal, temporal, and occipital cortex proceed to the pons [1, 5].

The *substantia nigra,* which is the largest nuclear mass in the midbrain, is so named because it contains melanin-pigmented cells. It is a motor nucleus situated between the tegmentum and basis pedunculi and extends the length of the midbrain into the subthalamic region of the diencephalon. Afferent fibers arise mainly from the caudate nucleus and putamen. Efferent fibers project to the corpus striatum and thalamic nuclei [1, 5]. The significance of the substantia nigra as a major pathway in the metabolic synthesis of norepinephrine has been discovered recently. The pigmented cells of the substantia nigra are rich in dopamine (dihydroxytyramine), which is the immediate precursor in the biosynthesis of norepinephrine.

TEGMENTUM

The tegmentum of the midbrain is a continuation of that of the pons and contains most of the same fiber tracts. The medial lemniscus traverses the midbrain in this area. Spinotectal fibers leave the spinal lemniscus to enter the superior colliculus and the lateral and ventral spinothalamic tracts continue into the diencephalon. The *red nucleus,* so called because it has a pinkish hue due to a particularly rich vascular supply, extends from the superior colliculus into the diencephalon. It is involved with pathways through which the cerebellum influences motor function by projecting either to lower neurons or motor regions of the cerebral cortex through thalamic relay. Afferent fibers come to the red nucleus from deep cerebellar nuclei and the cerebral cortex. Efferent fibers from the red nucleus project to the cere- bellum, parts of the facial nucleus, the lateral radicular nucleus of the medulla, and the spinal cord. Ascending afferent fibers project to the thalamus [5].

CRANIAL NERVES

Two of the twelve cranial nerves arise in the midbrain, the oculomotor or third and the trochlear or fourth cranial nerves. These two nerves, together with the abducens or sixth cranial nerve, supply motor fibers to the extraocular muscles to provide the coordinated movement of the eyes for binocular vision. The nuclei for these three nerves receive afferent fibers from the same sources [1].

The *oculomotor nerve complex* serves to innervate the inferior oblique, the superior, medial, and inferior rectus muscles, and the levator palpebrae muscles. It also provides parasympathetic fibers to the ciliary muscle and sphincter of the pupil. Nuclei of the oculomotor nerve are situated in the lower midbrain just above the pons. The fibers of this cranial nerve emerge as a series of roots at the junction of the upper pons and midbrain, along the interpeduncular fossa and between the superior cerebellar and posterior cerebral arteries. They penetrate the dura mater and enter the orbit via the cavernous sinus and superior orbital fissure. Crossed fibers supply the superior rectus muscle, which elevates the eyeball when it is adducted. Uncrossed fibers supply the medial rectus, which adducts the eyeball, and the inferior rectus, which turns the eyeball downward. The levator palpebrae muscles, which elevate the lids, receive bilateral innervation. The sphincter pupillae causes constriction of the pupils, and the ciliary muscle decreases tension of the lens capsule in order to increase the convexity of the lens for near vision. The change in contour of the lens is accompanied by convergence of the eye and constriction of the pupil [1, 5].

The *trochlear* or fourth cranial nerve is the smallest and the only one to emerge from the posterior aspect of the brainstem. The nucleus of this nerve is a small appendage to the oculomotor nuclear complex, and its fibers follow those of the oculomotor nerve. The trochlear nerve innervates the superior oblique muscle that rotates the eyeball outward and downward. These functions will be lost when there is damage to the trochlear nerve. Such damage will also cause double vision and difficulty in walking downstairs [1, 4, 5].

CEREBRAL CIRCULATION (See also Chapter 8)

Regulatory mechanisms

The total cerebral blood flow in a normal man averages 750 ml/min. This blood flow is kept fairly constant through control systems regulating the circulation. In addition to the basic regulatory mechanisms intrinsic to circulation the brain has a regulatory mechanism based on carbon dioxide concentration in the brain. When carbon dioxide, the most potent stimulus to cerebral circulation, is increased in the brain, the blood vessels dilate and there is an increase in blood flow and consequently in carbon dioxide removal, thereby reducing the carbon dioxide level toward normal. Conversely, with a decrease in carbon dioxide, the blood vessels constrict, causing an accumulation of carbon dioxide in the tissues and a consequent increase in the carbon dioxide level toward normal.

The oxygen deficiency mechanism for vasodilation also serves as a regulator of cerebral blood flow. The rate of oxygen used by the brain is constant under many different conditions, varying little with mental or physical exercise. If the blood flow to the brain is insufficient to supply the needed oxygen, the deficiency then serves as a potent vasodilator, allowing transport of oxygen to cerebral tissues to return toward normal. The function of these autoregulatory mechanisms in the cerebral circulation is to ensure constancy of cerebral blood flow, even with changes in arterial pressure. Cerebral blood flow suffers significantly only when the arterial pressure falls below approximately 60 mm Hg [10, 15].

Supplying major arteries

The cerebral blood supply is derived from the right and left internal carotid arteries and the right and left vertebral arteries (Fig. 2-10). The internal carotids are branches of the common carotid arteries. The right internal carotid artery arises from the right common carotid, which is one of the two branches formed by the bifurcation of the brachiocephalic artery. The left internal carotid artery arises from the left common carotid, which comes directly from the aortic arch. The common carotid arteries bifurcate at the upper level of the thyroid cartilage to form the internal and external carotid arteries. The vertebral arteries, which are branches of the subclavian arteries, unite to form the basilar artery. The basilar artery subsequently bifurcates to form the two posterior cerebral arteries [5].

The *internal carotid artery* is divided into four sections: the cervical, intrapetrosal, intracavernous, and supraclinoid. All the major branches of this vessel arise from the supraclinoidal portion. These are the ophthalmic, posterior communicating, and anterior choroidal arteries. The internal carotid bifurcates at the level of the optic chiasm to form the anterior cerebral artery and the middle cerebral artery. The *vertebral artery* arises from the subclavian artery and enters the posterior cranial fossa through the foramen magnum. The right and left vertebral arteries follow the anterolateral surface of the medulla and unite at the pons to form the basilar artery. Branches of the vertebral and basilar arteries supply (1) the medulla, (2) pons, (3) midbrain, (4) cerebellum, (5) posterior parts of the diencephalon, and (6) parts of the temporal and occipital lobes [5].

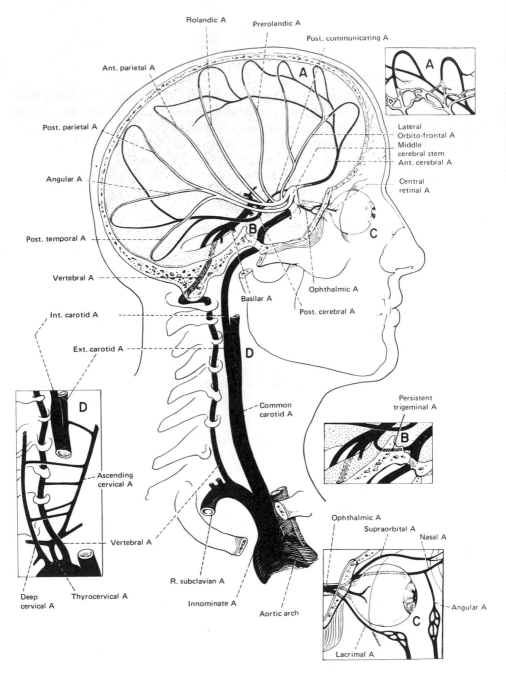

Figure 2-10
*Diagram of the upper chest, neck, and head, showing origin of the major arteries
that supply the brain. (From* Harrison's Principles of Internal Medicine *by Winetrobe
et al. [8th ed.]. Copyright © 1977 by McGraw-Hill, Inc. Used with permission of
McGraw-Hill Book Company.)*

CIRCLE OF WILLIS
The *circle of Willis* is an arterial anastomosis located at the base of the brain. It is formed by the junction of the basilar artery with the internal carotid arteries via the posterior communicating arteries and the anterior communicating artery (Fig. 2-11). The circle of Willis has three main branches for distribution of blood to the cerebral hemispheres — the anterior cerebral artery, the middle cerebral artery, and the posterior cerebral artery. Each vessel supplies a specific area of the brain. The *posterior communicating arteries* arise from the internal carotid arteries and anastomose with the posterior cerebral arteries, which are formed by the bifurcation of the basilar artery. The *anterior communicating artery,* located in front of the optic chiasm, connects the two anterior cerebral arteries, which also arise from the internal carotid arteries. The two *anterior cerebral arteries* originate at the bifurcation of the internal carotid arteries, pass below the optic nerve, and are joined by the anterior communicating artery. The anterior cerebral artery enters the interhemispheric fissure, passes over the medial surface of the cerebral hemisphere, and continues on the superior surface of the corpus callosum. The two *middle cerebral arteries* are actually a continuation of the internal carotid arteries from which they originated. They pass over

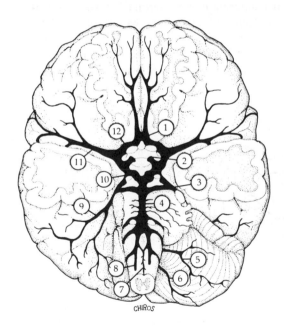

CHIROS

Figure 2-11
The circle of Willis. 1. Anterior communicating artery. 2. Internal carotid artery.
3. Superior cerebellar artery. 4. Basilar artery. 5. Anterior inferior cerebellar artery.
6. Posterior inferior cerebellar artery. 7. Anterior spinal artery. 8. Vertebral artery.
9. Posterior cerebral artery. 10. Posterior communicating artery. 11. Middle cerebral artery. 12. Anterior cerebral artery. (From M. Beyers and S. Dudas [3].)

the anterior perforated substance and enter the lateral cerebral fossa between the temporal lobe and the insula, where they divide into many branches. The two *posterior cerebral arteries* are formed by the bifurcation of the basilar artery. They pass over the crus cerebri and receive anastomoses from the posterior communicating arteries. The posterior communicating arteries then continue along the lateral aspect of the midbrain and along the medial and inferior surfaces of the temporal and occipital lobes [5] (Fig. 2-12).

Branches of the circle of Willis are classified as central and cortical arteries. The *central arteries* arise directly from the circle of Willis and the proximal portions of the major cerebral arteries. These branches penetrate the brain to supply its deep structures. *Cortical arteries* are branches of each of the major cerebral arteries. They pass into the pia mater to supply large areas of the cerebral cortex. These cortical arteries undergo subsequent branching to form many smaller arterial vessels, which penetrate the cerebral cortex [5].

Central branches.   The central branches supply the diencephalon, basal ganglia, and internal capsule. These arteries, which penetrate the structure of the brain, are classified into four groups — anteromedial, anterolateral, posteromedial, and posterolateral. The choroidal arteries are also central branches and will be discussed further. The *anteromedial branches* arise from the anterior cerebral and anterior communicating arteries. They enter the most medial portion of the anterior perforated substance to supply the anterior hypothalamus and the preoptic and supraoptic areas.

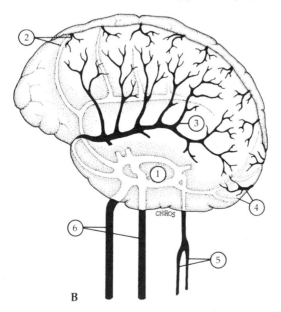

B

Figure 2-12
Lateral view of the cerebral hemisphere, showing the major blood vessels. 1. Circle of Willis. 2. Anterior cerebral artery. 3. Middle cerebral artery. 4. Posterior cerebral artery. 5. Vertebral arteries. 6. Carotid arteries. (From M. Beyers and S. Dudas [3].)

The *posteromedial branches* arise from the posterior communicating artery and the proximal portion of the posterior cerebral artery. These branches supply the hypophysis, infundibulum, and tuberal regions and parts of the thalamus, midbrain, tegmentum, and crus cerebri. Branches of the *posterolateral* group arise from the posterior cerebral artery. They supply the geniculate bodies and pulvinar of the thalamus. Vessels from the *anterolateral* group are usually referred to as the striate arteries. Most of them arise from the proximal portion of the middle cerebral arteries. However, the medial striate artery arises from the anterior cerebral artery. The anterolateral branches enter the anterior perforated substance to supply portions of the basal ganglia and internal capsule. The medial striate artery supplies part of the caudate nucleus and parts of the putamen and internal capsule. The lateral striate arteries supply portions of the caudate nucleus and putamen, the lateral portion of the globus pallidus, and the anterior limb and part of the posterior limb of the internal capsule [5].

The anterior and posterior *choroidal arteries* are also classified as central branches. The anterior choroidal artery arises from the internal carotid artery distal to the posterior communicating artery. This vessel has a long subarachnoid course, and its caliber is narrow. It passes across the optic tract toward the surface of the temporal lobe and enters the inferior horn of the lateral ventricle through the choroid fissure. The *anterior choroidal artery* supplies the choroid plexus, hippocampal formation, and parts of the globus pallidus, as well as the posterior limb and retrolenticular portion of the internal capsule. Smaller branches of this artery supply portions of the optic tract, amygdaloid complex, tail of the caudate nucleus, posterior putamen, and ventrolateral thalamus. The *posterior choroidal arteries* arise from the posterior cerebral artery. They include one medial posterior choroidal artery and two lateral posterior choroidal arteries. The *medial* vessel curves around the midbrain to the pineal body. Its branches supply the tectum, the choroid plexus of the third ventricle, and the superior and medial surfaces of the thalamus. The two *lateral* vessels partially encircle the brainstem and enter the choroid fissure to supply parts of the choroid plexus in the lateral ventricle [5].

Cortical branches. The cortical branches of the circle of Willis are derived from the anterior, middle, and posterior cerebral arteries. The *anterior cerebral artery* gives rise to the medial striate, orbital, frontopolar, callosomarginal, and pericallosal arteries. The *orbital branches* arise from the ascending part of the anterior cerebral artery ventral to the genu of the corpus callosum. They supply the orbital and medial surfaces of the frontal lobe. The *frontopolar artery* arises from the anterior cerebral artery, where it curves around the genu of the corpus callosum. Branches of the frontopolar artery supply the medial portions of the frontal lobe. Some branches extend into the convexity of the cerebral hemisphere. The *callosomarginal artery* arises from the anterior cerebral artery just beyond the frontopolar artery and passes into the callosomarginal sulcus. It supplies the paracentral lobule and parts of the cingulate gyrus. The *pericallosal artery* forms the terminal branch of the anterior cerebral artery. It follows the dorsal surface of the corpus callosum and supplies the medial surfaces of the parietal lobe.

The *middle cerebral artery* gives rise to branches that cover the lateral convexity of the cerebral hemisphere. These branches include the lenticulostriate arteries, the anterior temporal artery, the orbitofrontal artery, the pre-rolandic and rolandic arteries, the anterior and posterior parietal arteries, the posterior temporal artery, and the angular artery. This last vessel supplies the angular gyrus and is the terminal branch of the middle cerebral artery. These vessels supply the lateral parts of the orbital gyri, the inferior and middle frontal gyri, most of the pre- and postcentral gyri, the superior and inferior parietal lobules, and the superior and middle temporal gyri including the temporal pole.

The *posterior cerebral artery* gives rise to cortical branches that extend into the lateral surfaces of the cerebral hemisphere to supply parts of the inferior temporal gyrus, portions of the occipital lobe, and portions of the superior parietal lobule. Additional branches form the posterior temporal artery and the internal occipital artery. The posterior temporal artery supplies the occipitotemporal and lingular gyri via its posterior branches. This vessel also has an anterior temporal branch that supplies the anterior portion of the inferior surface of the temporal lobe and may anastomose with branches of the middle cerebral artery. The internal occipital artery bifurcates to form the parieto-occipital artery and the calcarine artery. Both of these vessels supply areas of the occipital lobe. The calcarine artery supplies the primary visual cortex [5].

VERTEBRAL BASILAR SYSTEM

The vertebral basilar system supplies the medulla, pons, mesencephalon, and cerebellum. The *vertebral arteries* give rise to the posterior spinal arteries, the anterior spinal arteries, and the posterior inferior cerebellar arteries and the posterior meningeal arteries. The *posterior spinal artery* supplies the fasciculii gracilis and cuneatus and their nuclei. The *anterior spinal artery* supplies the paramedian region of the medulla. This includes the pyramids, medial lemniscus, medial longitudinal fasciculus, most of the hypoglossal nucleus, parts of the solitary nucleus, the dorsal motor nucleus of the vagus nerve, and the medial accessory olive. The *posterior inferior cerebellar artery* supplies the retro-olivary region of the medulla, which contains the spinothalamic tracts, the spinal trigeminal nucleus and tract, the nucleus ambiguus, and the dorsal motor nucleus of the vagus. It also supplies part of the inferior cerebellar peduncle.

The *basilar artery,* which is formed by the union of the two vertebral arteries, gives rise to the following branches: (1) the anterior inferior cerebellar arteries, which supply the inferior surface of the cerebellum; (2) the labyrinthine arteries, which pass through the internal auditory meatus to the inner ear; (3) the superior cerebellar arteries, which supply the superior surface of the cerebellum; (4) the long circumferential arteries, which supply the lateral parts of the middle cerebral peduncle and the pontine tegmentum; and (5) the posterior cerebral arteries, which are the terminal branches of the basilar artery and supply the mesencephalon. These have already been discussed [5].

The mesencephalon and ventral portion of the pons are supplied mainly by four branches of the basilar artery. These are the posterior cerebral artery, the superior cerebellar artery, the posterior communicating artery, and the anterior choroidal artery. Branches from these four vessels are grouped as the paramedian arteries and long and short circumferential arteries. The *paramedian arteries,* which arise from the posterior communicating artery and the proximal part of the posterior cerebral arteries, form a plexus in the interpeduncular fossa. These arteries enter the brainstem through the posterior perforated substance to supply the oculomotor complex, the medial longitudinal fasciculus, the red nucleus, the medial portion of the substantia nigra, and the crus cerebri. The *long circumferential arteries* are derived mainly from the posterior cerebral artery. The most important one is the quadrigeminal artery, which encircles the brainstem and supplies the inferior and superior colliculi. The *short circumferential arteries* arise from the proximal portions of the posterior cerebral and the superior cerebellar arteries. They supply the central and lateral portions of the crus cerebri, the substantia nigra, and the lateral portion of

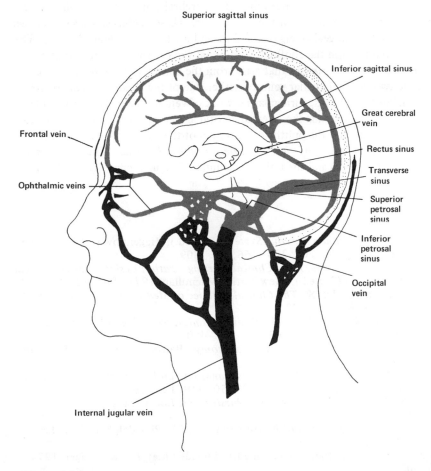

Figure 2-13
Lateral view of the head, showing the dural sinuses and their principal connections with extracranial veins. (From M. B. Carpenter [5].)

the tegmentum of the midbrain. Each of the two cerebellar hemispheres is supplied by one superior cerebellar artery and an anterior and a posterior inferior cerebellar artery [5].

Cerebral veins and venous sinuses

There are two sets of cerebral veins, the deep and the superficial, which are interconnected by many anastomoses. The *deep veins* drain the choroid plexus, periventricular regions, diencephalon, basal ganglia, and deep white matter and empty into the internal cerebral and great cerebral veins. The *superficial veins* drain the cortex and subcortical white matter and empty into the cavernous, petrosal, and transverse sinuses [5].

Fine veins that emerge from the substance of the brain to form plexuses within the pia drain into the larger cerebral veins. The cerebral veins pass through the subarachnoid space into the sinuses of the dura mater. These venous sinuses lie between the periostial and meningeal layers of the dura and are lined with endothelium. The dural sinuses join to form the confluens sinuum at the internal occipital protuberance. The two *transverse sinuses* that arise from the confluens sinuum carry the blood to the two internal jugular veins on either side of the head. The *cavernous sinus,* which consists of a large irregular network of venous channels on both sides of the sella turcica, surrounds the internal carotid artery, the oculomotor, trochlear, and abducens nerves, and the ophthalmic division of the trigeminal nerve. The cavernous sinus drains into the *inferior and superior petrosal sinuses.* These two sinuses enter the transverse sinus and the bulb of the internal jugular vein (Fig. 2-13) [4, 5].

REFERENCES

1. Barr, M. L. *The Human Nervous System* (2nd ed.). Hagerstown, Md.: Harper & Row, 1974. Pp. 82–207; 224–266; 282–309.
2. Beland, I. L., and Passos, J. Y. *Clinical Nursing: Pathophysiological and Psychosocial Approaches* (3rd ed.). New York: Macmillan, 1975. Pp. 232–247.
3. Beyers, M., and Dudas, S. *The Clinical Practice of Medical-Surgical Nursing.* Boston: Little, Brown, 1977.
4. Brock, S., and Kreiger, H. P. *The Basis of Clinical Neurology* (4th ed.). Baltimore: Williams & Wilkins, 1963. Pp. 128–450.
5. Carpenter, M. B. *Core Text of Neuroanatomy.* Baltimore: Williams & Wilkins, 1974. Pp. 1–6; 13–37; 68–244.
6. Clark, R. G. *Essentials of Clinical Neuroanatomy and Neurophysiology* (5th ed.). Philadelphia: Davis, 1975. Pp. 18–22; 50–119; 127–168.
7. Conway, B. L. *Pediatric Neurologic Nursing.* St. Louis: Mosby, 1977. Pp. 35–81.
8. Gardner, E. *Fundamentals of Neurology* (5th ed.). Philadelphia: Saunders, 1968. Pp. 256–338.
9. Goss, C. M. *Gray's Anatomy* (29th ed.). Philadelphia: Lea & Febiger, 1974. Pp. 802–829.
10. Guyton, A. C. *Textbook of Medical Physiology* (5th ed.). Philadelphia: Saunders, 1976. Pp. 694–709; 988–1004.

11. Guyton, A. C. *Organ Physiology, Structure and Function of the Nervous System* (2nd ed.). Philadelphia: Saunders, 1976. Pp. 54–71.
12. Martin, J. B. Hypothalamus and Releasing Hormones. In M. M. Wintrobe, et al. (Eds.), *Harrison's Principles of Internal Medicine* (8th ed.). New York: McGraw-Hill, 1977. Pp. 471–474.
13. Mitchell, G. A. G. *The Essentials of Neuroanatomy* (2nd ed.). Edinburgh: Churchill/Livingstone, 1971. Pp. 21–86.
14. Pansky, B. *Dynamic Anatomy and Physiology.* New York: Macmillan, 1976. Pp. 248–271; 294–296.
15. Raichle, M., and DeVivo, D. Disorders of Cerebral Circulation. In S. G. Eliasson, A. L. Prensky, and W. B. Hardin (Eds.), *Neurological Pathophysiology.* New York: Oxford University Press, 1974. Pp. 242–267.
16. Streeter, D. Disorders of the Neurohypophysis. In G. W. Thorn et al. (Ed.), *Harrison's Principles of Internal Medicine* (8th ed.). New York: McGraw-Hill, 1977. Pp. 490–501.

3. Standards of care for the stroke patient

Goals, and a methodical way of arriving at them, are necessary to any nursing care. In this chapter we attempt to set down the goals of nursing care of the stroke patient, the problems that typically arise, and the particular standards of care that should be maintained in order to combat each problem. Since the patient's capabilities, limitations, and behavior patterns will influence the goals that realistically can be set for him, the nurse must assess these factors before establishing goals to meet standards of care.

A standard is considered here to be a measurement of quality established by an authority and known by experience to produce, generally, a desirable outcome. Once a standard of care has been established, guidelines can be developed that specify the functions required to maintain the established standard. These guidelines, or working plans, are based on a knowledge of a specific condition and provide a logical sequence of actions necessary to attain specified goals.

The results of stroke can be seen in many areas of the patient's functioning. Because of the multiplicity of actual and potential problems facing patients who have suffered a stroke, measures must be instituted early to ensure that complications are minimized and potential for recovery maximized. A systematic approach to the identification of the patient's neurological deficits is essential to the prompt formulation of an appropriate plan of care. To guarantee a complete assessment, the nurse must evaluate all areas that are generally seen as problematic to the stroke patient. A thorough assessment should reveal the nursing care problems that must be dealt with to ensure provision of comprehensive care in keeping with established standards. As the patient progresses from one stage of his disease to another, alterations in the plan of care may be necessary to meet his changing needs. Plans must be continually reviewed, reassessed, and revised to ensure that the patient will reach his maximum state of well-being or rehabilitation.

In the following table, the "goals" are the hoped-for outcome of nursing care, the "problems" are those raised by the stroke patient's particular disabilities, and the "standards" indicate the level of care that must be maintained if the problems are to be overcome and the goals achieved or at least worked toward. Each of these critical factors in the care of the patient with stroke is discussed comprehensively in the chapters that follow.

Table 3-1
Standards of Care

Goals	Problems	Standards
Neurological function Maintenance of normal neurological function or identification and correction of any altered function	Change in neurological function secondary to cerebral edema or extension of the lesion	Evaluate neurological signs periodically to detect any significant alterations.
Language function Establishment of adequate means of communication	Aphasia Dysarthria Dysphasia	Assess ability to communicate and identify deficits. Initiate speech therapy when indicated.
Perceptual ability Establishment of methods of compensation for visual and perceptual loss	Hemianopsia Disorders related to perception of self and illness Disorders related to perception of space Disturbances of the recognition or identification of objects through vision, hearing, and touch Inability to carry out certain movements	Assess vision and perceptual awareness and establish a means of compensating for deficits. Initiate occupational therapy consult to establish a therapeutic program. Provide sensory input to stimulate the patient's awareness of self and awareness of space.
Respiratory function Maintenance or restoration of adequate ventilation	Respiratory failure secondary to airway obstruction, retained or aspirated secretions, disturbance in gas exchange, or damage to the respiratory center	Assess character, pattern, and rhythm of respirations and patency of airway, carry out necessary monitoring of laboratory evaluations, and provide needed respiratory/ventilatory assistance.

Maintenance of normal cardiac function and adequate systemic circulation

Cardiovascular function

Pneumonia or atelectasis secondary to aspiration or immobility

Position the patient so as to provide optimal lung function and to facilitate drainage of secretions.

Change his position periodically to aerate both lungs.

Institute a prophylactic program in pulmonary therapy to promote optimal respiratory toilet.

Cardiac disease

Thrombus formation

Adverse effects from medications

Assess cardiac status and perform necessary monitoring for laboratory evaluations.

Monitor vital signs as indicated.

Monitor patients closely for signs of side effects from medications.

Examine extremities periodically for any signs of peripheral stasis or thrombus formation.

Fluid and electrolyte balance

Maintenance or restoration of fluid and electrolyte balance

Successful feeding by mouth

Inability to take fluids and food by mouth secondary to coma, clouded sensorium, and paralysis

Difficulty in chewing and swallowing secondary to decreased gag and swallowing reflexes

Assess fluid and nutritional status, monitor necessary laboratory evaluations, and provide needed fluid and electrolyte replacements.

Evaluate gag reflex and swallowing ability periodically to determine when the patient is able to swallow safely.

Provide small feedings of a consistency that the patient can swallow safely.

Skin integrity

Maintenance of integrity of the skin and mucous membranes of the oral cavity

Potential pressure necrosis secondary to immobility, sensory loss, or perceptual deficits

Assess the integrity of the skin, establish a plan for regular skin inspection.

Change the patient's position regularly to avoid sustained pressure.

Protect skin from heat and irritation with particular attention to areas with diminished sensation and/or lack of awareness.

Provide regular bathing and lubrication of the skin.

Table 3-1 (continued)

Goals	Problems	Standards
Skin integrity (continued)	Poor oral hygiene secondary to improper care of the mouth and teeth	Carry out oral hygiene procedures approximately three times daily.
Bowel and bladder function Maintenance or restoration of normal bladder function	Incontinence or retention of urine Urinary tract infection	Assess bladder function and establish a bladder program when indicated.
Maintenance or restoration of normal bowel function	Incontinence or fecal impaction	Assess bowel function and establish a bowel program when indicated.
Neuromuscular function Maintenance of full active and passive range of motion in all joints.	Restricted passive and active ranges of joint motion	Assess active and passive range of motion of all joints and identify limitations.
Maintenance or improvement of strength in all extremities	Contracture deformities Weakness of affected and non-affected extremities Disuse atrophy	Initiate physical therapy to evaluate the patient's condition in preparation for an eventual therapeutic program. Give passive range of motion exercises to affected extremities and active exercises to unaffected extremities approximately four times daily. Position head, neck, and extremities to maintain proper body alignment and to support joints. Change the patient's position regularly to prevent sustained pressure and joint contracture.
Rehabilitation and long-term care Optimal level of performance in ADL	Impairment of motor function, sensation, visual acuity, and language Cognitive and perceptual deficits	Assess performance in ADL and identify deficits. Establish a program to teach the patient techniques of functioning optimally in mobility, transfers, and self-care.

Coordination of rehabilitation services to ensure a comprehensive program

Discharge of the patient with an appropriate therapeutic plan to follow at home, or discharge to a facility to provide continuation of rehabilitation program or long-term care.

Mental or physical disability preventing independent living

Initiate physical, occupational, and speech therapy to evaluate and assist in establishing a therapeutic program.

Periodically evaluate performance and adjust program as indicated.

Periodically evaluate rehabilitation potential to determine feasibility of independent living, living with supervision, or need for close observation.

4. Assessment of neurological functioning

This chapter outlines the basic elements included in a neurological history and physical examination, the observations to be made in an ongoing assessment of the patient's neurological functioning, and the ancillary diagnostic procedures commonly used in stroke. It does not intend to teach techniques of performing the neurological examination; for this, the reader should consult specific texts. Rather, the aim of this chapter is to give nurses and therapists a clearer understanding of the significance of the stroke patient's neurological deficits and to encourage them to interpret the findings recorded on neurological examination and incorporate this knowledge into their plan of care for the patient. This is important in the case of patients followed in outpatient rehabilitation programs as well as for acutely ill patients in specialized intensive care units. Emphasis will be placed on neurological deficits associated with stroke and on related differential diagnoses. It should be recognized that other neurological diseases have similar manifestations and that signs of other disease entities may be elicited from the neurological examination.

Assessment of neurological functioning is important during all stages of stroke. Initially it provides the physician with data for both the establishment of the diagnosis and the determination of size, location, and type of lesion that has occurred. While the patient remains acutely ill, close monitoring of neurological status can alert clinicians to subtle changes that may indicate deterioration. This is especially important for early recognition of signs of impending *herniation*. Herniation is the process by which the brain begins to shift downward due to increased volume, thereby causing compression of the brainstem. The skull, being inelastic, allows only minimal expansion of the brain. When the skull cannot accommodate swelling of cerebral tissue, the pressure exerted results in prolapse, with damage to the displaced tissue as well as to the compressed brainstem and blood supply, with increased edema, obstruction, and hemorrhage. The nurse is often the first person to observe an alteration in the neurological functioning of the acutely ill patient. It is most important that she or he recognize the significance of the changes noted and respond accordingly. As the patient's condition stabilizes, neurological signs can be monitored less frequently. However, continued neurological assessment is essential for identification of deficits, establishment of rehabilitation potential, and evaluation of functional restoration.

THE NEUROLOGICAL EXAMINATION

The neurological examination includes (1) a history, (2) assessment of mental status, (3) assessment of speech and language function, (4) examination of the cranial nerves, (5) examination of the motor system, (6) examination of the sensory system, and (7) testing of reflexes. The major objective of the neurological examination is to elicit the signs and symptoms of the patient's neurological dysfunction in order to acquire the clinical data necessary for analysis of the disease process. In the acute stage it is carried out with the purpose of arriving at a definitive diagnosis and initiating treatment. Throughout the course of hospitalization, the neurological examination may be performed to assess the patient's progress and modify therapy accordingly. *Symptoms* are the patient's subjective description of his illness, while *signs* are the objective manifestations of illness that the clinician observes. Findings on physical examination are correlated with the history of illness provided by the patient [4, 8] . Physical signs will indicate the site of the lesion, but the patient's description of his symptoms and their progression is most useful in determining the pathological process involved.

History

The history should be obtained directly from the patient. If this is impossible, as it often is in the acute stage of stroke, when the patient may be unconscious, aphasic, or unable to remember or appreciate his functional impairment, family or friends may be able to supply details of the course of events preceding the stroke and symptoms of which the patient may have complained. The history includes a statement of major complaint, a detailed description of the symptoms and course of the current illness, a chronological account of the development of this illness, and an outline of the past medical history and family history. The *history of present illness* should describe each symptom, including chronology of occurrence, character, mode of onset, precipitating or etiological factors, duration, treatment, and progression or regression [4, 8] .

A complete *past medical history,* including family history, should also be taken at this time, since conditions such as diabetes mellitus, hypertension, arrhythmias, atherosclerosis, valvular heart disease, thrombophlebitis, and cerebrovascular insufficiency are important etiological factors in the development of stroke. Since many of the disorders due to cerebrovascular disease are of a subjective nature, the examiner should inquire whether the patient has experienced convulsions, headache, weakness, numbness, vertigo, pain, bowel or bladder dysfunction, disturbance of speech or comprehension, visual alterations, or difficulty in walking or in performing any other physical activity that has not been specifically mentioned. Periodic lightheadedness related to postural changes may be indicative of cerebrovascular insufficiency, particularly when associated with weakness, numbness, vertigo, or disturbances of vision or language. Abrupt onset of a motor, sensory, visual, or language disturbance without headache or loss of consciousness is characteristic of an ischemic infarction. A progression of symptoms from headache to paralysis, stupor, and coma is more characteristic of a hemorrhagic stroke. When this is suspected, other conditions that cause increased intracranial pressure will be included in the differential diagnoses and diagnostic efforts will be directed to ruling them out. These include hemorrhage due to trauma, rupture of vascular malformations or vascular tumors, brain abscess, and encephalitis [5, 8] .

Assessment of mental status
LEVEL OF CONSCIOUSNESS
The first step in assessment of the patient's mental status is to determine his level of consciousness. The patient may be described as alert, lethargic, stuporous, semicomatose,

or comatose. The *alert* patient is awake, reacts spontaneously, and usually behaves appropriately. Unless he is aphasic, he will initiate and respond to conversation. Lethargy is a morbid state of drowsiness. The *lethargic* patient can be awakened and will appear completely aware and mentally intact. However, he will fall back to sleep as soon as the stimulus that awakened him is removed. The *stuporous* or semicomatose patient's level of consciousness is impaired. The degree of impairment will vary. He may be aroused with some difficulty for brief periods but show a slow and inadequate response. With a more profound degree of stupor the patient will respond only to painful stimuli. However, swallowing, coughing, corneal, and pupillary reflexes as well as superficial and deep tendon reflexes will remain intact. Pathological reflexes will not be elicited. The *comatose* patient is completely unresponsive, makes no voluntary movements, and reacts with only elemental reflexes. Frequently even the most powerful and painful stimuli, such as pressure on the eyeballs and pinching the skin, elicit no response. His pupils may remain either dilated or constricted, without reaction to light. His swallowing and coughing reflexes are lost. He may exhibit decerebrate or decorticate posturing.

In some cases there is only slight impairment of the patient's level of consciousness, his simple mental functions, elemental responses, and reaction to ordinary commands remaining intact. This is referred to as *confusion.* The usual manifestations are impairment of memory, attention span, perception, and orientation. Cerebrovascular disease is the most common cause of an impaired level of consciousness. When either thrombosis or hemorrhage occurs in the basilar artery, profound coma usually ensues [4, 5, 8].

GENERAL MENTAL STATUS

Once the level of consciousness has been established, the examiner will note the patient's general appearance and behavior and proceed with an assessment of his sensorium, memory for past events, general knowledge, arithmetic ability, and ability to comprehend abstract relationships. Observation of *appearance* and general behavior includes physical appearance, posture, facial expression, motor activity, manner of speech, attitude, conduct, and reactions.

A complete appraisal of *sensorium* includes assessment of level of consciousness, degree of orientation, personal identification, concentration, and comprehension. All these faculties may be disturbed to some degree with stroke. Assessment of level of consciousness has already been discussed. In order to test for *orientation* to time and place, the examiner asks the patient the date, day of week, and location of the building and city in which the examination is being performed. To test personal identification the patient is asked to give his name, age, residence, and various data concerning his education, employment, family, or medical history. The patient's capacity for *concentration* and ability to maintain interest and attention will be observed throughout the examination as he is called upon to perform the various tests and respond to specific questions. The most critical test of *comprehension* is how much insight the patient has about the impairments resulting from his illness and how willing he is to accept the medical recommendations for treatment. Patients lacking insight will be indifferent to their impaired functioning or ascribe the source of their signs and symptoms to some external cause [4, 7].

Testing of *memory* includes remote and recent events as well as immediate recall. Memory for remote events is usually tested by asking the patient about events of his own past life. Recent memory is tested by giving the patient several common objects to remember, then questioning him about them ten minutes later. Immediate recall is tested by having the patient repeat a series of six digits. *General knowledge* involves the patient's grasp of current events. He is questioned about history, science, geography, or local civic events to assess the amount and accuracy of his information. The patient's educational background must of course be considered in posing such questions and in assessing the responses. *Arithmetic ability* may be evaluated by having the patient complete simple addition, subtraction, multiplication, and division. Usually he is asked to subtract 7 from 100, then to continue subtracting 7 from each resulting remainder. Depending on the educational level and capability of the patient, problems involving more complex computation may be posed for solution. The *ability to comprehend abstract relationships* is ordinarily tested by quoting a well-known adage or proverb such as "a rolling stone gathers no moss" and asking the patient to explain what is meant by the statement. If the patient demonstrates concrete thinking by a failure to recognize the subtle abstract principle implied by the adage, detailed psychological testing may be ordered [4, 8]. For example, the patient who demonstrates only concrete thinking might reply, "Most turning things don't pick up anything." The patient who demonstrates abstract thinking might reply, "A drifter isn't burdened by responsibilities."

Assessment of speech and language functions

Disorders of speech and language are common findings in stroke. The examiner will listen to the patient's speech to detect dysarthria, dysphonia, or aphasia. Dysarthria is a defect of articulation, enunciation, and rhythm of speech, while dysphonia denotes the production of abnormal sounds from the larynx. Aphasia is an impairment of the use and understanding of spoken or written language. If the patient's history or findings on examination suggest a stroke in the speech area, a formal evaluation of speech and language functions will be carried out. This should include an assessment of the patient's ability to speak, read, write from dictation, copy, and comprehend what he has said, read, and written. Gestures may be used for communication when speech is absent. It is also important to ascertain that vision and hearing are intact before testing for aphasia. Disorders of speech and language and the assessment of these functions are discussed in detail in Chapter 5 [4, 8].

Examination of the cranial nerves

Examination of the cranial nerves is important and must be carried out in great detail. Usually each nerve is examined individually, in succession. The anatomical location and functions of the twelve cranial nerves have been described in Chapter 2. The procedure for testing cranial nerve function and some of the deficits associated with cranial nerve damage due to stroke will be described here.

OLFACTORY NERVE (I)
The sole function of the first cranial nerve is the sense of smell. A nonirritating volatile oil such as clove or lemon is ordinarily used to test this sense; coffee, vanilla, or tobacco may also be used. After checking to be certain both nasal passages are open, the examiner tests each nostril separately. With the patient's eyes closed, one nostril is occluded and the opposite side tested by bringing the substance up to the nose and asking the patient to identify it. Damage to the olfactory nerves may result from infarction of the adjacent brain tissue. The major manifestations of stroke in this area, however, are so life-threatening as to preclude testing of olfaction. Anosmia, the absence of the sense of smell, is sometimes noted following subarachnoid hemorrhage [4, 8].

OPTIC NERVE (II)
The major function of the second cranial nerve is vision. Visual impulses are carried by the optic nerves from the retina to the optic chiasm, where they enter the visual pathways leading to various parts of the cerebral cortex for recognition of the visual stimuli. Optic nerve fibers are the axons of ganglion cells in the retina. Other fibers of the optic nerves are involved in ocular reflexes. Ocular fixation is regulated so that any image that is looked at will be brought onto the macula, which is the area of most acute vision [10]. Each optic tract is composed of fibers from the temporal half of the retina of the same side and the nasal half of the retina of the opposite side. The decussation of the optic nerve fibers occurs at the optic chiasm, where left and right optic nerves unite. Abnormalities can result from lesions at any point in the extensive pathway from the retina to the cerebral cortex [4]. Testing of optic nerve function includes an examination of visual acuity, and range of vision as well as direct visualization of the optic nerve and retina by means of a funduscopic examination.

Visual acuity.   The ability of the eye to perceive detail, is tested for near and distant vision in both eyes. If the patient wears corrective lenses, the examination is usually carried out with and without the lenses. It should be noted that refractive errors for which corrective lenses are prescribed are not usually associated with neurological impairments. Near vision is tested by having the patient read from a set of sentences printed in varying sizes of type, and distant vision is tested by a Snellen chart. The chart consists of a series of letters of diminishing size designed to be read at distances varying from 200 feet to 10 feet. Each eye is examined separately. With the opposite eye covered, the patient is asked to identify the letters on the chart. The degree of visual acuity for each eye is expressed as a fraction in which 20 is always the numerator and the denominator is the distance in feet at which the smallest letters on the chart could be read by the patient. If the patient standing 20 feet from the chart can only identify with his right eye those letters which he should be able to read at 40 feet, his visual acuity for the right eye will be expressed as 20/40 vision. Obviously such testing cannot be carried out with an acutely ill or confused patient. If a patient has marked impairment of visual acuity, the examiner will note the distance at which the patient can distinguish gross forms and count the extended fingers of the examiner's hand. Lesions affecting the optic chiasm can cause a loss of visual acuity that may progress to blindness [4, 6, 8].

Range of vision. The patient is tested for his visual fields, i.e., the limit of his peripheral vision, or the space within which he can see an object while his eye remains fixed on another spot. When precise delineation of the periphery of visual range is necessary, a detailed study of the visual fields can be carried out using an instrument called a perimeter. This allows for testing of the field of vision through the arc of a circle that is concentric with the retina. For screening purposes the visual fields are usually tested by *confrontation.* Using himself as a control, the examiner compares his normal field of vision with that of the patient's opposite eye. To accomplish this he stands in front of the patient with his right eye closed. The patient is instructed to close the left eye, look straight ahead at a fixed spot on the wall and respond as soon as he becomes aware of the examiner's moving finger. The examiner then extends his arm and wiggles his index finger while bringing the hand in from the periphery of all four quadrants of the visual field at an equal distance between himself and the patient. This same procedure is then carried out for the opposite eye. If a defect is noted, the examiner can determine the configuration of the loss of vision by moving the finger in from several areas within the affected quadrant. When visual fields are tested, the examiner looks for the peripheral limits of vision and also the areas within these limits where vision is absent. A sketch of the defects noted should be placed in the patient's medical record.

The visual field defect seen most often with stroke is a homonymous hemianopsia, which is caused by lesions beyond the optic chiasm, in the optic tract and radiations. With cerebrovascular insufficiency of either the carotid or the vertebrobasilar systems there may be transient episodes of hemianopsia or brief recurrent loss of binocular vision. Occlusion of any of the arteries that supply cortical areas of the visual pathway can cause permanent defects of the visual field [4]. The loss of vision will occur in corresponding halves of the fields of both eyes, affecting either the right or the left half of the total visual field (Fig. 4-1). Lesions in the parietal lobe that interrupt the pathways from the superior portion of the retina to the optic radiations may result in a homonymous defect of the inferior quadrant of the visual field. Temporal lobe lesions that interrupt the pathway from the inferior portion of the retina may cause a homonymous defect of the superior quadrant of the visual field [4, 8].

The last stage of the visual pathway from the retina to the cortex starts at the lateral geniculate body. From here the optic fibers enter the posterior limb of the internal capsule. The fibers emerge from the capsule as the optic radiation or geniculocalcarine pathway, which runs to the area striata of the occipital lobe. The posterior portion of the optic tract and the anterior portion of the optic radiations are supplied by the anterior choroidal artery. The middle portion of the optic radiations is supplied by the middle cerebral artery, and the posterior part is supplied by branches of the posterior cerebral artery. The geniculate bodies are supplied by the anterior choroidal artery and branches of the posterior cerebral artery. The striate cortex of the occipital lobe receives its blood supply from cortical branches of both

Homonymous — blindness of the nasal half of one eye
and the temporal half of the other eye. This is the
form usually found in lesions of the cerebral hemispheres.

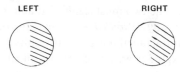

Bitemporal — loss of the temporal fields of vision in both eyes.

Binasal — loss of the nasal halves of the field of vision in both eyes.

Figure 4-1
Hemianopsia.

the posterior cerebral artery and the middle cerebral artery [4]. The main arterial
supply to the visual cortex comes via the posterior cerebral artery. Thrombosis of
this artery or infarction of the visual cortex will result in a crossed homonymous
hemianopsia [10]. Involvement of the optic tract from the chiasm to the geniculate
body will result in a contralateral hemianopsia. Lesions of the geniculate body or of
the optic radiations from that body to the occipital cortex will also produce a contralateral hemianopsia [4].

Funduscopic examination.   The retina and optic nerve can be visualized directly by
means of an ophthalmoscope — the *funduscopic examination.* The background color
of the normal retina is red-orange with black pigmented areas that vary in size with race
and complexion. The optic disc, which represents the entrance of the optic nerve
into the retina, is a pale pink and has a sharp border. It may be outlined by black pig-
mentation of the retina. Blood vessels diverge from the disc and spread out across
the retina. These arteries and veins usually occur in pairs. The veins are dark red and
solid and may be seen to pulsate. The arteries are a brighter red than the veins, are
approximately four fifths the diameter of their corresponding veins, and are pulseless.
In the temporal side of the optic disc is a white or pale yellow depression called the
physiologic cup. The examiner observes the color, size, shape, and borders of the optic

disc and studies the retina, blood vessels, and physiologic cup. The appearance of these structures is most important in neurological disorders.

Any abnormalities seen are described in the medical record. Retinal hemorrhages are characteristic of subarachnoid hemorrhage [5]. The two most significant abnormalities are papilledema (choked disc) and optic atrophy. *Papilledema,* a swelling of the optic disc, is usually associated with increased intracranial pressure. It results from obstruction of venous outflow caused by elevated pressure of cerebrospinal fluid against the optic nerve. As the subdural and subarachnoid spaces are continuous along the course of the optic nerve, any increase of intracranial pressure will be conducted to the optic nerve. The first signs of papilledema may be an absence of pulsations in the retinal veins or an increase in diameter of the retinal veins in relation to their corresponding arteries. As the condition progresses, (1) the margin of the optic disc will become indistinct, (2) the disc will be elevated above the surface of the retina, (3) the normal cupping in the center of the disc will disappear, (4) an arching of the arteries and veins will be seen where they pass from the retina over the margin of the optic disc, and (5) the physiological blind spot will be enlarged. With severe papilledema, hemorrhages will be seen in and around the retina. Papilledema requires immediate attention. If pressure on the optic nerve is not relieved, optic atrophy and eventually blindness will result. *Optic atrophy* is classified as (1) primary, when it results from disease that affects the optic nerve directly, and (2) secondary, when it is the result of papilledema due to increased intracranial pressure. With optic atrophy the disc will be a pale yellow or white with a sharp margin and an accentuated physiological cup [4, 6, 8].

THE OCULAR NERVES (III, IV, VI)
The oculomotor (III), trochlear (IV), and abducens (VI) nerves, which work together to regulate eye movements, are examined together. Through *conjugate function* these three cranial nerves control the extraocular muscles so that the two eyes remain parallel throughout their range of motion and thus maintain binocular vision. The oculomotor nerve also controls the levator palpabrae superioris muscle, which elevates the upper eyelid, and the muscle that constricts the pupil in response to illumination, or conversion and accommodation. Since the cervical portion of the sympathetic nervous system assists the oculomotor nerve in innervation of the eyelid and pupil, this function is also considered in assessing the ocular nerves [4]. Lesions that affect any of the three ocular nerves will result in weakness of the muscles innervated by these nerves, with deviation of the eyeball from the parallel position. Diplopia (double vision) and drooping (ptosis) of the upper eyelid will occur [8]. A lesion that interrupts the oculomotor nerve will paralyze all the extraocular muscles except the superior oblique and lateral rectus. Complete paralysis of the oculomotor nerve will result in ptosis of the upper eyelid, paralysis of the medial and upward gaze, and weakness of the downward gaze, accompanied by sustained dilation of the pupil and loss of power to vary the curvature of the lens for close and distinct vision. If a lesion affecting the oculomotor nerve is within the midbrain, only certain functions may be lost. When the lesion occurs

anywhere from the emergence of the nerve to the eye, paralysis of the nerve will be complete [4].

Examination of the ocular nerves includes (1) inspection of the eyelids; (2) examination of the size, shape, equality, position, and reflexes of the pupils; and (3) testing of ocular movements.

Eyelids.   The eyelids are inspected for drooping. The position of the eyelids is inspected with the patient looking directly at the examiner (elevation of the upper eyelid is a function of the levator palpebrae superioris). With partial drooping the patient can elevate the lid only partially, by voluntary effort; with complete ptosis, the patient will be unable to raise the lid voluntarily.

Pupils.   The pupils are inspected for size, shape, equality, and position. Their *size* can vary considerably with the surrounding illumination; in lighting of average intensity they are approximately three to four millimeters in diameter. Inspection of the pupils should be carried out in subdued light. Pupils of less than two millimeters in diameter are referred to as *miotic* and the condition as *miosis.* Pupils with a diameter greater than 5 millimeters are said to be *mydriatic* and the condition, *mydriasis.* Since certain drugs influence pupil size, the examiner should always inquire as to medications the patient may have taken or instilled into the eyes before assessing the significance of any alteration in pupil size. Brainstem stroke may cause marked miosis due to a bilateral interruption of the descending pathway of the nerves that dilate the pupils. Dilation of the pupil is an early sign of increased intracranial pressure, which causes the uncal portions of the temporal lobe to compress the midbrain and obstruct its circulation. When this occurs, dilation of the pupil will be followed by ptosis of the eyelid and paralysis of the extraocular muscles [4].

Normally the pupils are round and the outline regular. Any irregularity of *shape* or notching of the outline of the pupil is significant and should be reported. The pupils should appear approximately *equal* in size on inspection. A slight difference (approximately one millimeter) is found in approximately twenty percent of the normal population, however, and is usually not significant. Gross inequality between the two pupils is referred to as *anisocoria.* A dilated and fixed pupil in a comatose patient may be indicative of a lesion of the ipsilateral hemisphere, if there is direct pressure on the oculomotor nerve due to herniation of the hippocampal gyrus through the tentorial notch [4]. When a pupil is not in its normal position in the center of the iris, it is said to be *eccentric.* Eccentric pupils may result from trauma or iritis [4, 8].

Three pupillary reflexes are tested separately for each eye: the pupillary light reflex, the accommodation-convergence reflex, and the ciliospinal reflex. To evaluate the pupillary *light reflex,* a bright light is shone into one eye. Both pupils should constrict promptly when light is focused on the retina and dilate when the source of light is withdrawn (Fig. 4-2). Both the homolateral and contralateral pupils respond as a result of the semidecussation of the cranial nerve fibers. The response of the

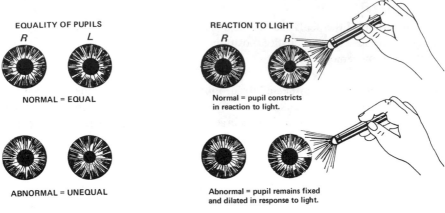

Figure 4-2
Normal and abnormal pupillary signs.

eye into which the light is shone is called the *direct light reflex* and that of the opposite eye, the *consensual light reflex*. Both reflexes should be tested for each eye and the responses noted as prompt, sluggish, or absent. When a lesion affects the oculomotor nerve, both the direct and the consensual light reflexes will be absent on the involved side, due to paralysis of the pupillary sphincter, but will remain intact on the uninvolved side. A blind eye will not respond directly to light and the opposite eye will not respond consensually. If the oculomotor nerve is intact, and the optic nerve of the opposite eye has not been affected, the blind eye will respond consensually to light. To test the *accommodation-convergence reflex,* the patient is instructed to gaze into the distance, then look quickly at an object placed about six to eight inches from his face. Normally both eyes adduct and the pupils constrict. Loss of this response is due to a lesion of the oculomotor nerve. The normal *ciliospinal reflex* is a dilation of the pupil on the same side when the skin of the neck is pinched. This demonstrates the integrity of the cervical sympathetic pathway [4, 8] .

Ocular movements.   The function of the extraocular muscles is examined to test the integrity of the ocular nerve pathways that innervate them. First the eyes are inspected for alignment. Any deviation of visual alignment is indicative of a weakness of one or more of the extraocular muscles and is called *strabismus.* The examiner then moves his finger into six different positions, having instructed the patient to follow it with his eyes, and observes the *oculomotor movements.* Each of the six positions emphasizes the activity of one pair of muscles:

1. Eyes to the left — right medial rectus and left lateral rectus
2. Eyes to the right — right lateral rectus and left medial rectus
3. Eyes to the right and upward — right superior rectus and left inferior oblique
4. Eyes to the left and upward — right inferior oblique and left superior rectus

5. Eyes to the right and downward — right inferior rectus and left superior oblique
6. Eyes to the left and downward — right superior oblique and left inferior rectus

As the eyes are turned to each of these six positions, the examiner notes whether the patient experiences diplopia and whether he exhibits signs of muscle weakness and nystagmus. Lesions affecting the abducens (VI) nerve will produce paralysis of the ipsilateral rectus muscle, causing an internal strabismus and inability to direct the eye laterally. As with any impairment of the extraocular muscles, the patient will experience diplopia. *Nystagmus* is a series of rhythmic, repetitive, jerking movements of the two eyes. A few beats are considered normal when the eyes are turned to an extreme position. Nystagmus is considered abnormal when it occurs with the eyes looking straight ahead or at a moderate angle of deviation. In describing a nystagmus the examiner will use the term "quick component" to indicate the direction toward which the eye moves [4, 8].

When voluntary movement is absent due to coma, it is possible to test for *reflex ocular movements* — the *oculocephalic reflex* or *doll's head phenomenon*. The examiner holds the patient's eyelids open and turns the head rapidly from side to side. If the oculocephalic reflex is intact, the eyes will move to the opposite direction from that toward which the head is turned. Failure of the eyes to move to one side indicates paralysis of conjugate gaze to that side, and dissociation of response indicates a brainstem disorder. The oculocephalic reflex is absent in deep coma and severe brainstem involvement and may be referred to as "doll's eyes" in the medical record.

Oculomotor nerve defects are commonly associated with aneurysms of the internal carotid and posterior communicating arteries [8], and may occur as isolated palsies of the oculomotor (III) and trochlear (IV) nerves [5]. Significant disturbances of ocular nerve function caused by stroke include paralysis of extraocular muscles, weakness or paralysis of conjugate gaze, pupillary changes, and nystagmus [4].

Conjugate gaze refers to the normal ability of the two eyes to gaze together in a given direction. Often lesions that destroy cortical areas of the frontal lobe anterior to the motor strip will prevent the patient from directing his gaze to the other side and can cause the eyes to deviate toward the side of the lesion. A lesion in the pons will impair the abducens (VI) nerve, preventing gaze toward the side of the lesion and resulting in a persistent conjugate deviation away from the affected side [8]. With hemianopsia resulting from subcortical infarction of the parietal and occipital lobes, the head and eyes will be deviated away from the blind visual field, and the patient will be unable to deviate the eyes voluntarily beyond the midline into the hemianopic field. This will be seen with lesions of either hemisphere in the area supplied by the middle cerebral artery. Each cerebral hemisphere directs the eye movement to the contralateral side. Conjugate defects that affect the movement of both eyes will therefore localize to the affected hemisphere [5].

Horner's syndrome is caused by lesions in the pathway of the sympathetic nerve fibers that assist the oculomotor (III) nerve in dilation of the pupil and innervate the smooth muscle of the eyelid. It occurs most often with vascular lesions of the brainstem [8]. The signs are a mild ptosis of the upper lid, constriction of the pupil, and absence of sweating on the affected side of the face.

TRIGEMINAL NERVE (V)

The trigeminal nerve has a motor and a sensory component. The principal function of the motor division is innervation of the muscles of mastication. The sensory component mediates general sensation for the intracranial cavity above the tentorium, face, scalp, paranasal sinuses, and nasal and oral cavities. It is also involved in the corneal reflex and jaw reflex [4, 6, 8].

Motor function. To assess the motor function, the muscles of mastication are tested as follows. The patient is instructed to clench his jaw while the examiner palpates the masseter and temporal muscles for abnormalities of size or contraction. The patient is then instructed to open his mouth wide so the examiner may note any asymmetrical movement of the jaw [6].

Sensory component. The trigeminal nerve has three divisions: ophthalmic, maxillary, and mandibular. The distribution of these three divisions has been described in Chapter 2. The patient is instructed to close his eyes while the examiner tests the sensation over the distribution of each division by touching each side of the face in the ophthalmic, maxillary, and mandibular area, first with a pin, then with a wisp of cotton. The findings on one side are compared to those on the other, and any abnormalities are noted. The mucous membranes are also tested. A sketch will be drawn in the medical record to illustrate any sensory loss or impairment. When the *corneal reflex* is tested, the patient is told to turn his eyes away to prevent involuntary blinking in response to the approach of the examiner's hand. The tip of a small wisp of cotton is then brought in from the side to touch the patient's cornea. The normal reaction is a bilateral blinking of the eyes. To test for a *jaw jerk reflex,* the patient's mouth should be partially open, with the muscles of mastication relaxed. The examiner places his thumb on the midline of the mandible below the lower lip and taps the thumb with the reflex hammer. Normally this reflex cannot be elicited. When it is present there will be a brisk elevation of the mandible. Presence of a jaw jerk reflex is indicative of a frontal lobe lesion [4, 8].

It should be noted here that, although the integrated movements of facial expression, chewing, and swallowing are mediated by cranial nerves, lesions occurring at any level of the motor pathway due to a unilateral hemispheric stroke will affect these movements [5]. Since the motor nuclei of the trigeminal nerve have a predominantly bilateral innervation, unilateral lesions occurring above the motor nuclei usually will not cause a marked degree of paralysis of the muscles of mastication, although there may be a contralateral weakness. With bilateral lesions above the motor nuclei, however, a marked paralysis quite often results. Supranuclear involvement of the trigeminal nerve may be due to vascular lesions that affect the cerebral cortex, internal capsule, basal ganglia, cerebral peduncles, or those areas of the pons above the trigeminal nerve nuclei. Vascular lesions affecting the pons in the area of the nuclei may result in sensory or motor impairment or both. With brainstem stroke there may be an impairment of sensation, loss of corneal reflex, pain over the distribution of the three divisions of the nerve, and profound weakness of the musculature served by the trigeminal nerve. Thrombosis of the posterior inferior cerebellar artery will also affect functioning of the trigeminal nerve [4] .

FACIAL NERVE (VII)
The functions of the facial nerve are to innervate the muscles of expression, mediate taste perception from the anterior portion of the tongue, and innervate certain salivary glands and the lacrimal glands. The *sensory function* is assessed by testing the patient's ability to identify the taste of vinegar or sugar placed on the tongue. The *motor component* is examined by observing the muscles of expression and testing their strength. Mild asymmetry of the face is normal. The examiner looks for drooping of one side of the mouth, flattening of the nasolabial fold, sagging of the lower eyelid, and asymmetrical movement of the sides of the face when the patient speaks. To test muscle strength the patient is instructed to raise and lower his eyebrows, wrinkle his forehead, smile, show his teeth, whistle, and close his eyes tightly while the examiner watches for loss of power or weakness in the involved muscles. It is important to note the distribution of any weakness observed. The degree of weakness can be assessed by having the patient hold his eyelids shut while the examiner attempts to open them [4, 8] .

The supranuclear connections of the nuclear center that controls the upper part of the face are both contralateral and ipsilateral, while those of the center that controls the lower part of the face are mainly contralateral. Consequently cortical and subcortical lesions due to stroke in one hemisphere will result in paralysis of the lower part of the face on the side opposite to the lesion but will leave the upper portion of the face relatively free of paralysis [4, 6] . When the nucleus of the facial nerve or its peripheral nerve fibers is affected, there will be a weakness over the entire half of the face on the side of the lesion. This is referred to as *peripheral facial weakness* and occurs when the lower motor neuron is affected. It must be distinguished from *central facial weakness,* which is a weakness of the lower half of the face on the side opposite the lesion resulting from an upper motor lesion in the corticobulbar tract [8] .

Lesions of the brainstem can involve the nuclei of the facial nerve and its fibers to result in facial paralysis and impairment of secretion from the submandibular, submaxillary, and lacrimal glands. In addition sounds will be heard as exceptionally unpleasant and undampened due to paralysis of the stapedius muscle [4] . Special attention must be given to the eyes in the absence of normal formation of tears. A solution of methylcellulose is usually instilled regularly to prevent corneal abrasion.

ACOUSTIC NERVE (VIII)
The acoustic nerve has two components, the auditory (or cochlear) and the vestibular. The cochlear component transmits nerve impulses from vibrations of the fluid in the cochlea to the brain and thus mediates hearing. The vestibular component

transmits impulses from the membranes of the semicircular canals of the inner ear and is concerned with balance, body position, and orientation in space [6, 8].

Cochlear component.   The ears are examined with an otoscope to determine whether the tympanic membranes are intact. The functioning of the cochlear component is then assessed by means of a variety of hearing tests. First the examiner whispers softly into each ear while the opposite ear is held closed. If this is understood clearly, there is obviously no hearing loss. The examiner should note the distance at which his voice can be heard and record any difficulty the patient has in hearing soft and loud noises and low and high pitches. If impaired hearing is detected, it is important to distinguish between conductive and neurogenic hearing loss. *Conductive hearing loss* is due to impaired transmission of sound through the external or middle ear. *Neurogenic hearing loss* is due to damage of the cochlear nerve.

The *Rinne test* is used to differentiate between conductive and neurogenic hearing loss. A positive test indicates neurogenic hearing loss. A vibrating tuning fork is placed on the mastoid process of the temporal bone and the patient is instructed to indicate when he no longer hears the sound. Then the fork is held next to the patient's ear. If he is able to perceive the sound better when the tuning fork is held on the bone than when it is held in front of the ear, the defect is one of conduction due to an abnormality of the middle or external ear. In this case the Rinne test is then considered negative. If the patient hears the sound better when the tuning fork is held next to the ear, the conduction mechanism is intact through the middle ear and the hearing defect is the result of the abnormally of the inner ear, or the cochlear nerve. In this case the result of the Rinne test is considered positive [4, 8].

The *Weber test* is also used to differentiate between conductive and neurogenic hearing loss. A positive Weber test indicates a conductive hearing loss. The handle of a vibrating tuning fork is held on the vertex of the skull or the middle of the forehead. Normally the sound is perceived equally in both ears and is usually described as coming from "all over the head." If there is a conductive hearing loss, the sound will be heard better in the affected ear. This is considered a positive finding. With a neurogenic hearing loss the sound will be perceived in the normal ear [4, 8].

Vestibular component.   The *vestibular* division of the acoustic nerve is not usually tested unless the history or findings (vertigo, ataxia) suggest involvement of the vestibular system. The *cold caloric test* is the standard method of evaluating vestibular function. An otoscopic inspection of the external auditory canal and tympanic membrane is always performed first to assure that an infection or perforation of the tympanic membrane will not be complicated by the test. The patient is placed in a supine position with the head elevated 30 degrees so that the semicircular canal is in a vertical position. Five milliliters of ice water are then introduced into the auditory canal through a soft-tipped rubber catheter. This is repeated for the opposite side. The normal response to this procedure is nystagmus of both eyes with quick movement toward the opposite side of the head. It may also induce nausea, vomiting, and vertigo. When there is no response or a decreased response, the vestibular system on that side is impaired [8].

Vascular lesions of the brainstem may involve the nuclei or the central connections of the cochlear and vestibular components. Subarachnoid hemorrhage can also damage the acoustic nerve. The pontine branches of the basilar artery supply the nuclei of the acoustic nerve. Therefore, aneurysms or thrombosis occurring in any of these vessels or causing infarction of adjacent areas can cause attacks of vertigo and deafness with impairment of equilibrium and nystagmus [4].

GLOSSOPHARYNGEAL (IX) AND VAGUS (X) NERVES

Cranial nerves IX and X are closely related anatomically and functionally. Both have motor and autonomic branches, with nuclei in the medulla, and they serve many structures in common. Therefore these two nerves are usually tested together. The *glossopharyngeal nerve* innervates part of the pharyngeal musculature, the carotid sinus and carotid body; conveys taste from the posterior portion of the tongue; and supplies sensation to the tonsils and mucous membranes of the pharynx. The *vagus nerve* innervates the thoracic and abnormal viscera, larynx, pharynx, and palate; and conveys sensory impulses from the digestive tract, heart, and lungs [4, 8].

The assessment of ninth and tenth nerve function includes inspection of the soft palate, examination of the oropharynx, and testing of the gag reflex and swallowing. If there is hoarseness or abnormal phonation, the vocal cords may be inspected by indirect laryngoscopy. The soft palate is inspected for symmetry. The patient is instructed to say "ah-h-h" while the examiner notes any deviation, lack of symmetry, or delay in rise of the soft palate. When there is a unilateral weakness of the soft palate, the affected side will be lower, without the characteristic arch. The posterior wall of the oropharynx is touched with a tongue depressor to elicit the *gag reflex*, which characteristically elevates the palate and constricts the muscles of the pharynx. If any weakness is apparent, the examiner should test both sides of the oropharynx for a gag reflex. To test swallowing ability, the patient is placed in a supine position with his head elevated, then asked to swallow some water. The examiner observes for any difficulty in swallowing or regurgitation of the water through the nose that would indicate an inability to close off the nasopharynx due to weakness of the soft palate [8, 10]. Testing of the gag reflex and swallowing are both extremely important for the patient with stroke, since aspiration of food, vomitus, and secretions can result in an acute airway obstruction or aspiration pneumonia, both of which are life-threatening.

Impairment of vagus nerve function can arise from vascular lesions of the brainstem that affect the nucleus itself as well as from supranuclear and infranuclear lesions. Nuclear involvement can result from thrombosis or hemorrhage causing infarction or compression of the medulla. This will cause a marked slowing of the heart and respiratory rates, projectile vomiting, and usually a significant rise or drop in blood pressure. The posterior inferior cerebellar artery supplies the lateral portion of the medulla, where the nucleus is located. Impairment of blood supply following thrombosis of this artery can produce the *Wallenberg syndrome*. This is characterized by an abrupt onset of hoarseness and dysphagia along with a clumsy arm and leg, loss of pain and temperature perception in the face, and Horner's syndrome, all of which occur on the affected side. Since the lesion is unilateral, the disability will be incomplete [8] . Supranuclear lesions affecting the vagus nerve are particularly significant when there is bilateral involvement [4] .

Complete paralysis of one vagus nerve will result in a paralysis of the soft palate, pharynx, and larynx on the involved side. While this paralysis will not be marked, the patient will have difficulty swallowing liquids and solids and may have a hoarse or nasal voice. Pharyngeal and palatal reflexes will be absent on the affected side. Extensive lesions, especially bilateral, will cause complete paralysis of the pharynx and larynx. Unless a patent airway is restored immediately, death will ensue from asphyxia. Complete paralysis of both vagus nerves is incompatible with life. It involves total paralysis of the soft palate, oropharynx, and larynx, as well as (1) marked dysphagia; (2) dysarthria; (3) rapid irregular heart action due to interruption of parasympathetic inhibitory influences; (4) slow, irregular, labored breathing; (5) loss of hunger and thirst; (6) abdominal pain; and (7) vomiting due to dilation and atonia of the stomach and intestines [4] . It should be noted that lesions due to stroke occurring in the area of the nucleus ambiguus, which supplies the ninth, tenth, and eleventh nerves, can produce complete laryngeal paralysis with these same life-threatening results.

SPINAL ACCESSORY NERVE (XI)
The eleventh cranial nerve innervates the sternocleidomastoid muscle and the upper portion of the trapezius muscle. The sternocleidomastoid, acting on one side, serves to turn the head so that the face is upward to the opposite side. The trapezius assists in lifting or shrugging the shoulders and in rotation of the scapula to allow raising of the arm beyond a horizontal plane. Both muscles act together to flex the neck and to brace and retract the shoulders [4, 8] . Assessment of eleventh nerve function involves an examination of the two muscles it serves. A contralateral paresis of these muscles will result from upper motor neuron lesions affecting the spinal accessory nerve. The examiner places his hands on either side of the patient's jaw and instructs the patient to turn his head from side to side. Thus the strength and bulk of the *sternocleidomastoid muscle* can be appraised by palpation, observation of the direction of rotation, and amount of resistance against the examiner's hands. To test the function of the *trapezius muscles* the examiner places the palms of both hands on the patient's shoulders and instructs the patient to shrug his shoulders in resistance as the examiner pushes downward. Continuing to hold down the patient's shoulders, the examiner then instructs him to raise both arms above his head [4, 8] .

With hemiplegia there will be no deviation of the head to one side, but a slight weakness may be noted when the function of the sternocleidomastoid is tested.

The patient will have difficulty in turning his face to the unaffected side. Moderate drooping of the shoulder and weakness of the trapezius on the affected side usually accompanies hemiplegia [4].

HYPOGLOSSAL NERVE (XII)
The function of the twelfth cranial nerve is innervation of the tongue muscles. The tongue is inspected at rest within the mouth for loss of symmetry, deviation to one side or the other, and presence of fasciculations. The patient is then instructed to protrude the tongue. Any deviation to one side indicates a weakness of the muscles on the side toward which the tongue deviates. The patient is then instructed to push his tongue against his cheek while the examiner presses against the outside of the cheek. This is repeated on the other side. The mobility and strength of the tongue muscles can be tested by having the patient open his mouth and touch his hard palate with the tip of his tongue. If the examiner has noted any dysarthria, coordination of the tongue muscles will be tested by having the patient open his mouth and move his tongue from side to side, then in and out, as rapidly as he can [8].

Vascular lesions that cause destruction of the hypoglossal nucleus or interruption of the nerve, which are classified as lower motor neuron lesions, will result in paralysis of the ipsilateral side of the tongue with loss of muscle tone and eventual atrophy. The tongue will deviate to the weak side on voluntary protrusion. A unilateral upper motor neuron lesion would cause a contralateral paralysis of the tongue because most of the afferent fibers are crossed, with the hypoglossal nerve receiving innervation from the cerebral cortex of both hemispheres via the corticobulbar tracts. Therefore, unilateral corticobulbar lesions will cause only slight weakness, resulting in an unbalanced action of the muscles that draw the tongue forward. Bilateral lesions, however, can cause serious impairment of speech and swallowing. Lesions of the nucleus due to stroke can cause paresis or paralysis of the tongue. Tongue paralysis or paresis can also follow lesions of the cerebral cortex, internal capsule, cerebral peduncle, or pons. Most often it is the result of infarction of the cortex or the pyramidal pathway [4, 8].

Examination of the motor system

The motor system includes those parts of the nervous system that are directly involved in initiating, maintaining, and controlling movement. Functioning of the motor system depends upon the coordination of a complex set of interactions between opposing muscles, the nerves that stimulate them, and impulses to and from the cerebral hemispheres and the cerebellum.

The terms *upper motor neuron* and *lower motor neuron* are used frequently in describing clinical signs of patients with neurological disorders. Understanding the distinction between the two terms is important for accurate interpretation of findings on physical examination. *Upper motor neuron* refers to a neural pathway that begins in the cerebral cortex and projects downward toward the brainstem and spinal cord. The *corticobulbar tract* ends in the various nuclei of the cranial nerves located in the brainstem. The *corticospinal tract* crosses the medulla and ends in the region of the anterior gray horn of the spinal cord at various levels from cervical to sacral. The *lower motor neuron* system includes motor cells of the cranial nerve nuclei with their axons and the anterior horn cells of the spinal cord with their axons. The axons of the anterior horn cells of the spinal cord form the motor portion of the spinal nerves responsible for innervation of the body musculature [4, 8].

Adequate functioning of the motor system depends on muscle tone, resistance to passive movement, muscle volume and contour, and coordination of movement, posture, and gait [4]. The examination of the motor system includes (1) inspection of the muscles for bulk, (2) testing of muscle strength, (3) observation of gait, (4) assessment of muscle tone, and (5) testing of cerebellar coordination. The examiner should observe for abnormalities and always compare the findings on the two sides of the body, noting any asymmetry. Before testing is begun, the examiner should inquire whether the patient is right- or left-handed. This is of particular importance with stroke because of its relationship to cerebral dominance and the difference in speech performance between patients with lesions in the dominant hemisphere and those with lesions in the nondominant hemisphere. The examination may need to be modified for a confused or stuporous patient. Often only a rough approximation of motor function can be made. Assessment of motor function in the comatose patient will have to depend on presence of spontaneous movements, position of extremities, asymmetry of voluntary movement, and withdrawal in response to painful stimuli [4].

MUSCLE BULK

The bulk of the muscle masses is examined for both volume and contour. The individual muscles as well as major muscle groups should be appraised by inspection, palpation, and measurement for signs of hypertrophy or atrophy and asymmetry between muscles of the two sides. Any abnormality should be noted. A muscle is described as atrophied when it is smaller than normal and has a wasted appearance. A tape measure may be used to document the degree of atrophy. Any flattening, hollowing, or bulging of muscle mass should also be noted. It is especially important to examine the muscles of the face, shoulder, and pelvic girdles and the distal parts of the four extremities [4, 6].

MUSCLE STRENGTH

Muscle strength or power is demonstrated by voluntary or active movement. It can be tested in two ways, (1) having the patient carry out movements against the resistance of the examiner and (2) having him resist the active attempts of the examiner to move fixed parts of his body. In testing muscle strength the examiner should include the various movements at each joint, testing the strength of each major muscle separately. It is impossible from a practical standpoint to include every muscle in testing for strength, but the musculature involved in the following movements should be tested always [8]:

1. shoulder abduction and adduction
2. elbow flexion and extension
3. wrist flexion and extension
4. hand grip
5. hip flexion and extension
6. knee flexion and extension
7. ankle dorsiflexion [8]

Muscles are always compared to those on the opposite side of the body and the presence or absence of involuntary movements is noted. The extent of testing will vary, of course, with the condition of the patient, his history, and other physical findings. Both active and passive movements should be tested. If movement causes discomfort or pain, this should be noted. If the patient is unable to move a limb normally, the examiner should have him rest the extremity on the bed or a table and attempt to move it in a direction that will not be affected by the forces of gravity. The proximal portion of a limb should be in a fixed position whenever movements of the distal portion are being tested, since the patient may compensate for a weakness in the distal musculature by using the muscles of the proximal portion of the limb [4]. This is particularly important in stroke, since return of muscle function is slower in the distal extremities. The examiner should note whether weakness is more marked in the distal or in the proximal portions. Distal weakness is indicative of nerve damage while proximal weakness indicates muscle damage [6].

Table 4-1 shows how muscle strength is graded on examination. The term *paresis* is used to describe an impairment of strength or power and is distinguished from *paralysis,* which is a loss of strength [4]. Recumbent or seated comfortably, the patient is instructed to resist the examiner's active attempts to move parts of the patient's body or else to initiate and carry out movements that are resisted by the examiner for the following set of screening procedures for muscle strength.

Screening procedure for the arms. The patient's *grip* is tested by having him squeeze the examiner's hand as firmly as he can. To test *shoulder* strength, the patient is instructed to stand holding his arms outstretched in front of him, palms up, for 20—30 seconds, while his ability to maintain this position is observed. The examiner then attempts to depress the patient's outstretched arms against the patient's resistance, noting the strength and any displacement of the scapula on either side. Next the patient is instructed to raise his arms over his head with the palms forward for 20—30 seconds. The examiner then tries to force the arms down against resistance. Any drifting or weakness of one side is an indication of hemiparesis. Flexion and extension of the *elbow* is tested by having the patient push and pull against the examiner's hands. Dorsiflexion of the *wrist* is tested by having the patient make a fist and resist the examiner when he attempts to push the fist down [2].

Table 4-1
Classification of muscle strength

Grade	Finding on Assessment of Muscle Strength	% of Strength
0	No contraction	0
1	Trace or flicker of contraction without actual movement	10
2	Poor strength, muscle moves through complete range of movement when gravity is eliminated	25
3	Fair strength, muscle moves through complete range of motion against gravity	50
4	Good strength, muscle completes motion against gravity with varying amounts of resistance	75
5	Normal strength, muscle goes through complete range of motion against gravity with full resistance and no signs of fatigue	100

Screening procedure for the legs.　The patient is told to walk across the room; the examiner observes his posture, balance, arm swing, and leg movement. Next he is asked to hop in place, first on one foot, then on the other; to do a shallow knee bend with each leg; and to walk on his heels and then on his toes. The ability to hop indicates overall strength of the legs. *Knee* bends demonstrate the strength of the quadriceps femoris muscle. Any weakness of this muscle will make it very difficult to bend the knee. Ability to walk on the toes demonstrates plantar flexion of the *ankle,* while ability to walk on the heels demonstrates dorsiflexion. To test flexion of the *hip,* the examiner places his hand on the patient's thigh and has him raise his leg against resistance. The examiner tests abduction of the hips by placing his hands firmly on the bed outside the patient's knees and having the patient spread his legs against resistance. To test adduction of the hips, the examiner places his hands firmly on the bed between the patient's knees and has the patient bring his legs together against resistance. To test *knee* flexion the patient is instructed to maintain a position with his knee flexed as the examiner exerts pressure to straighten the leg. Extension of the knee is tested by supporting the knee and having the patient straighten his leg against the resistance of the examiner's hand. Plantar flexion and dorsiflexion of the *ankle* can be tested by having the patient push his foot down and pull it up against the resistance of the examiner's hands [2].

A stroke patient in coma can be examined for hemiplegia in the following manner. The patient's upper arm is positioned with the flexed elbow resting on the bed. The examiner releases the patient's hand. A flail-like dropping of the wrist and forearm will occur with paralysis. The patient's leg is then flexed and placed with the heel resting on the bed. When the examiner removes his support, a similar dropping of the leg with extension and external rotation occurs, if paralysis is present. Pressure is then applied on the supraorbital ridge. With hemiplegia, contraction of the facial muscles in response to this stimulus will occur only on the unaffected side [4].

GAIT

The patient's *gait* is observed as he walks in to the examination. Posture, balance, and the relationship between steps and arm swing are also noted. Normal gait has a rhythm and regularity, whereas neurological lesions cause characteristic altera-tions in gait. The patient's gait is tested further by having him walk forward, back-ward, sideways, and around a chair, first with his eyes open and then with his eyes closed. He is also instructed to walk heel-to-toe (tandem walking), placing the heel of the foot being advanced down directly in front of the toe of the opposite foot. Since this reduces the patient's usual base of support, it shows up abnormal-ities of gait related to strength and coordination that might not be detected in casual walking.

With *hemiparesis,* the normal rhythmic swinging of the arms is reduced on the affected side. If the lesion is located in the corticospinal tract, muscle tone is increased so that the affected leg is held stiffly and circumducted as the patient walks with his toe scraping along the floor. The affected arm is held in a flexed position, since flexor tone predominates in the upper extremities. *Ataxia* is associated with lesions affecting the cerebellar pathways. The ataxic patient is unsteady on his feet, with great difficulty in maintaining his balance. To steady himself he walks with his feet placed wide apart, perhaps with high and slapping steps. The patient with a unilateral cerebellar lesion will sway and deviate toward the affected side. Any lesion that interrupts the pyramidal innervation to one half of the body will result in the *gait of spastic hemiplegia.* The leg will be held stiffly in extension, and with each step the pelvis will be tilted upward on the affected side to aid in lifting the toe off the floor. The patient can flex the affected leg only with great difficulty and may have to swing the entire leg around in a semi-circle from the hip to advance it. The affected arm will be held tightly to the body, rigid and flexed. It can be extended only with great difficulty and will not swing when the patient walks [4, 6, 8].

MUSCLE TONE

Tone refers to the tension or firmness of the muscles. The degree of muscle tone present is determined by the amount of resistance to passive stretching of the muscles. This is assessed by examining the passive range of motion of a joint, observing the extensibility of the musculature involved, and feeling the tension of the muscles and their resistance. It is essential that the resistance to passive manipu-lation be examined with no voluntary control or active muscle contraction by the patient. Disturbances of muscle tone include hypotonicity — a decrease or loss of normal tone, and hypertonicity — an abnormal increase in muscle tone. *Hypo-tonicity* or *flaccidity* is caused by lesions of the cerebellum, lower motor neuron disease, and interference with proprioceptive pathways. It is characterized by inert or flaccid muscles that offer no resistance to passive movement, do not check extremes of passive movement, and do not maintain a position into which they have been placed passively. A reduced muscle tone may be difficult to detect when it is not pronounced, since the normal degree of resistance is slight.

Increased muscle tone, *hypertonicity*, is easier to evaluate. There are two types, spasticity and rigidity. *Spasticity* is a state of slight to severe muscle tension or contraction in response to passive stretching. It is the result of upper motor neuron lesions, usually involving the pyramidal and extrapyramidal tracts with loss of the impulses that inhibit tone. *Rigidity* is characterized by increased tone in all the flexor muscles and involves a steady muscular tension. It is associated with lesions of the basal ganglia and their connections.

Before assessing muscle tone, the examiner instructs the patient to relax his arm or leg completely while it is being moved: "Don't try to move it yourself, just give it to me while I move it." All four extremities are tested for signs of flaccidity, spasticity, or rigidity. The arm is supported while the elbow is slowly taken through its complete passive range of motion, then the leg is supported while the knee is put through its range. The extremities may be moved through their range of motion at successively faster speeds to detect spasticity, since it will not always be apparent with slow passive movement [4].

With *flaccidity* no resistance to passive extension or flexion will be observed, even when the movement is carried out rapidly. Excursion of the joint usually is increased. If allowed to drop, the extremity will fall with a flail-like motion. The elbow joint will have increased flexibility and mobility, allowing it to be bent at an abnormally acute angle.

Spasticity due to lesions involving the pyramidal and related systems is characterized by sustained contraction, which involves certain muscle groups more than others. With upper motor neuron lesions, tone in the flexor muscles of the arms will be increased more than that of the extensors, while in the leg, the tone of the extensors will be increased over that of the flexors. This accounts for the characteristic posture and gait of the stroke patient with spastic hemiplegia. Usually the passive range of motion can be carried out successfully when done slowly and through a limited range of motion. Increased resistance is detected with a rapid or forceful movement, and any extreme movement such as complete flexion or extension of the joint will block further movement. The spasticity is not usually present through the full excursion of joint movement — only initially. The term "clasp knife phenomenon" is used to describe the elastic springlike resistance of the spastic muscles at the onset of movement followed by resistance to a point, then relaxation [10].

Rigidity is a state of steady muscle tension which is equal in opposing muscle groups. Flexor and extensor muscles are involved equally and show continuous resistance to passive motion in all directions through the entire range of motion [4, 6, 8].

CEREBELLAR COORDINATION
Coordination is the harmonious interplay of the motor and sensory systems to achieve balanced muscular activity and synchronization of movement. Coordination relies on the synergistic action of the systems involved for organization of a perfectly executed act. The cerebellum, which is essential to synergy, is considered to be the center of coordination. Both *equilibratory coordination* — the action of

the body as a whole — and nonequilibratory coordination — discrete intentional movements of the extremities — are examined.

Types of cerebellar dysfunction.   In assessing coordination the examiner is actually testing cerebellar function.   The principal manifestations of cerebellar dysfunction are disturbances of muscular coordination, locomotion, and equilibrium.   Voluntary movement is impaired, with loss of control and intermittent, irregular muscle contractions.   Abnormalities of cerebellar coordination are described as asynergy, dysmetria, and dysdiadochokinesia.

   Asynergy is a loss of the faculty for associating relatively complex movements that have a special function.   *Dyssynergy* is an impairment of this function rather than a loss.   With dyssynergy, there will be a lack of coordinated action between various groups of muscles or movements as components of an act, with impairment of the proper harmony and sequence required to perform the act smoothly and accurately.   Speed and skill in carrying out movements that depend on the synchronous activity of several muscle groups or a series of motions will be lost.   *Dysmetria* is an inability to gauge the distance, speed, or power of a movement.   This will cause the patient to stop an act before the goal is attained or overshoot the desired point.   *Dysdiadochokinesia* is an inability to carry out successive movements, to stop one act and follow it immediately with a completely opposite act.   It is a disturbance in reciprocal innervation of agonist and antagonist muscle groups.   Alternate movements will usually be carried out slowly, irregularly, and clumsily.   In testing the patient's coordination it should be kept in mind that any impairment of muscle strength, tone, or sensory input, even though there is no cerebellar dysfunction, can prevent the patient from carrying out the coordinated movements he is called upon to perform [4, 8].

Equilibratory coordination.   Testing of coordination of the body as a whole includes an examination of posture, station, and gait.   Besides the testing of gait and muscle strength already described, observation of the patient carrying out his usual activities such as lying down, standing up, sitting, walking, dressing, and eating will also give the examiner information about disturbances of coordination.   The supine or seated position will only show gross disturbances such as inability to coordinate spinal, trunk, pelvic, and shoulder muscles.   It is in the standing position that less apparent problems can be detected.   The patient is asked to stand with his feet close together, with his eyes first open, then closed.   The position of the head, shoulders, and feet is observed.   Any tremors, lurching, or swaying are noted.   Often the patient will have to separate his feet to maintain an upright position.   With a sensory ataxia due to an impairment in conduction of proprioceptive impulses through the spinal cord, the patient will be able to remain standing while his eyes are open but will sway to one side or tend to fall when he closes his eyes — the positive *Romberg sign.*   This test is used to distinguish sensory from cerebellar ataxia.   Difficulty with balance can be accentuated by having the patient stand with one foot in front of the other.   He may be given a slight push to one side, then to the other, and asked to stand on one foot at a time while the opposite knee is flexed. In order to differentiate between cerebellar and sensory ataxia, the patient is asked to carry out each of these procedures with his eyes open, then closed. During gait testing the patient is asked to walk back and forth with his eyes open, then closed, and perhaps to walk in tandem or to follow a straight line on the floor. Disturbances noted while the patient is standing will become more pronounced with walking [4].

Nonequilibratory coordination. The examiner looks for signs of asynergy, dyssynergy, dysmetria, and dysdiadochokinesia. First the upper, then the lower extremities are tested for ability to carry out discrete intentional movements. The examiner observes (1) the patient's ability to control muscles and movements that normally act in harmony; (2) his ability to judge and control distance, the speed and power of an act, and its component parts; and (3) his ability to carry out successive movements, then to stop and follow immediately with a completely opposite movement. As for equilibratory coordination, the patient completes each test first with his eyes open, then with them closed, to differentiate between sensory and cerebellar ataxia.

The patient is instructed to touch the tip of his index finger to the tip of his nose several times, first slowly, then more and more rapidly, while the examiner observes his smoothness, accuracy, and speed. With *dyssynergy,* the activity is not performed smoothly. The patient may stop frequently or be unable to complete the action at all unless it is broken down into its component parts. With *dysmetria,* the patient will overshoot or undershoot, touching another part of his face or body.

To test for dysdiadochokinesia the patient is told to alternately pronate and supinate his two hands together. This may be done with flexed elbows as well as with outstretched arms. It may also be performed in a seated position, the patient patting his thighs with both hands at the same time, alternating between the palms and the backs of his hands, with increasing rapidity. These activities require a reciprocal innervation and alternate action of agonists and antagonists. Therefore, with varying degrees of dysdiadochokinesia, the patient will be unable to perform these activities smoothly or at all. Especially when the disability is not marked, it is important to test the two hands simultaneously in order to compare the functions of the affected with unaffected side.

Normally the body uses a "checking factor," or braking mechanism, following any sudden release of a resistance to which it has opposed a strong voluntary movement and allows antagonistic muscles to contract immediately after relaxation of agonists. With cerebellar dysfunction there is a loss of this checking factor. The *rebound test* demonstrates ability to check movements quickly with the coordinated action of agonists, antagonists, and synergists. The patient is instructed to flex his arm at the shoulder and elbow and clench his fist. Then the examiner pulls on the patient's wrist and releases it suddenly. Under normal circumstances such a movement is checked rapidly and the displaced limb returns to its former position smoothly and accurately. The contraction of the biceps and other flexed muscles in the arm is followed almost immediately by contraction of the triceps. The tendency toward flexion is checked by a rapid action of the antagonists, which stops continued movement of the arm. The patient with impaired cerebellar function will have lost the ability to stop contraction of the flexors and to follow immediately with a contraction of the triceps when his flexed arm is released suddenly. Therefore his hand will fly up, striking his shoulder or face if not stopped by the examiner. Extension can be tested rather than flexion by observing the patient's response to a sudden passive displacement of his outstretched arms.

Tests similar to those used for the upper extremities are applied to the lower extremities. In the *heel-to-knee-to-toe test* the patient is instructed to place the heel of one foot on the opposite knee and slide the heel down along the shin in a straight line to the great toe. With dyssynergy this motion is uneven and jerky and usually has to be broken into its component parts. With dysmetria the patient overshoots the mark, having difficulty placing his heel on the knee and in hitting the toe. To test for ataxia the patient is asked to trace a circle or figure eight on the floor with his foot. The ataxic patient's movements will be unsteady and the figures formed irregular. To test for dysdiadochokinesia the patient is instructed to flex his feet alternately forward and backward or to tap the floor with the soles of his feet. The rebound test is carried out by the sudden release of the knee or ankle after the patient has been resisting either extension or flexion [1, 4] .

Examination of the sensory system

The function of the sensory system is to convey information about the condition of the body and its relationship with its external environment to the central nervous system. This function is carried out by means of three processes: enteroception, proprioception, and exteroception. *Enteroception* refers to those physiological processes that alert the brain to the status of the internal organs. *Proprioception* concerns the position of the limbs in relation to the rest of the body and awareness of the body and its parts in relation to space. *Exteroception* is the process by which stimuli from the body surface relay information about the body's interaction with the surrounding environment. The information gathered by means of these three processes is integrated and interpreted in the cerebral cortex.

The examination of the sensory system includes (1) an assessment of exteroceptive sensation, testing sensitivity to pain, temperature, and touch; (2) an assessment of proprioceptive sensation, testing sense of joint motion and of position; (3) testing of vibratory sense; and (4) testing of cortical sensory functions that require integration of exteroceptive and proprioceptive sensations. The purpose of the examination is to identify any increase, decrease, or alteration of sensation that would indicate neurological impairment. Enteroception cannot be adequately evaluated because sensations are poorly localized, and due to the origin of these sensations, clinical methods are not available for testing them.

Abnormalities of sensation involve increase, perversion, impairment, or loss of feeling. The most striking example of an increased sensation is pain, sometimes growing more intense with pressure. Perversion of sensation includes paresthesias, dysesthesias, and phantom pain. Impairment or loss of sensation may be a lessening of the acuity of the sense organ involved or a dysfunction of either the nerve fibers that conduct the sensation or those areas of the brain responsible for perception and interpretation of the sensation. The examiner will ask the patient to report any abnormal sensations or loss of feeling, specifically pain, loss of feeling, numbness, burning, pressure, tingling, and feelings of weight or absence of parts of the body. If there are no subjective complaints concerning the sensory system and no motor impairment has been noted, the examiner will restrict the examination to the major sensory nerve and segmental supply to the face, trunk, and extremities. When there are specific sensory symptoms and/or significant motor signs, the examination will focus on the involved area [4, 8].

EXTEROCEPTIVE SENSATION

Exteroceptive fibers originate in the skin and mucous membranes and respond to external agents and the environment. The three major exteroceptive sensations are pain, temperature, and touch. Response to superficial pain is usually tested with a pin. The patient is instructed to close his eyes and indicate whether what he feels is sharp or dull while the examiner exerts slight pressure over various areas of the body, first with the pointed, then with the blunt tip, of the pin. Any differences between the two sides of the body and between proximal and distal portions of the extremities are noted and, when there is an abnormality, the boundaries of the affected area are carefully delineated. Usually the findings are recorded graphically. Reduced sensitivity to pain is called *hypalgesia;* increased sensitivity, *hyperalgesia;* and insensitivity, *analgesia.* Since the pathways for perception of pain and temperature are closely related, *temperature perception* usually is not tested if no impairment of sensitivity to pain has been found. However, since perception of temperature may be altered sooner than that of pain with some lesions, it will be tested whenever the examiner has reason to suspect such a lesion. Any cold or warm stimulus may be applied to the various areas of the skin. Usually test tubes filled with warm and cold water are used. Tactile sensation or response to light *touch* is assessed in the same manner as pain, substituting a wisp of cotton for the pin. Various areas of the body are stroked lightly with the cotton, and the patient is instructed to indicate when he feels the examiner touching him. Changes in tactile sensation are *anesthesia,* a loss of sensation; *hypoesthesia,* a diminished sensation; and *hyperesthesia,* an increased sensation [4, 8].

PROPRIOCEPTIVE SENSATION

Proprioceptive sensations originate in the muscles, joints, tendons, bones, and other deeper body tissues. They provide the sense of motion and body position. The examiner tests this sense in all extremities by grasping the distal phalanx of one of the digits, slowly flexing and extending it, and asking the patient whether the joint is up or down. If position sense is severely impaired, the patient may not even be able to identify movement of the proximal joints such as the ankle or knee [8].

VIBRATORY SENSE

Pathways that conduct the sense of *vibration* have not been clearly identified but are thought to be related to those of proprioception. The vibratory sense is diminished in peripheral neuropathy and posterior column disease. This sense is tested by placing a vibrating tuning fork against a bony prominence of each extremity and asking the patient when he feels the vibration [8].

COMBINED SENSATIONS

The combined sensations, a variety of integrated exteroceptive and proprioceptive sensations that require cortical activity for perception, are required for perceptual and discriminative functions. These include the faculty of perceiving and understanding the form and nature of objects through the sense of touch, or *stereognosis;* the ability to differentiate between weights of various objects; and the ability to localize a sensation within the body, *topognosis.* Disturbances of these perceptual functions are discussed in detail in Chapter 6. Specific sensory functions can be evaluated to gain information about the functioning of higher cerebral centers of integration beyond the thalamus (cortical sensory functions). However, it must first be established that the transmission of sensory impulses from the periphery of the body to the cortex is unimpaired. For instance, if the primary sensations in the hand are normal, an inability to recognize an object by touch indicates a disturbance of parietal lobe functioning; but if the primary sensation in the hand is impaired by a peripheral nerve lesion, the result of testing will be misleading. The following tests are performed, therefore, after the integrity of the primary sensory modalities has been established.

In the test for *stereognosis,* perception through touch alone, the patient shuts his eyes and tries to identify a series of objects placed one at a time into each hand. *Graphesthesia* requires a highly discriminative cutaneous sensation, the loss of which indicates a cortical lesion. To test for this ability, the patient is instructed to close his eyes while the examiner traces several letters or numbers on his outstretched palm and asks him to identify the figures. *Two-point discrimination* is the ability to distinguish between stimulation at one location on the body and stimulation at two points. The examiner applies either one or two pointed objects to the skin in various areas, asks the patient if he feels one or two stimuli, and notes the minimum distance between two points that are felt separately. The clinical significance of this test is that loss of two point discrimination, when tactile sensation is intact, is an indication of parietal lobe lesions. *Double simultaneous stimulation* is used to assess the appreciation of two simultaneous stimuli on symmetrically opposite areas of the body. Impairment of this ability is indicative of parietal dysfunction on the side on which the stimulus is felt. Failure to recognize one of the stimuli is called *sensory inattention* or *extinction.* This faculty can also be tested for visual response: a moving finger is presented to both sides of the patient's visual field [4, 8].

Testing the reflexes

Reflexes are reliable indicators of the integrity of the motor and sensory systems. Often changes in the intensity and character of the normal physiological reflex activity are valuable clues to a disturbance of neurological function. Three categories of reflexes are considered in assessment of neurological function: muscle stretch reflexes, cutaneous reflexes, and pathological reflexes. The anatomical basis for all these is the *reflex arc,* which consists of (1) a receptor organ, (2) an afferent pathway from the receptor organ at the periphery of the body to the brainstem or spinal cord, (3) neurons within the central nervous system that relay impulses to efferent neurons, (4) an efferent pathway from the central nervous system via the lower motor neurons to the effector organ in the periphery, and (5) the effector organ [10]. The most basic definition of a reflex is a response to a stimulus. The eliciting stimulus may be a touch or pinprick, the sudden stretching of a muscle, or an event such as a glandular secretion or alteration of blood gases, which excites an afferent impulse in the reflex arc.

Physiological reflex activity is an integral part of normal functioning and protects the body from harmful stimuli. It depends upon the integrity of the reflex arc, however, to perform these functions. Lesions that interrupt the pathway at any point along this arc will abolish the normal reflexes. Pathological reflexes, as their name implies, are seen only when neurological functioning has been impaired [4, 8]. Only those reflexes that are important in assessment of neurological function for the stroke patient will be presented here. Reflexes related to the cranial nerves have already been discussed in Chapter 2 and in this chapter under Examination of Cranial Nerves.

MUSCLE STRETCH REFLEXES

Muscle stretch reflexes are usually referred to as tendon reflexes or deep tendon reflexes ("DTR's"). They are elicited by a sudden blow with a percussion hammer to the tendon of insertion for the muscle to be tested. These reflexes consist of an afferent arc, which carries the impulse produced by the stretching of the muscle; a synapse within the spinal cord; and an efferent pathway carrying an impulse back to the muscle being tested [8]. All these reflexes are produced by indirect stimulation of the muscles and their response to a sudden stretch imposed upon them. The various reflexes are identified by the muscles involved rather than by the tendon, site of stimulation, or nerves involved.

Before striking the tendon, the examiner places his hand over the muscle to be tested in order to feel it contract. He then stretches the muscle slightly by positioning the extremity or by pressing his thumb against the tendon of insertion. To help relax the extremity, the patient may be instructed to concentrate on a voluntary act that does not involve the muscle being tested, for example, clenching his fists or holding onto the bed or examining table.

A grading system with a range of 0—4 is used to classify the reflex response. *Grade 1* indicates a diminished or minimal response. *Grades 2 and 3* both reflect normal reflex response. They are used according to the examiner's judgment for intermediate responses. *Grade 4* indicates a brisk, hyperactive response often with associated clonus. *Clonus* is a rhythmic series of contractions that occurs in response to maintained tension in a muscle. The response for each reflex is compared with the corresponding reflex on the opposite side, since asymmetry may be indicative of a pathological condition. With upper motor neuron lesions, such as stroke, the deep tendon reflexes will be exaggerated on the opposite side, since the corticospinal tract crosses the midline in the medulla.

Three muscle stretch reflexes or DTR's are tested in the arms — the biceps, the triceps, and the brachioradialis. Two are tested in the legs — the quadriceps, often referred to as the patellar or knee jerk reflex; and the gastrocnemius, commonly called the Achilles reflex. To elicit the *biceps reflex,* the examiner places his thumb on the tendon of insertion of the biceps muscle to create tension in it, then taps his thumb with the percussion hammer. The response is flexion of the arm. To test the *triceps reflex* he supports the patient's partially extended arm under the elbow and taps the tendon of insertion for the triceps muscle with the percussion hammer. This will result in extension of the arm. If the patient is in a supine position, the examiner flexes the patient's forearm slightly, then taps the tendon just above the olecranon process. The *brachioradial reflex* is elicited by tapping the lower third of the radius when the forearm has been positioned midway between pronation and supination. Flexion of the forearm results, frequently accompanied by flexion of the hand and fingers as well. Usually the *quadriceps or patellar reflex* is tested with the patient sitting in a chair or on the side of the bed. The examiner places his hand over the quadriceps muscle and taps the patellar tendon. Extension of the knee results. If the patient must be supine, this reflex can be tested by supporting his leg. To obtain the *gastrocnemius or Achilles reflex,* the patient's foot is placed at a right angle to the leg to create tension of the gastrocnemius muscle, and the Achilles tendon is struck. Plantar flexion of the foot is the normal response [1, 8].

CUTANEOUS REFLEXES

Cutaneous or superficial reflexes are elicited by stroking the skin and observing a response in the related muscle group. Two reflexes are commonly tested, the abdominal and, in males, the cremasteric. The *superficial abdominal reflex* involves a contraction of the superficial abdominal musculature in response to a light, rapid stroke of the skin in each upper and lower quadrant of the abdomen. Usually a pointed instrument such as an applicator stick, the end of a percussion hammer, or a pen is used. The *cremasteric reflex* is an elevation of one side of the scrotum resulting from contraction of the cremaster muscle. This is elicited by a stroke applied to the inner aspect of the thigh [8].

PATHOLOGICAL REFLEXES

Pathological reflexes can be obtained only in the presence of disease. The most common is the *Babinski reflex,* which is important because it indicates the presence of an upper motor neuron lesion. The lateral border of the sole of the foot is stimulated by one continuous stroke from the heel to the toes with a pointed instrument such as a pen, applicator stick, or key. The *Babinski sign,* or abnormal response is a dorsiflexion of the great toe, sometimes accompanied by fanning of the other toes. Because of the sensitivity of the sole of the foot, it is sometimes difficult to evaluate the response to this test. An identical response with the same significance can be obtained by stroking the lateral aspect of the dorsum of the foot, which is less sensitive, from the heel to the toes. In this case a response of dorsiflexion of the great toe is referred to as *Chaddock's sign* [8].

MONITORING OF NEUROLOGICAL STATUS

The preceding section described the elements of the neurological examination and the deficits that might be identified by the examiner. The record of this initial assessment should be referred to when planning care for the acutely ill patient, and the findings should be used as a baseline for comparison with subsequent findings. While the patient's condition remains unstable, he will require continued monitoring of his neurological status. This next section is intended for quick reference and provides a brief overview of the neurological signs that should be measured regularly at the bedside, so that any deviation from the baseline or alteration in the pattern of responses that might herald an impending herniation can be identified readily.

The following should be monitored: (1) orientation, (2) level of consciousness, (3) eye signs, (4) motor signs, (5) speech, and (6) vital signs. Each of these has been discussed in detail in the previous section.

Orientation

Orientation is the awareness of person, place, and time. When oriented, the patient is aware of who he is, where he is, and the time of the day, week, or month. It is important to remember that a patient may be aware of himself and his environment but incapable of responding to questions because a lesion has caused loss of speech or hearing. If the patient has lost the faculty of speech, his orientation may be tested by having him shake his head or move his eyes in response to questions.

Level of consciousness

Level of consciousness refers to the patient's degree of awareness, which may range from the extremes of alert to totally unresponsive, with intermediate stages of lethargy and obtundation. A change in level of consciousness may be the first sign of increasing intracranial pressure. A declining level of consciousness is frequently the most important indicator of decreasing neurological function. While it is not difficult to differentiate between alertness and unresponsiveness, the gradations of change occurring between these two extremes may be overlooked or minimized. The levels of consciousness are defined as (1) alert; (2) lethargic, drowsy, or sluggish; (3) stuporous; and (4) comatose. The *alert* patient is awake, reacts spontaneously, and usually demonstrates appropriate behavior. Unless aphasic, he will initiate and respond to conversation. The *lethargic* patient is less responsive to questions, appears disinterested in his surroundings and usually displays reduced spontaneous activity. His attention span may be decreased. Once lethargy is first noted, it is important to observe the patient closely for any deepening of this state. A patient who is *stuporous* can be aroused, but only with great effort. He may withdraw from stimuli, grimace, and/or utter unintelligible sounds. It may be necessary to apply painful stimuli to rouse him when evaluating his state of awareness. The patient in *coma* does not respond even to the most noxious stimuli except with elementary reflex responses such as a decerebrate or decorticate posture. Painful stimuli, such as substernal pressure or pinching the skin, must be applied before it can be decided that a patient is in coma.

Eye signs

Monitoring of eye signs involves comparing the equality of pupil size, checking the regularity of the pupils, and testing the reaction of the pupils to light. To examine the pupils properly, the light in the room should be subdued. After noting the size, shape, and equality of the pupils, the examiner directs a flashlight from the side into one eye at a time, noting whether the eyes react to light briskly, sluggishly or not at all. When the pupil does not react to light, but remains dilated, it is referred to as *fixed*. Figure 4-2 illustrates both normal and abnormal findings on monitoring of eye signs. Normally both pupils will be equal in size, and the pupils will constrict rapidly in response to a bright light directed onto the retina. However, in the early stages of cerebral edema, the reaction of the pupil on the side of the lesion will be less and slower than normal. As intracranial pressure increases, the pupillary response will become increasingly slower, and the pupil will begin to dilate.

Motor signs

In caring for the patient with stroke, movement as well as strength and muscle tone should be assessed regularly. Any difference in motor signs between the right and left sides of the body is significant, as is any progressive change in motion, strength, or muscle tone. If the patient is unable to respond to verbal commands, painful stimuli, such as pinching the skin, may be used to elicit a motor response.

To test for movement, the patient should be instructed to wrinkle his brow and smile — which demonstrates movement of the facial muscles — and to move all four extremities. It is important to note any facial asymmetry and to determine whether the patient's movements are purposeful or not. *Purposeful movement* signifies a normal motor response to a given command — such as "grasp my hand" or "raise your right leg" — or a normal reaction to a painful sensation. The stuporous patient may push the examiner away or withdraw an extremity. *Nonpurposeful movement* demonstrates reflex activity. This may involve generalized spastic movement or decerebrate or decorticate posturing. In *decerebrate posturing* the arms are in rigid extension, adduction, and internal rotation, with the hands flexed at the wrist and the legs in extension and plantar flexion. In *decorticate posturing* the arms, wrists, and fingers are flexed, and there is rigid extension of the legs with internal rotation and plantar flexion of the feet. Decorticate posturing follows an interruption of the corticospinal pathway.

To test for *strength,* the patient is instructed to grasp both the nurse's hands simultaneously and then to release the grip. The nurse should note whether one hand is weaker than the other or whether the patient has any difficulty releasing his grasp. The patient is then instructed to raise and then lower each arm and leg, singly, then both together. Any difference in strength between right and left sides should be noted. If one extremity is weaker than the other, the patient may not be able to raise it as high or may let it fall. If the patient is unable to follow the nurse's instructions, it should be noted whether or not his movements are appropriate and spontaneous.

Any changes in *muscle tone* may also be significant and should be noted. *Spasticity* will be characterized by an increased resistance to passive movement followed by release of this resistance. The release may be sudden or gradual. *Rigid* muscles, also characterized by increased muscle tone, will have an even, steady resistance to passive movement. Although at times the rigidity will be of an intermittent type, resulting in jerky movements, the muscles in the extremities will give the impression of a lead pipe. *Flaccidity* is characterized by a decrease in or loss of muscle tone. The muscles will be toneless at rest.

Speech

In checking the patient's neurological status it is important to note the presence of aphasia or of any change in speech pattern such as dysarthria or anarthria. (Disturbances of speech and language are discussed in detail in Chapter 5.)

Vital signs

Monitoring of vital signs includes temperature, pulse, blood pressure, and respiratory pattern. Any fluctuation or change in one or more of these signs may reflect an alteration of the patient's neurological functioning. Except in the terminal stages of herniation, when body *temperature* rises, temperature is not a particularly sensitive indicator of neurological deficit. Slowing of the *pulse* to less than 60 beats per minute may represent increased intracranial pressure. When there is cerebral edema, the increased workload on the heart to supply blood to the brain makes the *blood pressure* rise. Abnormal breathing patterns almost always accompany brainstem lesions. The character, rhythm, and quality of the *respirations* should be noted. The following patterns may be seen. *Cheyne-Stokes* respirations are characterized by a rhythm progressing from apnea to hyperventilation. They imply deep bilateral hemisphere dysfunction or dysfunction of the diencephalon or brainstem. *Central neurogenic hyperventilation* is rapid, deep breathing seen in brainstem stroke. *Apneustic breathing* is characterized by a prolonged inspiratory cramp followed by expiratory pause. It is seen most often with a pontine infarction. *Ataxic breathing* is irregular and uncontrolled respiration and is seen in the dying patient. Table 4-2

Table 4-2
Neurological observation sheet

Patient Name _____

Date ___ / ___ / ___

Time	Orientation	Consciousness	Pupils		Movement				Strength						Speech				Vital Signs					Comments
	A=Aware I=Impaired	A=Alert L=Lethargic S=Stuporous C=Comatose	Size (mm.)	Light Reflex	N=Normal O=None D=Abnor.				N=Normal O=Unconscious W=Weak						Normal	Aphasic	Dysarthric	Anarthric	Temperature	Pulse	Respirations	B. Pressure		Describe any change in character or rhythm of pulse or respirations, nausea, vomiting, headache, restlessness, diplopia, seizures, abnormal movement, change in behavior
AM PM	Person	Place	Time		R	L	R	L	ARM R	LEG L	R	L	ARM R	LEG L	GRIP R	L									

KEY: Gauge for Pupil Size

2 3 4 5 6 7 8 9 mm.

Light reaction: R=reacts; SR=sluggish; BR=brisk; NR=nonreactive.
Abnormal movements: Indicate decerebrate or decorticate posturing, myoclonus, or tremors in Comments column.

is an example of a nursing observation sheet that can be used to record findings of neurological and vital signs.

ANCILLARY DIAGNOSTIC PROCEDURES

The characteristic syndrome of stroke due to vascular lesions is usually diagnosed on the basis of the history and physical examination. However, certain ancillary diagnostic procedures may be used to clarify the etiology of stroke, to differentiate non-vascular brain lesions, to localize the area of infarction and, in some instances, to establish a diagnosis of stroke when the history and physical findings are equivocal. The diagnostic procedures used most frequently are (1) lumbar puncture and analysis of cerebrospinal fluid, (2) angiography of the head and neck vessels, (3) computerized axial tomography (CAT scan), (4) skull x-ray, and (5) electroencephalography (EEG) [7, 9].

Lumbar puncture

Lumbar puncture involves withdrawal of cerebrospinal fluid through a needle inserted between the lumbar vertebrae into the subarachnoid space. This procedure allows for visualization and laboratory analysis of the cerebrospinal fluid as well as measurement of pressure. It is not without significant risk, however, as withdrawal of cerebrospinal fluid can increase the likelihood of herniation when there is increased intracranial pressure. With cerebral *thrombosis* cerebrospinal fluid is ordinarily clear, and the pressure is usually normal but may be increased when there is a large area of infarction with edema. *Embolic stroke* does not ordinarily cause bloody spinal fluid unless there is an extremely large hemorrhagic infarct. In most cases of *intracranial hemorrhage* the cerebrospinal fluid will be grossly bloody and under increased pressure. With massive hemorrhage, temporal lobe herniation may be aggravated by the lumbar puncture. *Ruptured saccular aneurysms* will produce extremely bloody fluid under greatly increased pressure.

Following completion of the lumbar puncture, the patient should be observed closely for any change or deterioration in neurological status. This is a nursing responsibility. It is important to note that, in the presence of cerebral edema, slight leakage of cerebrospinal fluid following this procedure can continue undetected over a period of hours, since the fluid will be absorbed into the surrounding tissues rather than flow out from the puncture site. This continuous leakage of cerebrospinal fluid can act as a siphon, drawing on the brain tissue and gradually increasing pressure on the brainstem. Herniation as a complication of lumbar puncture, therefore, does not necessarily occur immediately during or after completion of the procedure but sometimes several hours later [7, 9].

Angiography

Angiography of the head and neck vessels is a radiological procedure that allows visualization of the vasculature and identification of occluded vessels, areas of infarction, and structural anomalies. A radiopaque substance may be injected after puncture of the vessel to be studied, or a flexible, radiopaque catheter may be introduced through a distal artery. Angiography is considered a definitive procedure for demonstration of arterial stenosis or occlusion and competence of the collateral circulation. Carotid and vertebral angiography is the only method available for positive identification of the site of an aneurysm. There is some risk involved. The procedure may enlarge an infarction already present when the vessels studied have been narrowed by atherosclerosis. The nurse should always check the patient's neurological status and vital signs before angiography is performed, in order to establish a baseline to which the patient's condition following the procedure can be compared [7, 9].

Angiography is a long, frightening and sometimes painful procedure. If the patient is able to comprehend, the physician will have provided a brief explanation of the technique and of the risks involved and will have obtained an *informed consent*. The nurse should understand the procedure as well as its purpose, the risks, and the sensations that the patient may experience during this procedure. It is her responsibility to prepare him by allaying his fears of the unknown and above all accepting the reasonableness of these fears. Her knowledge of the procedure and its consequences should enable her to plan care and monitor neurological status in an informed and intelligent manner. Although a sedative or tranquilizer usually is prescribed before the patient is taken to the radiology suite, the complexity of the equipment, noise, unfamiliar personnel, exposure of the groin, for a femoral approach, and use of restraints that may be necessary for immobilization will all add to the patient's fear and anxiety.

Often when contrast material is injected into the carotid artery there is a transient burning or painful sensation in the head or behind the eyes, which may be accompanied by transient nausea. The patient should be told that this is expected and will pass. Complications of angiography include (1) bleeding and hematoma formation at the puncture site, (2) airway obstruction resulting from compression of the larynx and trachea by an enlarging hematoma at the site of arterial puncture in the neck, (3) embolization to a distal cerebral artery, and (4) embolization to a peripheral artery. To decrease the possibility of hematoma formation, a cold pack is applied to the puncture site as soon as the procedure is completed. For the first twelve hours following angiography of the head and neck the patient must be observed closely for bleeding from the puncture site, development of a hematoma, seizures, and other signs of deterioration of neurological, cardiovascular, and respiratory status. Vital signs and neurological signs must be monitored often and very carefully [7, 9].

CAT scan

In contrast to lumbar puncture and angiography, the *computerized axial tomography (CAT) scan* is a noninvasive procedure usually tolerated by the patient with relative ease. It is a fairly new diagnostic tool available at most large medical centers. Because of the low risk and relatively limited exposure to radiation involved, it is becoming more widely used. This procedure makes use of a computer to calculate the resistance of the skull and intracranial structures to x-ray beams directed at the head as an x-ray tube makes a 180-degree scan, one degree at a time, in three or four planes. The density of the various tissues such as skull, meninges, brain, vessels, and ventricles, at different planes within the head, are assigned *absorption coefficients,* which are numbers ranging from −500 for air to +500 for bone. The computer calculates and records the tissue densities at each point and supplies a printout of the absorption coefficients. The printout is in the shape of the head at each plane studied. Images showing the density of the various structures at each plane studied and each degree are projected onto a viewing screen during the procedure. Bone appears as white, air as black, and the soft tissues as various gradations of gray depending on their density. Polaroid photographs can be taken of any of these images. The configuration and degree of shading in the images and on the computer printout assist in identification of intracranial lesions. A contrast medium can be injected if necessary to intensify the density of an abnormality [7, 9].

Blood and tumor tissue have measurably different absorptive values. Mass lesions and vascular lesions can therefore be distinguished readily. Infarction is usually demonstrable within the first few days following *thrombotic* stroke, but will be more apparent in the chronic state once cavitation has occurred. Since lacunar infarcts usually do not show up on the CAT scan, this procedure may be used to differentiate between embolic and thrombotic stroke. Unless there is a hemorrhagic infarct due to the embolus, the CAT scan will be normal. This procedure is most useful in the diagnosis of *intracranial hemorrhage.* According to Mohr, Fisher, and Adams the CAT scan "has revolutionized the diagnosis of intracerebral hemorrhage and has proved totally reliable in the detection of hemorrhages 1.5 cm or more in diameter situated in the cerebral or cerebellar hemispheres" [7, p. 1857]. These same authors found that this technique could localize hemorrhages with an accuracy far surpassing that of angiography and that the CAT scan was particularly helpful in demonstrating small hemorrhages that were not clinically recognizable. In cases of *ruptured saccular aneurysm,* diagnosis is established on the basis of grossly bloody cerebrospinal fluid, and the aneurysm itself can only be demonstrated by angiography. However, the CAT scan will show a localized clot adjacent to the aneurysm and/or a coexisting hydrocephalus [7].

The nurse is responsible for informing the patient about the procedure. He must be told that the top of his head will be placed within the scanning unit, reassured that the procedure is painless and simple, but impressed with the necessity for complete immobility to ensure accurate pictures. The unfamiliar surroundings and elaborate machinery can be extremely frightening to the patient, particularly if his sensorium is clouded or if he has receptive aphasia or visual or perceptual difficulties. Often such patients require sedation.

Skull x-ray

With stroke due to thrombosis or embolism, *x-ray of the skull* will not show a shift of the pineal body unless there is severe swelling of the cerebral tissue. When the stroke is the result of hypertensive intracranial hemorrhage, skull films taken early on may show a pineal shift away from the side of the lesion. Unless an intracerebral or subdural clot has formed, causing displacement of the pineal, skull x-ray will be negative, with ruptured saccular aneurysms [7].

EEG

Electroencephalography (EEG) is another diagnostic procedure that poses little threat of risk to the patient. The electroencephalogram provides a visible record of the electrical potentials generated by the neuronal activity of the brain. The procedure involves application of electrodes to specified locations all over the scalp. Each electrode is connected to an amplifier and pen that records the electrical potentials for that area of the brain in the form of waves on a moving strip of paper. The patterns created by potentials from various areas of the brain then can be compared and interpreted [8]. A normal range of EEG patterns has been established. Abnormal patterns are associated with (1) destruction of brain tissue due to tumor, infarction, or abscess; (2) seizure disorders, and (3) various metabolic diseases [8]. Electroencephalography may be helpful in differentiating mass lesions from transient ischemic attacks and stroke due to occlusive cerebrovascular disease.

The nurse is responsible for instructing the patient about the procedure and the various activation techniques that the EEG technician may use to elicit and record abnormal electrical activity, for example, asking the patient to hyperventilate, projecting flashing lights into his eyes, and administering a medication that will induce sleep or an intravenous stimulant that will cause a subclinical seizure. It is important to reassure the patient that no electrical shock is associated with any portion of the test. When needle electrodes are used rather than discs that are attached to the scalp with collodion or paste, some patients may feel as though a hair is being pulled out with the insertion of each electrode. In most instances this is not felt. If collodion is used, the nurse should see that the hair and scalp are thoroughly cleansed following the procedure. Brushing the hair removes much of the dried collodion; the remainder should be removed with careful use of a solvent such as acetone followed by a shampoo [9]. If the patient appears drowsy following the EEG, it is important to determine whether this reflects a change in neurological status or the continued effect of a medication administered during the procedure.

REFERENCES

1. Alpers, B. J., and Mancall, E. L. *Clinical Neurology* (6th ed.). Philadelphia: Davis, 1971. Pp. 17–20.
2. Bates, B. *A Guide to Physical Examination.* Philadelphia: Lippincott, 1974. Pp. 263–293.
3. Carpenter, M. D. *Core Text of Neuroanatomy.* Baltimore: Williams & Wilkins, 1974. Pp. 79–120.
4. DeJong, R. N. *The Neurological Examination* (3rd ed.). New York: Harper & Row, 1967. Pp. 1–54; 55–105; 107–341; 445–567; 583–631; 949–988.

5. Levy, L. Examination and Diagnosis. In S. Licht (Ed.), *Stroke and Its Rehabilitation.* Baltimore: Williams & Wilkins, 1975. Pp. 78–107.

6. Mechner, F. Patient assessment: Neurological examination. *Am. J. Nurs.* Vol. 75, No. 9.

7. Mohr, J. P. Fisher, C. M., and Adams, R. D. Cerebrovascular Diseases. In G. W. Thoru, et al. (Eds.), *Harrison's Principles of Internal Medicine* (8th ed.). New York: McGraw-Hill, 1977. Pp. 1832–1868.

8. Simpson, J. F., and Magee, K. *Clinical Evaluation of the Nervous System.* Boston: Little, Brown, 1973. Pp. 1–163.

9. Skydell, B., and Crowder, A. S. *Diagnostic Procedures.* Boston: Little, Brown, 1975. Pp. 15–45.

10. Walton J. *Brain Diseases of the Nervous System* (8th ed.). New York: Oxford University Press, 1977. Pp. 51–59, 65–89, 118–119.

5. Disorders of language

Language is a system by which man makes use of words as symbols to communicate his thoughts. This complex system includes rules for organization of these symbols in such a manner that their meaning and logic is expressed with precision. The basic components of any language are (1) a system of sounds, (2) a vocabulary, (3) a grammar, and (4) a semantic system. Speech sounds are referred to as *phonemes.* Combinations of phonemes, which are the smallest units of speech, serve to formulate words. Combinations of words are used to formulate sentences and convey ideas. This activity is the highest form of cerebral function. It occurs only in man [16].

The development of language in a child begins with auditory recognition of words. After he has learned to repeat them, he gradually masters the understanding of these words in appropriate context. In time he learns to combine them into sentences to formulate and communicate verbally thoughts which are increasingly more complex. The ability to read begins with recognition of individual letters and clusters of letters. As the child is taught the symbolic significance of various clusters of letters and the sounds they represent, he eventually recognizes them, in combination, as words. Once he is able to grasp the context of the word combinations, structured as sentences, he has learned to read. While he is learning to read, the child will associate the sounds with their symbols and thus also learns to spell. When he is able to associate the symbols that represent the sounds he wants to express with cursive movements of the hand, he learns to write. The end point of language development is the formulation of ideas in both the spoken and written language. Language serves as the vehicle for acquisition of almost every form of knowledge [1, 16].

Visual and hearing problems will alter significantly the process of language development. Physical impairments of the structures that produce voice and facilitate articulation of the spoken word will influence the quality of speech patterns developed in the child. Clarity of thought and ease of expression will vary from individual to individual on the basis of intelligence, maturity, cultural influences, and the degree of stimulation he receives from his environment. Mastery of language can range in degree from the ability to communicate one's most basic needs to production of literary work as an art form.

Man has devised various means of communication. According to Brain, "speech is a mode of communication in which symbols are used to convey ideas, to arouse feelings, or to excite actions" (cited in [14]). The symbols of the spoken word are sounds and those of written speech are visual patterns. Those who are blind must rely on tactile impressions to replace visual patterns, and those who are deaf and mute must substitute gestures, signs, and finger spelling for the spoken word [14].

COMMUNICATION DISTURBANCES

Communication difficulties are a common result of stroke. In addition to hindering some of the modalities of treatment required for other manifestations of stroke, the inability to express him- or herself or to comprehend instructions and explanations can be an extremely frightening and frustrating experience for the patient. Ease of expression and a good command of the language are interpreted as signs of intelligence in our society. The feeling that his inability to communicate adequately reflects a lack of intelligence can be devastating to a patient. The fear that a loved one's mental capacity has been severely altered can be equally devastating to family and friends. One of the primary goals in caring for the patient with speech and language problems is to help him to establish a means of communication. While working with the patient to achieve this, the nurse must also work with family members and friends to be certain they understand the nature of the deficit, are able to help reinforce the therapeutic approach, and can provide support and encouragement.

There is an important distinction between disorders of language and disorders of speech. *Speech* disorders imply an impairment in verbal expression that results from a weakness or lack of coordination in the musculature used in articulating words (dysarthria). Patients with *language* disorders may be able to articulate words properly, but the words they produce are linguistically incorrect. When the patient has a language disorder that affects comprehension, he will be unable to grasp the meaning of spoken or written words even though there may be no impairment of his hearing or vision [5].

For those unfortunate patients with severe *aphasia* (disorder due to brain damage), the ability to convey thoughts through writing or even the use of conventional gestures, such as nodding the head for "yes" and shaking it for "no," may be lost. Efforts must be made to anticipate such a patient's needs, and family members will require considerable support. They must be reassured that the capacity to understand what is said may still remain intact. They must be encouraged to visit frequently and to talk to the patient, speaking distinctly and at a comfortable conversational pace, even though he appears completely unable to follow their conversation or even acknowledge their presence. An understanding of the process of language development and of the neurological functions which govern language are essential in planning care for the patient with stroke.

The patient's premorbid level of intelligence and personality traits can have an important effect on his reaction to illness, acceptance of disability, and motivation to overcome his handicaps. These factors must be considered in planning care for all patients. In spite of this, however, it cannot be emphasized too strongly that speech and language disorders resulting from stroke are primarily manifestations of a diseased brain and not necessarily reflections of the patient's basic personality or level of premorbid intellectual functioning. Clinicians caring for patients with derangements of speech and understanding due to stroke must never lose sight of the fact that the patient's behavior is the result of a physiological loss over which he has no control. One must not be too hasty to label these patients as difficult, uncooperative, unable to learn, or unmotivated. Socially unacceptable speech patterns are as indicative of a pathological condition that can be localized to damage in a specific area of the brain as are incontinence, paralysis, and impairment of cardiovascular function.

CEREBRAL DOMINANCE

Cerebral dominance refers to the greater importance of one side of the brain over the other for certain learned behaviors. Certain functions are located mainly within one of the two cerebral hemispheres. This issue is particularly important with regard to language function, since damage to the dominant hemisphere will result in a different deficit than damage to the nondominant hemisphere. Most of our knowledge about the control of the capacity for speech by one half of the brain has been derived from the study of patients who have suffered strokes or other brain damage. It has been demonstrated by Geschwind and Levitsky [9] that there are striking anatomical differences, visible to the naked eye, between the two cerebral hemispheres. The area of the temporal lobe attributed to speech function was larger in the left hemisphere, which is most frequently the dominant, than it is in the right hemisphere. These studies support the original work of Carl Wernicke in 1874, which described the differences in aphasia occurring with lesions in different areas of the brain [5].

Cerebral dominance is related to "handedness," that is, preference for use of one hand over the other. The higher nervous pathways for speech are usually located in the left hemisphere of the brain in persons who are right-handed (approximately 93% of the population). Their left cerebral hemispheres are thus classified as dominant. Conversely, the speech pathways of left-handed persons are ordinarily situated in the right hemisphere, which is then considered dominant. It is important to note that while 7% of the population is left-handed, about 60% of these people have speech centers located in the left hemisphere and only 40% have their speech centers located in the right hemisphere. It is thought by some that handedness is a hereditary trait, with right-handedness inherited as a mendelian dominant and left-handedness as a recessive [2].

HISTORICAL BACKGROUND

In 1861 Paul Broca, a French surgeon, observed that two patients with lesions in the posterior part of the left inferior frontal convolution had lost the power of speech. In Germany thirteen years later, Wernicke expanded this concept and distinguished three forms of aphasia [2]. (1) *Sensory aphasia* was due to damage of the auditory center in the temporal lobe and resulted in an inability to understand words and a lack of recognition of this speech defect on the part of the patient. (2) *Motor aphasia* was due to a lesion of the third frontal convolution and resulted in loss of images for articulated speech. When the lesion was in the pathway between the auditory and the speech center, *conduction aphasia* occurred. The patient would still show comprehension, would use words inappropriately but know he had erred.

(3) *Total aphasia,* due to destruction of both centers, resulted in a loss of both the ability to comprehend and the expression of speech. Current concepts of disorders of speech are based upon this scheme. It should be kept in mind, however, that brain lesions do not necessarily occur precisely within the prescribed boundaries of the areas classified within this scheme, nor does the strict subdivision of motor and sensory functions for language provide an accurate reflection of the clinical picture in all instances. There is much inconsistency in the degree of speech impairment among patients with lesions located in the same area of the brain [2, 12, 14].

Research today continues to try to establish correlations between various disorders of language and the location of lesions in the brain as well as to clarify the neural basis of speech itself. The relationship of cerebral dominance to other functions is also being investigated [5].

AREAS OF THE BRAIN ASSOCIATED WITH DISTURBANCES OF SPEECH AND LANGUAGE FUNCTIONS

Stroke may result in lesions that destroy areas of the cerebral cortex or impair conduction between cortical areas that govern language and speech. The following cortical areas of the brain have been associated with such disturbances (see Figure 2-5):

WERNICKE'S AREA
Wernicke's area is located in the temporal lobe between Heschl's gyrus, which is the primary receiver of auditory stimuli, and the angular gyrus, which relays stimuli between the auditory and visual areas [7]. Areas 41 and 42 (as classified by Brodmann) are related to recognition of spoken language. Comprehension of spoken language is associated with areas 21 and 22. Lesions in these areas will result in auditory-verbal agnosia [1]. The patient will be unable to recognize or understand the words he hears. Although he can speak, his words convey little or no thought content.

BROCA'S AREA
Broca's area is in the frontal lobe adjacent to the region of the motor cortex that controls movement of the lips, jaw, tongue, soft palate, and vocal cords [7]. It corresponds to area 44, as classified by Brodmann, and contains the engrams for memory of motor patterns of speech. Damage to this area can result in motor aphasia. The patient will have difficulty in articulating the words he wishes to use. Speech will no longer be fluent and may be labored.

AREA 37 AND POSTERIOR PART OF AREA 21
Area 37 and the posterior part of area 21 in the temporal lobe are associated with formulation of language and recall of words. Lesions here may produce anomia, amnesic aphasia, or defects in language formulation. The patient will be unable to recall familiar words and phrases or names of known persons, objects, and places [1].

ANGULAR GYRUS

The angular gyrus in the parietal lobe is related to visual recognition of the symbols used in such activities as reading, writing, and arithmetic. Damage to this area can cause alexia (impaired reading ability), agraphia (impaired ability to write), and acalculia (impaired calculation ability). The patient may have difficulties with the use of numbers, letters, or other symbols. All these problems can occur in a variety of combinations [1, 19].

It is thought that auditory patterns from repetition of words are relayed from Wernicke's area to Broca's area via the bundle of nerve fibers called the *arcuate fasciculus,* which connects the two areas. In the same way the angular gyrus, which connects the visual cortex with the speech areas, serves to permit comprehension of written language. Upon these assumptions Geschwind has described the following model for the production of language [7].

1. When a spoken word is *heard,* the stimulus is relayed from the auditory area in the cortex to Wernicke's area.
2. For a word to be *spoken,* the auditory pattern must be relayed from Wernicke's area to Broca's area so that it can be articulated.
3. When a spoken word is to be *spelled,* the pattern must be transmitted from the auditory area to the angular gyrus to produce a visual pattern.
4. When a word is *read,* the stimulus to the visual center in the cortex must be transmitted via the angular gyrus to Wernicke's area to arouse the auditory form of the word in order to assure comprehension [7].

According to this model, when a lesion occurs in Wernicke's area, comprehension of spoken as well as written language will be impaired. The patient is able to speak fluently as long as Broca's area has not been affected, but he will not use the correct words and his speech will lack content, since the proper information cannot be transmitted to Broca's area. When the lesion occurs in Broca's area, the ability to articulate words will be affected, although the patient's comprehension will be spared. In this case, speech is no longer fluent and may be labored. The patient will have difficulty with certain words and phrases, often with very simple statements [7].

TYPES OF APHASIA

There are many terms that qualify aphasia, and some are used interchangeably. They may classify the disorder in terms either of the location of the cerebral insult that precipitated it or of the functional impairment that results. Localization of the lesion and identification of the underlying pathological and etiological conditions are essential to the physician who is responsible for establishing a diagnosis and instituting an appropriate plan of treatment for the patient with aphasia. Reference to the various types of aphasia will be encountered frequently in the physician's progress notes, in the medical literature, and during patient rounds or care conferences. Nurses, therapists, and other health care practitioners responsible for providing care appropriate to the patient's needs must understand the nature of the patient's language disorder in order to discharge this responsibility. Various terms used to classify types of aphasia are presented in the following paragraphs. It must be emphasized that, regardless of the nature and exact location of the lesion causing aphasia, care should be planned according to the resultant deficit.

One of the most important descriptors used in reference to all types of aphasia is *fluency*. With *fluent aphasia,* speech is well articulated and follows normal intonational patterns. The patient is able to produce long phrases or sentences with a preserved grammatical skeleton. When one listens to them carefully, however, these sentences convey very little meaning. Patients with *nonfluent aphasia* produce very little speech. Words are spoken slowly, with great difficulty in articulation. Sentence structure lacks small grammatical words. Nonfluent aphasia results from lesions in Broca's area. Since lesions in this area usually involve the adjacent motor cortex, nonfluent aphasics generally have a hemiparesis or hemiplegia as well. With fluent aphasia, Broca's area remains intact, and the patient does not usually have hemiparesis or hemiplegia. Fluent aphasia may be further qualified on the basis of the patient's ability to comprehend spoken language and repeat it [6].

BROCA'S APHASIA

Broca's aphasia is also referred to as *expressive, motor, anterior,* or *nonfluent aphasia.* When a patient has a lesion in Broca's area, his or her ability to transform sounds into articulatory patterns is impaired or lost. The deficit ranges from a slight difficulty with articulation to an almost complete loss of power for expression of spoken words, although the musculature necessary for formation of speech may still function for other purposes. Usually such a patient speaks haltingly, and the great muscular effort entailed in forming each word is most apparent. The patient frequently makes obvious facial and hand articulatory gestures when trying to speak. Since he may consistently omit small grammatical words, the resulting speech pattern is sometimes referred to as "telegraphic." Comprehension of both spoken and written language is not altered. Therefore, in spite of the deficit, he is able to communicate by means of single word responses to questions in most cases and can name objects correctly. However, penmanship is usually affected, and the same language difficulties are manifested in writing as in speech. Handwriting, therefore, cannot be used as a means of communication. Patients with a more severe deficit may be able to produce only one or two words. Frequently such patients repeat their few remaining words over and over, even though they are usually quite aware that these are not correct. This can be most frustrating for the patient, since he understands what is said and going on around him, and he knows precisely what he wishes to say. As recovery takes place, speech may be slow, laborious, slurred, and mostly agrammatical, with omission of small words such as conjunctions, adjectives, and adverbs. The same deficit may result when there is a subcortical lesion that interferes with the connection between Broca's area and the lower end of the rolandic cortex [5, 8, 12].

WERNICKE'S APHASIA

Wernicke's aphasia, also referred to as *receptive, sensory,* or *fluent aphasia,* occurs when the connection between the primary auditory cortex and the angular gyrus region is destroyed. When this happens, associations to spoken words cannot be aroused in other areas of the brain. As a result, the patient's comprehension of speech is impaired. Since the area of the brain that controls the articulation of words (Broca's area) is not affected, the patient can still talk. He usually does so volubly and at great length, seemingly unable to stop in spite of many errors in the use of words. Often he is unaware of these errors and appears somewhat euphoric. His speech will have normal intonation and rhythm, but, since he is not always able to produce the correct words, he will substitute circumlocutory phrases, nonspecific words, or incorrect words. These incorrect words are called *paraphasias.* There are three types, literal, verbal, and neologistic. *Literal or phonemic paraphasias* are incorrect sounds or syllables inserted into words that would otherwise be correct to express the patient's thought. Sometimes the distortion created is slight enough that one can recognize the meaning intended. At other times, completely unintelligible words are produced. For example, the patient may say "Toofuf" for toothbrush. *Verbal paraphasias* are substitutions of one word for another. Sometimes the meaning of the two words is related in some way; at other times, there is no relationship whatever. *Neologistic paraphasias* involve substitution of an undecipherable expression which is nonsensical. For example, the patient may say "ferbish" for toothbrush.

With Wernicke's aphasia, the patient neither comprehends the examiner's words nor is able to repeat them. Such patients have difficulty naming objects, and, although their penmanship is unaffected, their writing manifests the same lack of content as their spoken language or content will not be pertinent to the discussion and they therefore cannot be expected to express their needs in writing [5, 6, 12].

GLOBAL APHASIA
When stroke results in a massive lesion affecting both the anterior and posterior speech areas, the patient manifests a combination of Broca's aphasia, with inability to transform sounds into words, and Wernicke's aphasia, with impairment of comprehension. All language modalities are affected, and impairment is so severe that the patient may be unable to communicate on any level. The patient with global aphasia has been likened to a visitor in a foreign land who does not recognize the local alphabet, cannot read or comprehend a single word he sees or hears, and although rational, able to retain the sum of his experiences, and in full possession of sound judgment, remains absolutely cut off from all communication with the world around him. The global aphasic generally suffers a severe hemiplegia [1, 6, 12].

CONDUCTION APHASIA
Conduction aphasia occurs when a lesion of the arcuate fasciculus disrupts the connection between Broca's and Wernicke's areas. Although the patient may produce many words, very little of his speech conveys meaning. He may make errors of syntax and grammar and even use nonexistent words. His use of written language will reflect his problems with speech. He will not be able to write from dictation, although, since penmanship is preserved, he can copy the words if they are written down. Basically he cannot perform those tasks that require having been previously taught to recognize the relationship between two different types of stimuli: for

example, the relationship between the sound of the word "apple" and the sight of the combination of letters that form the word "a-p-p-l-e".

Some patients with conduction aphasia may be quite alert and able to comprehend everything they see and hear, but remain incapable of self-initiated speech or repetition of words. They may be very much aware of their deficits. Because there has been a disruption of the connection between the auditory and speech motor areas, these patients will have extreme difficulty with repetition of words, even if they understand them completely. They will have problems reading aloud for the same reason, even though they may comprehend the written words [2, 8, 12].

ISOLATED SPEECH AREA

The syndrome of the isolated speech area occurs when the connection between Wernicke's and Broca's areas remains intact but all other connections between the speech areas and the rest of the brain have been destroyed. The patient's oral and written comprehension are severely impaired, since no associations can be aroused in other areas of the brain. Although he can still speak, he is unable to transfer any information from other areas of the brain to Wernicke's area, to be translated into verbal form. Thus, his speech is usually rapid and marked by paraphasias. He will have no difficulty in repeating words said to him and, in fact, echolalia, which is an automatic and compulsive repetition of words without any understanding of their meaning, may be noted [8, 12].

AMNESIC APHASIA

With less severe lesions in the temporal lobe amnesic or anomic aphasia may arise. The patient retains the ability for repetition and has good comprehension of both written and spoken language but shows difficulty naming objects or evoking words for certain conditions or qualities. The degree of difficulty can vary from a groping for the correct word to complete loss of ability to name familiar objects shown to him. Often he will substitute a description of how the object is used [12, 19].

PURE ALEXIA

Pure alexia without agraphia occurs with destruction of the left visual cortex and the posterior section of the corpus callosum. This is usually the result of an infarction in the area supplied by the posterior cerebral artery. Since the right visual region is cut off from the speech area, the sight of a written word cannot be translated into the spoken word form. Thus, the patient will be unable to read. When the lesion involves the angular gyrus and interferes with the connection between the speech area and the visual association cortex, the patient will have *pure alexia with agraphia* – that is, difficulty with both reading and writing, since written words cannot be translated into spoken word form, nor can spoken words be translated into the written form [8, 19].

PURE WORD DEAFNESS

Pure word deafness is the result of lesions in the temporal lobe or bilateral cortical lesions in the superior temporal region that prevent auditory stimuli from reaching

Wernicke's area. The patient is unable to comprehend, write to dictation, or repeat what is said. However, his speech demonstrates correct thinking and use of language. The ability to read and write, remains intact [12].

PURE WORD BLINDNESS
With pure word blindness the patient loses the ability to read and name certain objects, although his power to comprehend, write, and repeat spoken language remains intact [12].

EVALUATING THE PATIENT'S LANGUAGE ABILITY

In caring for patients with stroke, it is essential that those providing care understand any existing language deficits so that a means of effective communication with the patient can be established. Once the patient's medical condition has become stabilized, a standardized list of the patient's deficits and residual language function should be drawn up by the speech therapist. However, since the nurse is the professional responsible for constant supervision of the patient's condition, she must be able to perform a preliminary assessment of the patient's language ability as soon as possible after the stroke. This informal bedside evaluation should include the patient's ability to speak spontaneously, to understand the spoken word, to understand written language, to express himself in writing, and to name objects. The nurse should first consider other deficits that can hinder the production of language, such as mental confusion, diminished visual acuity or a visual field deficit, primary hearing loss, dysarthria that inhibits use of the muscles for speech, or unfamiliarity with the English language. As each of the different aspects of language use is assessed, the nurse must be careful not to provide the patient with clues that can be perceived by a sense other than the one being tested. For example, if the patient's ability to understand the spoken word is being tested, gestures should not be used. Conversely, if visual-verbal recognition ability is being tested, the examiner should not inadvertently speak the words or allow her hand movement to be seen as she writes the test words [1].

The following techniques may be used by the nurse to gain information concerning the patient's expressive and receptive language abilities.

ABILITY TO SPEAK SPONTANEOUSLY
Note whether or not the patient produces any speech whatsoever. Note if there is a deficit in production of words. Then listen to hear if the speech is meaningful, and note the extent of vocabulary used and the clarity of speech. If the patient has no speech, attempt to stimulate speech by asking some open-ended, uncomplicated questions such as, "Tell me about your work," or "Tell me about your family."

ABILITY TO UNDERSTAND THE SPOKEN WORD
A simple method of testing comprehension is to ask questions of increasing complexity that require yes or no responses. Note whether he is able to answer "yes or no" questions appropriately. If the patient cannot speak, note whether he is able to

respond "yes" or "no" by nodding or shaking his head or to fulfill commands appropriately through gestures.

The patient may be given a series of commands of increasing complexity. Observe and listen. If he is able to respond verbally, establish whether or not the response is appropriate to the command.

ABILITY TO UNDERSTAND WRITTEN LANGUAGE
Give the patient a series of written requests or instructions. Observe and listen to determine whether he is able to comprehend and carry out the instructions appropriately or respond by saying or nodding "yes" or "no."

ABILITY TO EXPRESS IDEAS IN WRITING
Provide the patient with paper and pencil and observe what he does with them. If he is able to write, ask him to write out a request — for example, what he would like for dinner — or to give an account of the weather, his complaint, or his name, address and phone number.

ABILITY TO NAME OBJECTS
Show the patient a series of pictures and commonly known objects and ask him to name them. This is important, since it allows for identification of even very slight degrees of dysphasia.

This preliminary language assessment is essential to establishing some means of communication between the asphasic patient and the nurse. It cannot, however, substitute for the standardized comprehensive testing performed by the speech therapist, nor is it intended to do so [4, 17, 19].

STANDARDIZED TESTING

Aphasia can affect all language modalities and may be accompanied by perceptual, sensory, and motor deficits, which further complicate the patient's problems of communication. Perceptual deficits are discussed in Chapter 6. This complexity together with the wide variety of aphasic disorders caused by stroke and the basic differences between individual patients, makes standardization of language testing very difficult. Various methods have been developed by different investigators. According to Weisenburg, fundamentally the test should "provide a satisfactory analysis of the performance in question" [20], and according to Sarno, it should assess both the deficits and whatever residual language function remains [16]. Some of the standardized tests available are based upon a theoretical model of how language is organized in the brain, while others are derived from traditional cognitive achievement tests. Most language tests are designed to evaluate ability to understand written and spoken words and ability for expression through speech and writing. Testing must also include an evaluation of mental awareness, vision, hearing, perceptual discrimination, and speech musculature, since impairment in any one of these areas can interfere with performance on the test [1, 4, 16, 20].

ABILITY TO UNDERSTAND THE SPOKEN WORD
When auditory comprehension is tested, an attempt is made to (1) evaluate the patient's ability to *understand the meaning of common, single words* and (2) to determine whether there is a reduction in the *auditory retention span.* The patient is given a series of verbal commands to see if he confuses words that sound alike. Initially the commands are quite simple, such as "close your eyes," and gradually they become more complex. A short factual paragraph is read to the patient to determine whether he can retain what is said to him and retell the facts. Gradually the length of the paragraph is increased to determine whether the patient's comprehension is reduced, and language errors increase as the length of conversation or material increases. Some patients will have a reduction in auditory retention span as materials increase in length [17].

ABILITY TO UNDERSTAND WRITTEN WORDS
The aim of testing visual recognition and comprehension is to evaluate the patient's ability to recognize letters, words, numbers, and sentences. To be certain that results will be accurate, the degree of the patient's visual acuity and ability to read line by line must be established. If the patient is able to speak, he will be asked to read aloud specific letters, numbers, or words pointed to by the examiner. If he is unable to speak, the examiner will read a letter or word and the patient will be instructed to point to the appropriate letter, number, or word written on a chart. He may also be asked to match objects with the appropriate written word or to pantomime their meaning. For numbers, he may hold up the appropriate number of fingers. Since the patient may be able to read a sentence aloud but not comprehend its meaning, he is given a written instruction and asked to read it to himself, then carry out the instruction. Sentence comprehension is assessed according to how well he follows the instruction. The length and number of sentences will be increased to see whether he confuses words that look alike, whether errors increase with the length of the paragraph, and whether his reading vocabulary is appropriate to his cultural and educational background [1, 17].

ABILITY TO EXPRESS ONESELF IN SPEECH
The examiner will want to assess the language still at the patient's command, the amount of vocabulary reduction that has occurred, and how much functional speech remains. Before initiating testing, the speech musculature must be examined in order to detect dysarthria that may cause errors in articulation. In testing the language at the patient's command, reactive speech (e.g., prayers or profanities), and serial responses (e.g., days of the week, months) will be elicited. An attempt will be made to obtain responses to simple, direct questions. To determine the extent of vocabulary reduction, the patient will be asked to name objects. In determining the amount of functional speech available, the examiner will look for word-finding difficulties, defective grammar or syntax, use of jargon, ability to express meaningful ideas, and use of phrases and full sentences. The patient will be asked to give simple biographical information, describe a picture, explain similarities between two objects, and retell a story [17].

ABILITY TO EXPRESS ONESELF IN WRITING

Before attempting to assess writing ability, the examiner must check for visual, motor, or spatial disturbances that might make it difficult for the patient to hold or guide the pencil and must find out whether or not the patient is able to write with his accustomed hand. The patient is tested on ability to copy, to write from dictation, and to write spontaneously. The examiner watches to see if he has difficulty in knowing where to start writing on the page or what direction to write in, and whether there is any reversal or distortion in letter formation. Letters and numbers are dictated in random order to determine whether the patient confuses those that look alike. Shorter to longer sentences are dictated to see if errors increase with the length of the sentence. To evaluate spontaneous writing, the patient is given a topic or shown a picture and asked to write a description. Spelling accuracy is assessed in relation to the patient's experience and education [17].

In some cases testing also includes an evaluation of mathematical skills, from simple arithmetic to complex computations [17].

Once the therapist has completed the standard tests, a summary of the patient's language assets and liabilities is prepared and a plan initiated to work with the existing assets to overcome the liabilities. Table 5-1 shows the disabilities that may result from disruption of language function due to stroke, and the language training required to correct them.

According to Sarno, a basic problem inherent in testing patients with aphasia is that standard test measures cannot take into account all the various nonlinguistic elements of communication and that some patients perform poorly on all levels of formal testing but do quite well in informal conversation. To assure the most accurate and objective assessment possible of the patient's potential for using whatever residual language skills he has, Sarno identifies two environments for observation of language performance outside the test situation: the *clinical,* in which information is obtained from observation during task-oriented test conditions; and the *functional* — observation of the patient's performance in a more natural context [16].

LANGUAGE RETRAINING

It is not within the scope of this book to present the details of language retraining. However, various techniques and approaches used in speech therapy are presented here in the belief that a clearer understanding of the patient's deficits and the speech therapist's goals for retraining will enable nurses and other clinicians to reinforce the learning process, assist the patient to achieve successful communication, speed up rehabilitation, and thus reduce the patient's frustration.

Reaction to loss of language function, as with all disabilities, is influenced by the patient's premorbid personality and life-style. No two patients will manifest their loss in quite the same way. Any therapy must be geared to a particular patient's situation and based upon use of the undamaged portion of his brain. Language retraining is not the same as teaching language to children and should never be patterned on behavioral approaches that will only cause the patient to regress and add

Table 5-1
Disabilities that may result from disruption of language function due to stroke and the language training required

Language Function	Defect	Disabilities	Training Required
Arithmetic	Acalculia	Inability to count, recall numbers, or perform the four basic arithmetic processes.	Counting, copying numbers, adding, subtracting, multiplying, dividing.
Handwriting	Motor agraphia	Loss of memory patterns for movements of handwriting.	Teaching of motor patterns of handwriting.
Written spelling, sentence formulation	Amnesic agraphia	Inability to spell or formulate sentences in writing.	Training in written spelling and sentence formulation.
Reading	Alexia	Inability to recognize letters or words and to understand simple or complicated written statements.	Practice in associating names with and words, silent reading for comprehension.
Recall of language	Anomia, amnesic aphasia	Inability to recall words and phrases on intent. "I know what it is, but I can't tell you."	Practice is associating names with objects, people, places, and in formulating language.
Auditory recognition of spoken language	Auditory-verbal agnosia, paraphasia, jargon	Inability to recognize or understand spoken language. Patient often does not detect errors in own speech, thus unknowingly uses wrong words.	Auditory training: recognition and comprehension of individual sounds, words, sentences.
Ability to pronounce sounds and words	Motor aphasia	Inability to recall placement of organs of speech (tongue, teeth, lips, etc.) in pronouncing sounds and words. Patient knows appropriate word, but cannot form it.	Practice in making individual sounds. Drills in front of mirror and in imitation of therapist.

Adapted from A. Agronowitz, and M. R. McKeown. *Aphasia Handbook for Adults and Children.* Springfield: Charles C. Thomas, 1964. P. 36.

to his sense of frustration and rejection. All materials used should be geared to adult interests, and the patient should always be addressed as a mature, experienced person [1, 16, 18]. Throughout the speech therapy sessions the therapist can provide significant emotional support to the patient who must adjust to this exceedingly frustrating handicap.

Overview of techniques used

The primary objective of speech therapy is to facilitate communication. The goals that various patients strive for, however, may differ significantly. While some patients may be satisfied with making their most basic needs known, others may wish to return to a career situation that relies heavily on expertise in both verbal and written expression of the most complex sort. Furthermore techniques of learning and teaching are not equally effective for all patients, and retraining should start for each patient at the level where language breaks down. Generally therapy begins with the patient repeating and reading in unison with the therapist and writing from dictation. This provides auditory stimulation, elicits responses for feedback information, and gradually increases the patient's retention span. The complexity of the material can be systematically increased as fast as the patient progresses. Attempts are made to provide a frequently used frame of reference for eliciting responses by word association to stimulate language and to provide the patient with an opportunity for success early on in therapy [16, 17]. For example, the therapist may say "apple pie and . . ." expecting the patient to add "ice cream" or "hotdog with mustard and . . ."

Schuell's treatment approach is based on the premise that auditory processes are always impaired in aphasia. She believes that "auditory stimulation is crucial in control of language processes and recommends it as the first principle of therapy. However, since feedback from more than one sensory modality contributes to behavior, she recommends that auditory stimulation be combined with visual stimulation at progressive levels of complexity, starting with the most basic material the patient can respond to [16, 17].

If the patient has a decreased auditory retention span, stimulation should begin with short words and phrases, progressing to longer words and sentences. When the patient is perplexed by a new word, he usually will come to recognize it after he has heard it repeated about six times. When there is a visual problem, the patient is instructed to copy a letter or word while naming it until he is able to produce it without looking at the copy. It should be remembered that recovery of reading and writing ability will be slower than recovery of speech for patients with visual impairment [17]. Patients with milder forms of language disability will be instructed to define words, write sentences or brief paragraphs, and report on current events described in the newspaper or on the radio.

For exercising reading skills, the therapist generally uses current newspapers and magazines that are of interest to the patient but are written in a simple style and appear in large print. Word games are useful when there is a deficit in naming objects. The therapist often constructs flash cards for letters, words, or pictures designed to assist the patient with his specific problem. Word fill-in and multiple choice exercises help patients relearning to read, and tape recorders and mirrors may help teach articulation of words.

Retraining for specific defects

If a patient has auditory-verbal agnosia and can no longer understand spoken language or interpret words, the therapist works on teaching him to carry out oral instructions of increasing complexity. A person with a severe auditory deficit may not understand verbal instructions but may receive nonverbal clues from the environment that provide him with some understanding of what a particular situation calls for. The therapist may point to particular picture cards and to objects, indicating by her gestures that she wants the patient to match them. The patient will also be called upon to identify objects, pictures, or word lists placed in front of him and identified verbally by the therapist.

Naming and recall techniques are used when the patient has *anomia* or *amnesic aphasia,* which prevents him from recalling names for the most common objects even when he recognizes them. The therapist shows a picture of an object to the patient, writes the word on the blackboard, pronounces it, and has the patient write the word and practice pronouncing it several times. The series of pictures can be expanded to increase the number of words in the patient's vocabulary.

If the patient continues to perseverate (repeat a word over and over, as though unable to stop) during the practice session, as is often the case with anomia, the therapist interjects another word to break off the pattern of perseveration [1].

As the patient with amnesic aphasia progresses and develops a larger vocabulary, the therapist will employ oral formulation techniques to help him develop more complete sentences that include descriptive words and phrases. Some patients become quite fluent and may be taught to formulate their thoughts into complete sentences, while others may only be capable of achieving the most basic vocabulary [1].

When the patient has *motor aphasia, dysarthria,* or *apraxia,* he is given motor speech pattern exercises. With motor aphasia the patient is unable to execute the proper movements to produce words because he cannot recall the motor patterns for speech. This defect can vary from complete inability to produce any intelligible sound to "telegraphic speech," utterance of key words only. With dysarthria the patient who has no aphasia recalls the motor speech patterns for the various sounds but is unable to form words because he has weakness and/or incoordination of the musculature involved in speech and voice production. With apraxia the patient is unable to protrude his tongue or purse his lips on command for speech, although he can perform these same movements spontaneously for other activities such as chewing or whistling. The exercises used include protrusion, lateral rotation and elevation of the tongue, whistling, pursing the lips, and blowing out matches.

Most patients with aphasia have some problem in understanding written language. With *alexia,* reading recognition and comprehension techniques are initiated. To establish word recognition, pictures are used along with word cards. To develop comprehension, patients are encouraged to define words by matching or circling the appropriate nouns or action words described on the word cards. As the patient progresses in comprehension, more complex materials are used [1].

Since writing depends on a combination of both motor and mental skills, two types of agraphia may occur. With *motor* or *apraxic agraphia,* the patient is unable to write because he no longer knows how to form the letters. *Agnostic* or *amnesic agraphia* involves an inability to spell. The patient is able to form letters but doesn't know how to put them together in sequence. With *paragraphia,* which is comparable to paraphasia, the patient will write the wrong words because he cannot recall the correct ones. For these patients with paragraphia, therapy starts with basic handwriting exercises and use of alphabet and numbers. If the patient has motor agraphia the therapist will help him to trace and copy lines, curves, and numbers. The patient gradually progresses to copying with the use of a picture card and corresponding word card until he is able to recall and write the appropriate word with just the picture card. Spelling exercises include recalling a word after the therapist has presented it, writing it, and saying it. The patient is then encouraged to progress to writing simple phrases, sentences, and finally paragraphs [1].

Patients with *acalculia,* or difficulties with numbers, have to relearn the concept of numbers and how to calculate orally as well as on paper. Exercises include placing numbers in chronological order, learning to use money, reading a calendar, and telling time. Eventually the processes of addition, subtraction, multiplication, and division are introduced. Some patients may progress to more advanced mathematical lessons [1].

When the patient can only produce *jargon, paraphasias,* or *dysarthric* oral speech, retraining is directed to helping him recognize his errors and correct them. Such patients ramble, are unable to explain clearly what they are trying to say, and are generally unaware of their inappropriate language. Their thought processes remain intact, but they cannot summon up the words to express them. This type of aphasia is the most difficult to correct. Auditory training is often employed: A tape recorder is used to help the patient identify his errors of speech. The therapist may also repeat his errors to him [1].

PROGNOSIS

The prognosis for recovery from aphasia depends on a variety of interrelated factors that include the site and extent of the lesion responsible for the language deficit, the age and general health of the patient, and his premorbid personality, intellectual capacity, and educational background [11]. It is not unusual for a remarkable recovery to occur within several months of a major stroke; it has been demonstrated that additional improvement at a very high level can take place for two or more years following onset of aphasia [10, 14]. The most dramatic and quantitatively spontaneous recovery occurs in the first three months following stroke. However, at this point the patient's ability to read, write, and speak may be far from adequate, and these activities usually require a great effort [11, 17, 18].

When the patient has suffered a loss of recognition in either the visual, tactile, or auditory areas, one of the other avenues must be used to help him to communicate. The prognosis for recovery is always better for patients with visual or tactile agnosias than for those with an auditory agnosia. When there is a loss of recognition in the auditory area, the visual and tactile must be used for retraining. When all three areas — visual, tactile, and auditory — are damaged, prognosis for recovery is poor, since the speech therapist has no viable avenue of approach to the patient [11].

LONG-TERM PLANNING

Because of the complexity of aphasia, the process of recovery must be considered in terms of years rather than months. Language skills are regained only gradually. It is important to realize, therefore, that, as recovery progresses, the patient's needs and capabilities will change. Treatment should be planned as a series of steps. Since some form of speech therapy usually continues following discharge from the hospital, careful discharge planning and family counseling is essential. Family members should be helped to understand and accept the limitations that result from the patient's aphasia. It is important that they realize how reading and writing skills have been affected, and, if the prognosis for return of language function is poor, that they be made aware of this. They should also understand that, although there may be little or no further improvement of speech, the patient is neither mentally ill nor retarded [17].

In helping the family to understand the patient's disability and special needs with regard to communication, the nurse should keep the following principles in mind. The aphasic patient may not understand everything that is said to him. He will understand best if short, simple statements are used and ample time is given for him to grasp one idea before the person speaking proceeds to a new idea. Do not over-articulate words or speak to him as though to a baby. What is more important is to use noncomplex speech forms. He should be allowed plenty of time to formulate a reply to each question. A second question or a repetition of the first can interrupt his thought process and prevent him from forming an answer. It will be much easier for him to follow a conversation when only one person speaks to him at a time. It is most important to speak slowly and distinctly. Often patients who have recovered from aphasia complain that everyone spoke so rapidly that all they could hear was a jumble of noise. They find any additional source of external noise, such as a radio, television, or stereo, extremely disruptive and frequently describe it as actually having caused them physical pain. It is most important to remember that a lack of response does not necessarily indicate a lack of understanding. Frequently patients who were unable to respond in any way during an early stage of their illness have later reported the anguish and loneliness they experienced when loved ones who visited talked about them rather than to them when they longed for some form of contact [17, 18].

Family members should be encouraged to work with the patient for some time each day to improve his speech and to help him live as normally as possible in spite of his language disability. For patients who cannot discriminate or retain auditory patterns, it may be useless to schedule weekly visits to a speech therapist. In such cases, family members can be instructed by the therapist to work with the patient at home. This continued stimulation may help alleviate the patient's depression by encouraging him to respond to what is going on around him [17, 18].

PSYCHOLOGICAL ASPECTS OF APHASIA

Throughout this chapter we have commented on the psychological implications of aphasia for the patient, his family, and his friends. The psychological impact of this loss of function is so overwhelming that certain aspects of it will be emphasized here. Contact with the world around him has been broken for the person with aphasia. He may be reduced to complete dependence on others, incapable of responding or making his needs known, often unable to comprehend what has happened to him or what is going on about him, and powerless to express his frustration and terror. His behavior will be affected by this. Thwarted by losses he does not understand, the person suffering from aphasia may lash out impulsively, throwing objects and striking those around him. Such behavior is an expression of the anger and fear he feels at being unable to carry out his wishes independently or respond to situations as he formerly did. His inability to explain why he is so perturbed with the turn of events only serves to heighten his anxiety and rage [11].

Those caring for the patient with aphasia must understand how the stroke has affected the patient's thought processes in order to deal with his behavior. Quite often the ability for abstract thinking is lost. The patient is able to think only in concrete terms. His thoughts relate solely to himself. Conceptual thinking relies on the ability to form abstractions, and in normal conversation a person must carry out a combination of abstract and concrete thinking to grasp the meaning of words as used in context. Attempts to help the aphasic person socialize are made extremely difficult because of his impaired ability for abstract thinking. Brain damage resulting from the stroke will have destroyed his ability to evaluate situations as a whole. Memory span may also have been affected. Usually response to any stimuli is delayed due to the insult to the brain. Most patients with aphasia exhibit considerable inconsistency in behavior, since they may have lost the ability to exercise practical judgment. With only an expressive deficit, the patient is usually somewhat aware of his problem and will experience a genuine concern about improvement of his behavior and mental capacity. The patient with a receptive deficit, however, lacks insight into his problems and will be much more prone to fits of rage and unacceptable behavior in social situations that are trying to him [11].

Patients with severe receptive deficits present many problems in management that are secondary to their inability to understand what has happened to them and what is currently going on around them. Since there is virtually no way to explain to them through written or verbal language, one must rely primarily on visual and tactile clues to communicate with them. The nurse should never lose sight of the fact that, no matter how severely impaired a patient's comprehension may be, he can still understand and respond to the reassurance of a warm smile, a soothing tone of voice, or a gentle touch. It is not uncommon for patients with receptive aphasia to suffer from severe sensory deprivation. They also may have visual defects such as hemianopsia, paralysis, and impairment of tactile sensation.

When a patient is isolated in a hospital room, deprived of any means to orient himself or to provide for normal bodily functions such as eating and elimination, his world can become one of total chaos. Such patients often become extremely restless and resist all diagnostic, therapeutic, or comfort measures because they do not understand what is being attempted or what the beneficial effects of such action might be. Procedures that are familiar to hospital personnel and thus looked upon as quite benign, such as placing an intravenous line, inserting a nasogastric feeding tube or indwelling catheter, placing an oxygen mask, or adjusting a humidifier, may be absolutely terrifying to the patient. Without any knowledge of its purpose and fearing the direct consequences, he will make every attempt to remove or prevent the insertion of this foreign object which he can only interpret as a source of pain or discomfort. To further immobilize the paralyzed patient will only compound his fear and aggravate his restlessness and combative behavior. There are times when it is absolutely essential to use physical restraints for the patient's protection, but they should not be applied indiscriminately. The nurse must weigh the benefits of such a procedure against the possible untoward outcome of the patient's continued state of agitation in response to the restraints. It is often safer to insert a nasogastric tube with each feeding, or to dispense with an indwelling catheter, than risk extension of the cerebral infarction.

Providing nursing care for the patient with dense global aphasia presents a real challenge. All too often these patients end up in the back wards of state mental hospitals because families are usually too bewildered to cope with their complex problems and their behavior will not be tolerated in nursing homes. This need not necessarily be the case. We feel strongly that a larger proportion of these patients could lead much more comfortable lives if staff and families responsible for their care had a better awareness of their abilities and the limitations imposed by their handicap.

The prognosis for recovery of functional speech for patients with global aphasia is practically nil. We have no firsthand information from patients on how best to deal with this situation. Therefore, we must rely on reports of families who have learned to cope and managed to provide an environment in which the patient appears to function as normally as possible within his limitations.

We feel that the key to success in this area lies in the ability of staff and family to provide a structured environment in which the patient feels secure. This must include a system of nonverbal communication, and it must be initiated immediately. So often, mismanagement of these patients during the initial phase of stroke renders all further attempts to communicate with them fruitless. It has been observed that many patients with global aphasia exhibit paranoid behavior. Not infrequently these patients suddenly become combative toward a staff member who has applied physical restraints or administered particularly unpleasant procedures in an earlier phase of the patient's illness. It is not a simple matter to communicate with a critically ill patient who can neither comprehend a word that is spoken to him nor convey in any manner what he thinks or needs and for whom all sound is but an unintelligible noise. Imprisoned within his aphasia, the patient can only perceive the messages conveyed by facial expressions, tone of voice, eye contact, touch, lack of physical contact, anticipation of his basic needs, and respect for his modesty. Is it any wonder, then, that in our busy medical institutions where staff and patients alike are expected to state their case histories as rapidly and succinctly as possible, and technology has placed more and more equipment between the patient and the staff caring for him, that the patient with global aphasia frequently perceives the ministrations of staff as torture rather than as care and reacts in kind? Well-intentioned staff often insist on forcing these patients to comply with an institutional routine or order which does no more than to instill terror.

Every attempt should be made to structure the patient's day so that he can anticipate what is coming and rest secure that either his needs will be met or he will have the opportunity to take care of them himself. Such an environment can only be established in a setting where the attitude and approach of the staff are flexible enough to create a safe and securely structured environment for each patient. Staff responsible for care of patients with global aphasia must make every effort to be aware of their nonverbal communication which will undeniably belie their attitude toward the patient. Not every family will have the maturity, strength, devotion, or financial resources to take a loved one home, knowing that they must provide a predictable routine, conduct all his business affairs, and anticipate all his potential problems without any direct input from the patient. Those who do will need much encouragement, support, and guidance from the nursing staff.

During the acute stage of stroke, many patients with aphasia are emotionally labile, with frequent outbursts of laughter and/or tears. These episodes are thought to result from tension or embarrassment and usually stop once the patient's neurological state stabilizes. Sometimes mannerisms such as a silly laugh or repetition of a stereotyped expression will be used excessively. Persistent euphoria, may be an indication of regression or an underlying depression. The aphasic patient may deny his problems because brain damage has deprived him of insight, or he may deny his problems because the losses are too threatening for him to face.

Psychosis can, of course, develop in the person with aphasia and it is important to be able to differentiate between the difficult behavior that may be manifested by the aphasic patient and the bizarre behavior of the psychotic patient. The abnormalities of aphasia are confined to language. The responses of the person with aphasia who is not psychotic, although they may be disruptive and difficult to handle, will be appropriate to the situations and persons he is dealing with. Even when his comprehension is impaired, he does not respond with bizarre behavior. Unfortunately psychotherapy is not useful for most patients with aphasia because of their inability to verbalize their feelings and their frequent misinterpretations of how others respond to them [17].

Speech improvement varies for individual patients and with the particular situation. In general they can talk more readily when they are rested and in a relaxed atmosphere, and with a single individual rather than group conversation. As with all people, they find that some individuals are easier to talk to than others. Usually this difference is related to the listener's concern for the speaker and interest in the subject of conversation. Patients with aphasia are usually very much aware of nonverbal communication from busy hospital staff, friends, and relatives. They are quite sensitive to looks and gestures of annoyance and impatience with their delayed or seemingly inappropriate responses. Many have been devastated by the apparent total lack of interest and concern for them as persons that results from their inability to initiate or participate in verbal communication with staff who invade their privacy and hurriedly proceed with treatment without explanation and, seemingly, without regard for their feelings [17, 18].

THERAPEUTIC ATTITUDE AND APPROACH

Research completed by Skelly at St. Louis University has demonstrated that the aphasic patient's inability to respond may be more closely related to his environment than to the brain damage he has suffered [18]. The nurse is in a key position to assure that the aphasic patient's environment is a therapeutic one and that professionals responsible for his care maintain an approach that will stimulate early recovery of language skills and reduce frustration. To accomplish this, she must have a clear understanding of the therapeutic goals for the patient and the techniques available for helping him develop understandable speech, reading, writing, and spelling skills. Most importantly, she should develop a therapeutic approach that incorporates the following principles in the care of the patient with aphasia.

1. Maintain a relaxed and calm manner with the patient.
2. Always speak *to* the patient and explain all diagnostic, therapeutic, and comfort measures before initiating them.
3. Maintain a quiet, uncluttered environment in the patient's room.
4. Encourage other staff and visitors to talk *to* the patient.
5. Explain what has happened to him and reassure him about the plans for his care.
6. Speak slowly and distinctly when addressing the patient, allowing him ample time to respond before interrupting or posing any additional questions or thoughts, but do not overarticulate.
7. Make every effort to understand what he tries to communicate through words, syllables, and gestures.
8. Encourage him to speak, rather than try to speak for him.
9. If he requests help with a word, say it slowly and distinctly.
10. Do not exhibit disapproval of emotional utterances or spontaneous use of profanity.
11. Avoid forcing him to do things he does not wish to, whenever possible.
12. Accept his statements of essential words without pressuring him to produce a complete sentence.
13. Whenever handing an object to him, state what it is, since hearing language is necessary to stimulating language development.
14. Never reprimand or scold the patient.

15. Never address the patient as though he were a child or mentally incompetent.
16. Explain to him the purpose of all assessments of his communication skills and the relearning exercises that are assigned.
17. Instruct family and friends concerning the approach that is most conducive to reducing frustration and fostering return of speech.

REFERENCES

1. Agronowitz, A., and McKeown, M. R. *Aphasia Handbook for Adults and Children.* Springfield, Ill.: Thomas, 1964. Pp. 25–45; 77–165.
2. Brain, W. R. *Speech Disorders, Aphasia, Apraxia, and Agnosia.* Washington, D.C.: Butterworth, 1961. Pp. 1–175.
3. Dahlberg, C. C., and Jaffe, J. *Stroke: A Doctor's Personal Story of His Recovery.* New York: W. W. Norton, 1977. Pp. 9–200.
4. Denny-Brown, D. *Handbook of Neurological Examination and Case Recording.* Cambridge: Harvard University Press, 1957. Pp. 55–59.
5. Geschwind, N. The organization of language and the brain. *Science* 170:940, 1970.
6. Geschwind, N. Aphasia. *N. Engl. J. Med.* 284–654, 1971.
7. Geschwind, N. Language and the brain. *Sci. Am.* 226:76–82, 1972.
8. Geschwind, N. Language, Aphasia, and Related Disorders. In P. Beeson and W. McDermott (Eds.), *Textbook of Medicine.* Philadelphia: Saunders, 1975. Pp. 555–556.
9. Geschwind, N., and Levitsky, W. Human brain: Left-right asymmetries in temporal speech regions. *Science* 161:186–187, 1968.
10. Hodgins, E. *Episode: Report on the Accident Inside My Skull.* New York: Atheneum, 1964. Pp. 3–72.
11. Longerich, M. C., and Bordeaux, J. *Aphasia Therapeutics.* New York: Macmillan, 1954. Pp. 9–60; 89–96; 97–108; 157–167.
12. Mohr, J. P., and Adams, R. D. Affections of Speech. In G. W. Thorn et al. (Eds.), *Harrison's Principles of Internal Medicine* (8th ed.). New York: McGraw-Hill, 1977. Pp. 135–145.
13. Nielson, J. *Agnosia, Apraxia, Aphasia.* New York: Hafner, 1965. Pp. 63–73.
14. Penfield, W., and Roberts, L. *Speech and Brain Mechanisms.* Princeton: Princeton University Press, 1959. Pp. 89–101; 192–235; 235–251.
15. Ritchie, D. *Stroke: A Diary of Recovery* (2nd ed.). London: Faber & Faber, 1965. Pp. 13–184.
16. Sarno, M. T. Disorders of Communication in Stroke. In S. Licht (Ed.), *Stroke and Its Rehabilitation.* Baltimore: Williams & Wilkins, 1975. Pp. 380–408.
17. Schuell, H., Jenkins, J., and Jimenez-Pabon, E. *Aphasia in Adults.* New York: Hoeber Medical Div., Harper & Row, 1964. Pp. 134–156; 159–176; 211–228; 275–296; 315–386.
18. Skelly, M. Re-thinking stroke, aphasic patients talk back. *Am. J. Nurs.* 75:1140, 1975.
19. Strub, R., and Black, W. *The Mental Status Examination in Neurology.* Philadelphia: Davis, 1977. Pp. 39–60.
20. Weisenburg, T., and McBride, K. E. *Aphasia: A Clinical and Psychological Study.* New York: Hafner, 1964. Pp. 132–140.

6. Perceptual disorders

Perception is the ability of the mind to analyze and integrate all the impressions that come to it through the senses in order to extract psychologically meaningful information. It is a complex intellectual process that relies on proper neurological functioning to assure that stimuli coming to the brain from all the senses can be recognized and interpreted in light of the person's present situation and past experience. It has been demonstrated that the parietal lobe of the brain carries a large responsibility for this integrative function. The blood supply to the parietal lobe is provided by all three of the major cerebral arterial systems — the middle cerebral, which supplies the major portion of the parietal lobe, anterior cerebral system, which supplies the anterior and medial portion of the parietal lobe, and posterior cerebral arteries, which supply a small part of the posterior portion of the parietal lobe. Stroke in any one of these arteries can damage the parietal area and consequently interfere with the patient's perceptual ability [36].

Motor and sensory defects resulting from stroke are usually quite evident. Perceptual defects are not so readily recognized and may leave the patient with a much greater handicap. Disorders of perception include disturbances of body image, spatial judgment, and sensory interpretation, all of which can contribute to an inability to carry out skilled or purposeful movements. Staff caring for patients with stroke must be able to assess the patient's perceptual abilities, identify deficits, and design a plan of care that will help the patient who has perceptual problems to reorient his sensory system and compensate for his deficits. This chapter includes a description of the various forms that perceptual disorders can assume, a methodology for assessing perception, and a program of care for the patient with perceptual problems.

FORMS OF PERCEPTUAL DISTURBANCE

Perceptual disturbances may be divided into the following categories: (1) difficulties pertaining to the patient's perception of himself and his illness, (2) disorders related to the patient's perception of space and his misconceptions concerning the relationship of his body image to the space around him [36], (3) agnosias, which are disturbances in recognition or identification of objects perceived by a sense, and (4) apraxia, which is an inability to carry out learned movements. Sensory data for vision, touch, pain, and joint sense are interpreted and integrated within the parietal lobe to establish an awareness of the body and its parts and a sense of spatial relationships. Evidence suggests that this activity is largely the function of the nondominant hemisphere, which for most people is on the right side [1, 10].

Disorders related to perception of self and illness

The impression or concept of the body as it presents itself to consciousness is referred to as the *body image* or *scheme* [33]. A variety of distortions of body image and awareness of self may follow lesions of the parietal lobe. The degree of impairment that results from damage to the parietal lobe will depend upon the location and extent of the lesion. An impaired awareness of one's own disability or disabled parts is called *anosognosia* [19]. It frequently is applied to hemiplegia but is not restricted to it, applying as well to other motor deficits and to such sensory defects as blindness or deafness [10]. Anosognosia is frequently applied to a spectrum of degrees of denial ranging from mild inattention to total denial of one side of the body or of an affected limb. Those abnormalities that are not clearly separable as clinical entities may be classified under four categories, inattention, unconcern, unawareness, and denial [3].

INATTENTION

Inattention is recognized as the mildest form of neglect and is usually demonstrated through the sensory examination by a technique called double *simultaneous stimulation. Tactile inattention* can be demonstrated by application of two simultaneous touches on symmetrically opposite areas of the body; an appreciation of this requires normal functioning of the parietal cortex. When there is cortical damage resulting in inattention to one half of the body, the patient will be able to perceive a single touch on the affected side but will not be able to perceive the stimulus on the affected side when both sides of his body are touched simultaneously. *Visual inattention* and neglect can be demonstrated by simultaneous activation of distance receptors. Two stimuli, such as moving fingers, are presented to the patient, one in the right and one in the left half of his visual field. A lack of perception of one finger when individual testing of visual fields has been normal is an indication of a perceptual defect involving a unilateral visual inattention. With inattention the patient may fail to use the involved side of his body unless his attention is drawn to it by someone else [10, 37].

UNCONCERN

Some patients exhibit a lack of concern over their disability, appearing quite complacent about their paralysis or other defects and fail to attach any importance to them. In addition to indifference they may also show evidence of inattention and/or unawareness. When questioned about their condition, these patients will admit to the presence of the disability, but their affect may be inappropriate in light of the magnitude of their handicap [3, 10].

UNAWARENESS

Some patients may lack any awareness of their hemiplegia, loss of power, or other faculties. When questioned about their condition, they usually do not refer to their disability unless prompted to do so. This problem is usually noted immediately after a stroke has occurred and is associated with a clouding of the sensorium. The problem is usually transitory and subsides as the patient's sensorium clears. These patients demonstrate a decrease in the use of the involved body part but may attempt to perform activities beyond their capabilities [3, 10].

DENIAL
Denial is the most severe form of unilateral neglect. Patients may totally deny the presence of paralysis or other deficits. When questioned about their disability they may, for example, attribute it to arthritis or a muscle sprain. If pressed for further explanation they may proceed with an elaborate and bizarre account of the origin and nature of the problem [3, 10].

Disorders related to perception of space and body image

DISORDERS OF SPATIAL UNDERSTANDING
Many of the disorders that involve the patient's perception of his body and of the effects of his stroke upon his body extend to his environment. *Spatial perception* is the process through which impressions coming from the various senses are synthesized and interpreted to provide an understanding of how the body is related to its environment. A person's conception of space is an explicit awareness of space, of the location of objects in his three-dimensional environment, and of the relationship of his body to its surroundings [10].

Unilateral spatial neglect. Neglect or lack of perception of one half of external space is, in reality, a disregard of the objects occupying that space rather than a neglect of the space itself. Unilateral spatial neglect manifests itself in a number of ways. The person usually bumps into objects located on his affected side and will always select doorways on his unaffected side or turn toward that side rather than toward the affected side. He may neglect all sensory input from the affected side and consequently will not be aware of people approaching from that side or alerted to activities there. He may injure his affected hand or foot in getting out of bed because he is not paying attention to proper placement. Unilateral neglect can be demonstrated through the use of drawings. When these patients are requested to draw a symmetrical object such as a daisy or clock, imperfections can be seen on one side; for example, they may omit the petals or the numbers on the affected side or produce a drawing with poorly formed or distorted petals or numbers on the affected side [10, 18].

Patients with unilateral neglect may also have visual field defects. Homonymous hemianopsia, defective vision or blindness in the corresponding halves of the visual fields of both eyes, is seen most often with stroke. However, it is believed by many that the visual defect is not the determinant of the neglect, because not all persons with homonymous hemianopsia show unilateral neglect, and unilateral neglect has been reported in persons with no quantitative field defect. It is also well known that patients with hemianopsia can compensate for their visual deficit by learning to scan their environment visually. Objects seen on the intact side will be a factor in determining whether objects on the other side are neglected or not, thus the patient will look for objects on that side [5, 10].

Hemianopsia. A patient with hemianopsia may neglect all sensory input from the affected side. He may not see people approaching from the neglected side. He may only see half of the items placed in front of him, such as dishes on a meal tray. Reading will present a problem, since lines will be cut in half longitudinally. With writing there will be difficulty in judging the transition from one line to another. The patient must be taught to compensate for this impairment by learning to scan the affected side visually. He must now learn to view directly what he once was able to see peripherally.

In the early stage of stroke the patient may be too lethargic to follow instructions in visual scanning, and consequently he may become frightened or confused. Therefore it is advisable for the nurse to make certain that the patient is always in a position where he can see his surroundings without having to compensate for his deficit. The placement of the patient's bed will have a direct effect on his interaction with the environment. It should allow for his limited field of vision to be directed toward the door of the room, so that he will see people coming and be alerted to the activities of his environment. If his affected or "blind" side is facing the door, he will be unaware of staff and visitors entering and may become startled at their approach. The patient with a stroke should never be unnecessarily isolated, with perhaps only a wall or window to look at.

DISORDERS OF SPATIAL ORIENTATION

Defects of spatial orientation include a number of disabilities having to do with the recognition of spatial relationships among objects. These interfere with the patient's ability to judge position, distance, movement, form, and the relationship of his body parts to objects surrounding him [5, 18, 22]. Luria states that "perception of spatial relationship and orientation in space are among the most complex forms of reflections of the outside world" [26]. At times patients may confuse the concepts of up and down, forward and backward, inside and outside. Because of these spatial-visual problems, patients may bump into objects, have difficulty negotiating their way down a straight corridor in a wheelchair, or have problems following the lines of written material.

Benton has outlined six categories of defective spatial orientation [5].

Defects in localizing objects in space, estimating their size, and judging their distance from the observer. To determine ability to localize an object accurately, the patient may be requested to touch or point to it. A more sensitive measure for accuracy is the task of bisecting a horizontal line. The patient is instructed to divide a horizontal line drawn on paper by placing an X at the center point. This will demonstrate any difference between the patient's estimated center from the actual center. Errors in estimating distance can also be seen — for example, the distance of a remote object may be underestimated while the distance of a nearer object is overestimated. The relative distance of two objects in relation to the observer may be misjudged, a distant large object appearing to be nearer than a near small object [5, 22].

Impaired memory for recall of spatial location of objects or places. Patients who show no defects in spatial localization or discrimination when the object is before them may show defects when the object has been removed and they are requested to match a design with the original object. Patients may fail to recall spatial positions of objects with which they have had repeated experience — for example, the arrangement of furniture in a familiar room [5].

Defective route finding. Patients may have difficulty learning new routes and following a route from one place to another and may even get lost in areas that were once familiar. They fail to appreciate the spatial schema of routes and consequently become confused at certain points along the path and may omit critical turns. It is not uncommon to find a directional trend; some patients fail to make left turns, some, less frequently, fail to make right turns. This tendency has been mentioned in the literature as "neglect or unawareness of the left half of space."

The patient's ability to find routes can be assessed by observing his behavior in everyday situations — for example, finding his way from one room to another. If this task is not feasible, he may be requested to sketch a route between his room and another room or building. A faulty representation may demonstrate omissions of one-sided turns or discrepancies in length of corridors or stairs [5].

Defective topographical memory. This defect represents a failure to retrieve long-established memories. Patients will have difficulty in attempting to recall and describe familiar routes, spatial aspects of familial surroundings and will also lose former geographic knowledge. This can be demonstrated by requesting the patient to describe routes and places that should be familiar to him. He may be given a map of his country and asked to locate some of the major cities [5].

Reading and counting disabilities. Spatial dyslexia is a reading disability that is related to a defect in recognizing the placement of words rather than one of comprehending the letters and words as symbols. Letters and words are recognized, but there is a disorganization in directional control of eye movements. One type of spatial dyslexia is related to unilateral spatial neglect. The patient fixes his attention on a point to the right of the beginning of the line, reads to the end of the line, and returns to a point to the right of the next line. A more severe form of spatial dyslexia is demonstrated by inability to move from one fixation point to another. The patient may begin reading at any point on a line and even skip lines. In a test situation he may select words at random, skip one or two words in a line, or even supply words in an attempt to make sense of what he is reading. As reading continues, it is common to see a patient's performance deteriorate.

Impairment in counting and in oral or written calculations is also seen with spatial disorientation. Patients will frequently make errors in calculations that require correct spatial placement and proper alignment of numbers. Figures may go unnoticed in a particular visual field, just as words are ignored in reading. As the patient proceeds from one mathematical unit to another, he may forget whether items have already been counted [5].

Visual constructive disabilities. It is known that patients with disturbances in spatial orientation frequently manifest impairment in visual constructive activities as demonstrated in drawing and block assembling. The following failures are considered to be related to spatial disorientation: (1) all the components of a simple structure are not integrated into the design; (2) only one half of a design or drawing is completed; (3) part of the design used as the model is taken and incorporated into the patient's design; and (4) the completed design may be rotated as compared with the model [5].

To Benton's list can be added an important defect: the inability to distinguish between left and right.

Right-left disorientation.   Right-left orientation is the ability to distinguish right from left in oneself and in the environment and includes the capacity for spatial orientation and the ability to apply the terms "right" and "left" to the respective sides. Confusion of right-left orientation is commonly noted in patients with hemiplegia following a left hemisphere stroke. When testing for right-left orientation the patient may be requested to identify right and left on himself and on the examiner, for example, (1) "point to your right ear"; (2) "point to your left hand"; (3) "point to my left arm"; (4) "point to my right ear." Cross-commands may also be given for both patient and examiner: (1) "touch your left ear with your right hand"; (2) "point to my left ear with your right hand" [7, 37].

It is especially important for those caring for patients who have lost the ability to distinguish right from left to be aware of this deficit, since many instructions to the patient will include a reference to right and left extremities or sides of the body. If the nature of the patient's problem is clearly understood by the staff, rehabilitation can be facilitated for the hemiplegic patient through avoidance of the words "right" and "left." The patient can understand the terms, "good leg," "paralyzed arm," and "affected side," and use of these terms may enable him to comply with the rehabilitation program more effectively.

GERSTMANN'S SYNDROME
Gerstmann's syndrome consists of four major deficits: *finger agnosia* (inability to recognize, name, or point to individual fingers on oneself and others), *right-left disorientation* (inability to distinguish right from left), *dysgraphia* (acquired disturbance in writing, referring specifically to errors of language), and *dyscalculia* (impaired calculation ability). Some neurologists consider this syndrome to be indicative of damage to the dominant parietal lobe and to be of diagnostic significance. Others question its significance, and some even believe that the individual elements do not necessarily constitute a true syndrome. The literature reports arguments for and against its diagnostic value [4, 11, 37, 38].

Agnosias

In order for the process of perception to take place, the mind must recognize the impressions that come to it through the senses. Only then can integration of these sensations occur. Recognition is that capacity of the mind that matches an observed, heard, or felt object with the memory picture, or mental image, that has been retained of a previously observed, heard, or felt object. *Agnosias* are disturbances of the recognition or identification of objects that have been perceived by a single sense function: either vision, hearing, or touch. They must not be confused with blindness, deafness, or loss of the sense of touch. Agnosias must also be distinguished from *aphasias,* which are defects of symbol formulation and comprehension [10, 33, 37]. Emphasis will be given here to visual, auditory, and tactile agnosias.

VISUAL AGNOSIA

True blindness can result from damage to the eye itself, to the optic nerve, or to the primary visual cortex. *Visual agnosia,* sometimes called "mind blindness," is a defect of visual perception and is generally the result of damage to the visual association areas [22]. When asked to identify an object, a patient with visual agnosia either describes its properties or identifies its component parts. He cannot recognize the object completely and identify it as a whole through the sense of sight. *Visual agnosia for objects* is a loss of the ability to recognize either objects or pictures of objects and may be accompanied by inability to identify colors [33]. *Prosopognosia* is a disturbance of recognition of faces and sometimes also mirror images and photographs. Patients with this defect must rely on the voice or a characteristic mannerism to recognize people familiar to them [10]. Prosopognosia is associated with bilateral lesions of the parieto-occipital cortex.

Any assessment of visual agnosias can be complicated by coexisting visual defects, such as decreased acuity, limited visual fields, or presence of metamorphopsias (visual distortions); by cognitive disorders and other perceptual disorders; and by the patient's inability to appreciate his defects. All these factors would contribute to an inadequate response to visual stimuli. Some practitioners feel, therefore, that visual agnosia as such does not exist. This defect of recognition would then be due to the visual defects that make identification of objects more difficult, or to a defect that prevents the patient from directing his gaze at will (visual scanning). Visual inattention is also thought to play a part. This means that the patient does not notice more than one object at a time unless his attention is directed to it by someone else [10, 22]. In spite of the controversy, the term visual agnosia is still considered useful for classifying visual defects resulting from damage to the parietal and occipital lobes.

AUDITORY AGNOSIA

A person who is deaf cannot hear sounds. If the patient has the ability to hear sounds, but is no longer able to recognize that he has heard them before, he is said to have an *auditory agnosia.* This results from a lesion of the temporal lobe, often both temporal lobes. It has two forms, acoustic *verbal* agnosia and acoustic *musical* agnosia. The latter is quite rare. With acoustic verbal agnosia, the only portion of the word which is not recognized is the sound. With word deafness, the patient may only recognize the voice as a voice, may recognize language but not understand it, or may be able to hear and repeat but not understand what he says. Pure word deafness, although technically an acoustic verbal agnosia, is classified as aphasia [33]. This is discussed in detail in Chapter 5.

An evaluation of the patient's hearing function is an important part of the general nursing assessment, since behavior difficulties may be caused by a patient's inability to communicate effectively due to loss or impairment of hearing. The nurse should refer to the history or ask a family member about the patient's previous hearing ability. If he requires a hearing aid, one should be made available to him and it should be checked regularly to assure that it is functioning. It is important to bear in mind that if the patient appears to have difficulty comprehending instructions or conversation, this may be the result of receptive aphasia rather than hearing loss. Auditory agnosia and word deafness are recognized by the intactness of visual input. The patient reads and understands words that cannot be appreciated verbally.

TACTILE AGNOSIA
Tactile sensibility is perceived in the thalamus. Recognition and localization of the sensation occurs in the parietal cortex. Destruction of the cortical area or destruction of the connections between the thalamus and the cortex will result in *tactile agnosia*, or *astereognosis*. This is the loss of ability to recognize, through the sense of touch alone, an object that has been placed in the hand. The patient will still be able to name the object if it can be seen or heard. This defect is usually due to a lesion of the parietal lobe opposite to the affected hand. There is no major or minor side for tactile agnosia. Astereognosis presupposes that the sensations for touch, pain, joint sense, and vibratory sense are all intact [10, 33].

Stroke results in impaired sensation for some patients. Those sensory deficits that most commonly interfere with the patient's performance of the activities of daily living involve cutaneous sensation and proprioceptive sensation. *Cutaneous sensation* is felt by the body surfaces. When a neurological dysfunction impairs his cutaneous sensation, the patient's reaction to touch, pain, or temperature may be increased, decreased, or totally lacking. This reaction can be tested by stroking the skin surfaces with a piece of cotton. Pain is tested by pricking the skin with a pin, and temperature may be tested by placing test tubes filled with hot and cold water on the skin surfaces. *Proprioceptive sensation* is felt in the joints, joint capsules, and ligaments and gives rise to sensations of body position and movement. With a neurological deficit the patient may be unaware of where his extremities are in space, or he may not be able to place them appropriately. Proprioception for the upper extremities is tested by grasping the sides of the patient's thumb, moving it gently up and down, and asking the patient to identify its position. The lower extremities are tested in the same manner, using the great toe.

How the patient perceives sensation will also affect how he carries out the activities of daily living. Impaired sensation may interfere with motor performance, such as transfers and ambulation, even though the patient is not paralyzed. The patient may be unable to judge distances adequately or unable to place his extremities in the position he chooses, and thus injure himself by falling or by failing to protect an extremity. Accurate movement is required in the performance of activities of daily living and self-care. Therefore, the patient may perform poorly in such activities as bathing, dressing, feeding, because he handles objects awkwardly, places them inaccurately, or drops them. Often impaired sensation and resulting lack of control may be more of a handicap to the patient than paralysis.

Apraxias

Apraxia is an inability to carry out a learned movement voluntarily. The apraxic patient may understand the task to be performed and have the necessary strength and innervation of musculature but be unable to carry out the required movements when he attempts the task voluntarily. At another time, however, he may perform the identical movements unconsciously. It is believed that this disturbance is caused by lesions in the following areas: (1) left parietal lobe, (2) precentral gyrus, (3) parieto-occipital region, and (4) corpus callosum [33]. It is firmly established that the dominant hemisphere for language is also dominant for learned motor skills. This can be supported by the fact that most people show a strong hand preference for such tasks as writing, throwing a ball and so forth [20, 37].

Apraxia is subdivided into three types based on the nature of the movement disorder. They are (1) limb kinetic apraxia, (2) ideomotor apraxia, and (3) ideational apraxia [14, 33, 37].

LIMB KINETIC APRAXIA

Limb kinetic apraxia is a disturbance of the ability to control limb movement and is caused by lesions in the motor cortex [14, 37]. These disturbances are characterized by clumsiness in performing simple tasks such as selecting objects from a jar to more complex movements such as writing or walking.

IDEOMOTOR APRAXIA

Ideomotor apraxia is a disturbance in the ability to accurately carry out previously learned motor acts. When asked to perform a simple task or one that the patient has performed automatically for many years he will fumble and make mistakes, or be entirely incapable of carrying out the task. When handed a toothbrush he may fail to grip it properly, fail to open his mouth or miss his mouth entirely. Impairment can be seen in mouth, limb or trunk musculature. Apraxic movements can be elicited through any number of tasks. The patient may be tested on his ability to perform a task in response to verbal command, in imitation of the examiner (examiner first performs the task), and on performance using an actual object, for example, the patient is presented with a book of matches and requested to strike a match [10, 14, 37].

IDEATIONAL APRAXIA

The disturbance in ideational apraxia appears to be either in the conceptualization of the act or formulation of the motor pattern required [32, 37]. Movement is characterized by a breakdown in the performance of a task which requires the integration of parts for its completion. The patient may be unable to follow the necessary sequence for the task of brushing his teeth as removing the cap from the toothpaste, taking the brush from the container and placing the paste on the brush. While the component parts may be carried out, they do not coalesce into a coordinated purposeful act. The resulting activity is disjointed. Many of the manifestations of ideational apraxia appear as extreme absentmindedness. These patients will need supervision in the activities of daily living because they may not be able to perform self-care safely. They may have difficulty with cooking a meal, making a bed or performing everyday chores that they were once able to do without problems. They may present a danger to themselves with handling ordinary appliances. Ideational apraxia is usually seen in patients with bilateral brain disease, especially diffuse disease affecting the parietal lobes [10, 37].

CONSTRUCTIONAL APRAXIA
Constructional ability is defined as the capacity to draw or construct two or three dimensional figures or shapes from one and two dimensional units. It is considered a high level, complex cognitive function which involves the integration of occipital, parietal and frontal lobe function, the parietal lobes playing the dominant role [37].

   Constructional apraxia is a disturbance of the ability to arrange, build, or draw simple figures. The patient has no apraxia for the various movements involved; his difficulty lies in the spatial aspect of the performance. This form of apraxia occurs with lesions of either hemisphere but more commonly with the nondominant one and is more severe with the nondominant [10, 32].

   Two tests are usually administered at the bedside to determine whether or not a patient has constructional apraxia — a paper and pencil test and a matchstick test. These are tests of the patient's ability to put together one-dimensional units to form two-dimensional figures or patterns. First the patient is given a paper and pencil and asked to copy a series of designs of increasing complexity. Then the examiner forms a design with a set of sticks or wooden matches and asks the patient to copy the pattern using an identical set of sticks. The matchsticks can be arranged in designs of increasing complexity. The patient is observed for the method he uses to accomplish the assigned task, any errors in performance, and any hesitancy, comments, or changes in approach. Usually the same defects are apparent regardless of which hand the patient uses.

   The following defects are typical of the paper and pencil test completed by a patient with apraxia [10].

1. The figure or drawing is crowded into one corner of the paper.
2. The figure is drawn much smaller than the model, or, occasionally, much larger.
3. The lines are very light and wavy, with significant gaps between them. (This is usually seen only in severe dementia.)
4. The patient superimposes his copy of the figure on the model drawn by the examiner.
5. Vertical lines are unduly long, and oblique lines are exaggerated.
6. The direction of the lines in the model is reversed to form a mirror image.
7. Large sections of the model figure are omitted in the patient's copy.

Similar errors are seen in the matchstick test [10].

1. The pattern is usually constructed in one corner rather than in the center of the space provided.
2. The patient reconstructs the pattern either on top of the examiner's model or crowded close to it.
3. The matchsticks are placed obliquely, rather than vertically and horizontally as in the model.
4. The entire pattern, or sections of it, is reversed to form a mirror image.
5. The matchsticks have large gaps between them.

Two other bedside tests of ability to form two-dimensional figures are (1) to hand the patient a sheet of paper and an envelope and ask him to fold the paper and insert it into the envelope and (2) to show the patient a picture of a geometrical figure and ask him to bisect it. Handwriting, calculations, and setting the hands of a clock or watch may also be tests of constructional apraxia. The handwriting of a person with constructional apraxia will show many oblique lines, with letters set on top of each other. In carrying out calculations, the patient will not place the numbers in proper order. Usually such patients are unable to place the hands of a clock in the position requested. To assess the patient's ability to construct *three-dimensional* patterns, the examiner may use blocks or bricks to create figures and patterns for the patient to copy.

Most patients with constructional apraxia will be unaware of the inadequacy of their performance in any of these tests, just as they are usually unaware of difficulty in performing such everyday tasks as writing, household chores, calculations, and manipulation of tools, radio and television sets and dial telephones.

DRESSING APRAXIA

There are two specific types of apraxia for dressing. One, described by Denny-Brown, is related to unilateral neglect: the patient ignores one side [14], and attends to dressing and grooming on one side and not the other. Essentially he fails to dress the neglected half of the body. This is found in lesions of either hemisphere. The second is related to spatial disturbance: the patient cannot orient his clothing in space and consequently tangles himself in the clothing when attempting to dress. He has difficulty in matching the garment to the appropriate body segment, and he may attempt to place a foot in the sleeve of a shirt. This is described by Brain and is seen predominantly with lesions of the right hemisphere [32].

PROGRAM FOR ASSESSMENT OF PERCEPTUAL DISORDERS
AND INITIATION OF THERAPY

It is a well-documented finding that patients with hemiplegia due to right hemisphere strokes more often incur perceptual disorders than patients with lesions of the left hemisphere. Since patients affected in the right hemisphere retain the power of speech, and since their paralysis involves the left side rather than the right, the full

Table 6-1
Perceptual problems commonly occuring with stroke

Perceptual Problem	Example	Therapeutic Approach
A. Disorders related to perception of self and illness		
1. Inattention to one side of the body that can involve motor, tactile, and visual modalities.	The patient will be unable to perceive touch on the affected side when both sides of the body are touched simultaneously but will be able to feel a single touch on the affected side only.	Remind the patient of any motor, tactile, or visual inattention that might interfere with functional activities.
2. Lack of concern for hemiplegia or other motor or sensory defects	Tendency to leave extremities in awkward or dangerous positions. The patient may allow arm to dangle over side of bed or may run over foot with wheelchair.	Teach patient to position the affected extremities carefully, using his unaffected hand to do so. Use sling for an affected arm that has little or no muscle tone.
3. Lack of awareness of hemiplegia or other motor and sensory deficits	Attribution of the problem to some minor somatic complaint. The hemiplegic may insist upon getting out of bed unassisted.	Observe the patient closely and anticipate his needs. In spite of repeated explanations, he will have difficulty retaining information about his deficits.
4. Denial of hemiplegia or other motor and sensory defects	Attempt at walking on the paralyzed leg. The patient may insist that his affected extremities have adequate strength.	Encourage handling the affected limbs to reinforce awareness of the affected side. Teach patient methods of performing activities that will ensure safety.
B. Disorders related to perception of space and body image		
1. Unilateral spatial neglect. Lack of awareness of one side of the body that can involve motor, tactile, and visual modalities.	Failure to recognize people approaching from affected side. On the neglected side the patient may bump into objects, fail to use his limbs, and ignore visual and tactile stimuli. He may walk to one side and turn only to the right.	Increase stimulation to affected side and encourage interaction of staff and visitors with neglected side. Have patient handle neglected limbs and teach him to bathe, dress, and position them. Place TV on that side.
2. Hemianopsia	Neglect of input from the affected side, for example, visitors, staff members, food or objects on a tray located on the affected side.	Place objects on his unaffected side. Instruct him to visually scan his physical environment.

3. Defects in localizing objects in space, estimating size, judging distance	Difficulty in abstracting one object from others surrounding it, e.g., in distinguishing food on tray from rest of background.	When working with the patient, close the curtain or door. Eliminate objects except those that the patient is using, e.g., soap and washcloth. Do not have flowers, etc., on the table, for these will distract him.
	Difficulty in focusing attention on one object or activity, letting attention jump from one stimulus to another.	Provide a quiet environment; eliminate clutter and any stimuli that will distract from the activity being performed at the present time.
	Difficulty in retrieving objects he has dropped or placing items down because of inability to judge distances accurately.	
4. Impaired memory for recall of location of objects or places	The patient will be unable to recall placement of furniture in his room once he leaves it. He may not recall where his bed is or where to locate his drinking glass or urinal if it is not placed where he can see it.	Place items patient will need to use regularly where he can see them. He will not remember even if you tell him when they are placed in a drawer, bedside stand, or closet.
5. Defects in route-finding	The patient will have difficulty learning new routes. He may get lost even finding his way on once familiar routes because he has no sense of direction or awareness of the relationship of turns to the point he is trying to reach.	The patient should never be sent alone on a new route, or allowed to leave familiar, safe surroundings unattended. In familiar territory, he should always have clearly written instructions with identification of landmarks that will help him identify the direction he should follow to a given destination.
6. Defective topographical memory	Difficulty in recalling and describing routes or spatial characteristics of familiar surroundings. For example, arrangement of furniture in a room, location of doorway to a room. Inability to become oriented to changes in environment while going from one place to another. Frequently the patient gets lost.	Provide a clue to routes or objects, for example, a colored piece of tape on the patient's bed to distinguish it from other beds. Since this impairment may extend to loss of previous geographic knowledge, the patient should not be allowed to wander unattended.

Table 6-1 (continued)

Perceptual Problem	Example	Therapeutic Approach
7. Reading and counting disabilities. Inability to align columns and rows of digits	When counting, the patient gets lost in proceeding from one unit to another, and may forget items that have already been counted.	Provide the patient with exercises in copying figures and placing them in columns for computation.
Inability to tell time	Inability to read the time or set the hands of a clock or watch.	When establishing schedules, orient the patient to time frequently by associating passage of time with the arrival of visitors, serving of meals, or appointments for scheduled therapy.
Reading and counting	Loss of directional orientation with respect to printed material. Patient may begin reading anywhere on the line.	Assist in directional orientation. Have patient use finger or ruler to follow the printed line.
8. Right-Left disorientation Inability to discriminate between the concepts of "right" and "left"	The patient will be unable to distinguish right and left sides of himself or others. Patient is unable to follow directions or instructions that rely on comprehension of the concepts "right" and "left."	Use descriptive adjectives such as the "weak" arm or the "good" leg to refer to the body, and descriptive phrases such as the "blue" room, the door "next to the bed" in directions.
C. Agnosias Failure to recognize and identify objects or configurations through a sense otherwise intact		
1. Visual agnosia Inability to recognize objects or people or to view the whole at once	Loss of recognition of objects and pictures, which may appear distorted. The patient may see part of an image only, as a handbag but not the person carrying it.	Simplify environment to eliminate hazards. Remove unnecessary furniture, objects, etc.
	The patient may get lost around the house or ward.	Place one object at a time in front of the patient, such as a dish. Add another dish when the patient has finished with the first. Tell the patient what he is eating.
	Inability to read symbols.	
	Inability to fixate normally on an object.	Encourage the patient to use touch to identify objects.
	Foggy and misty-appearing environment, objects blurred and devoid of contour.	
	Difficulty in finding objects, over- or under-estimation of distances; patient spills food, bath water, falls over objects.	

	Difficulty with household chores, as cooking, sewing, ironing.	
	Inability to recognize familiar faces, photographs, or one's image.	Teach the patient to rely on voices, familiar mannerisms, or uniforms to identify his family, friends, and staff caring for him.
2. Auditory agnosia Difficulty recognizing verbal sounds such as words, or sounds of bells, automobiles, whistles	The patient may be unable to recognize and differentiate environmental sounds. Words may sound like gibberish to him.	May respond appropriately to written words or lip-reading cues. When approaching the patient for treatments, explain verbally what is to be done and show him any equipment that will be used. Do not expect patient to recognize the sound of horns, alarms, warning devices, or the ring of a phone. Try to keep noise from radios and television to a minimum so as not to distract him.
3. Tactile agnosia Astereognosis – inability to recognize objects through tactile sense only	Inability of the patient to recognize objects that are placed in his hand, with ability to recognize them through the other senses.	Encourage the patient to look at objects he cannot identify through touch.
Impaired cutaneous sensation	The patient's reaction to touch, pain, and temperature may be absent, decreased, or increased.	Approach the patient gently and cautiously before administering any treatment or comfort measure to assess his reaction to touch, the temperature of water, or lotions and any other stimuli that might inflict pain. If reaction to pain or temperature is impaired, special measures must be taken to prevent burns, frostbite, or other injury to the insensitive area.
Impaired proprioceptive sensation	The patient may be unaware of where his extremities are. He may fall or fail to protect them from injury.	
Vertical–horizontal deviation	Difficulty in maintaining correct posture, balance, and locomotion. Patient leans to affected side to align with perceived vertical.	Provide sitting and standing balancing exercises. Use mirrors to assist in identification of the vertical and horizontal.
Judgment of median plane	Displacement of median to hemiplegic side. Difficulty in ambulating, transferring, and sitting because of distortion.	Use mirrors to assist in identification of the midline.

Table 6-1 (continued)

Perceptual Problem	Example	Therapeutic Approach
D. Apraxia 1. Inability to perform a learned movement voluntarily	Difficulty in using the hand, as in eating, threading a needle or writing. The patient may demonstrate extraordinary delays and be clumsy.	Encourage the patient to feed himself independently; if necessary, guide his hand to his mouth, but have him complete the action. With repetition, some patients improve in performance.
	Difficulty with movements of the mouth; this may interfere with speech, chewing, and swallowing. The patient may begin to feed himself by picking up food with an eating utensil, but may not complete the act. He may sit with the utensil in his hand but not bring it to his mouth, or he may return the utensil to his plate.	Speech, occupation, and physical therapy can provide some exercise to improve or to compensate for some of the deficits.
	Difficulty in initiating purposeful actions; for example, walking, rising, and sitting.	Teach individual components of an activity separately. Then proceed to integrate component parts into a completed activity.
2. Constructional apraxia Inability to put together 2-dimensional units to form 3-dimensional figures and patterns	Difficulty in assembling apparatus requiring interpretation of directions, as "do-it-yourself" kit.	Instruct the patient to rely more on touch than on vision when arranging objects. This is also a safety measure, for example, in handling sharp objects.
Inability to analyze visually, piece by piece, in order to construct a whole	Difficulty in arranging objects according to clear spatial awareness, for example, setting a table with dishes and silverware.	
Inability to reproduce simple patterns through arrangement of separate parts or through drawings	Inability to place hands of clock, appropriately.	
3. Dressing apraxia	Inability to put on clothes properly. The relationship of parts of garments is disturbed. The patient may put clothes on backwards or have difficulty finding a sleeve or he may neglect to clothe one-half of the body.	Instruct patient in dressing himself; for some patients repetition of an activity results in improved performance. Sometimes visual clues are helpful, e.g., colored labels sewn on the neck or sleeve of a garment.

significance of their perceptual problems may be overlooked and unrealistic goals may be set for their rehabilitation. The perceptual problems resulting from a stroke in the nondominant hemisphere involve visual and spatial deficits primarily. These patients suffer a far greater handicap from their inability to interpret sensory stimuli adequately and to perceive themselves accurately in space than they do from their hemiplegia. Furthermore their efforts to move and position their paralyzed limbs may be hampered by inability to sense the position of their extremities. The various perceptual disorders discussed in this chapter pose a serious barrier to the patient's recovery of independence. It is most important, therefore, that perceptual problems be identified as soon as possible so that appropriate therapy and nursing approach may be initiated [36, 39].

When efforts to rehabilitate patients with nondominant hemisphere strokes concentrate primarily on return of motor function to the paralyzed limbs, the outcome usually falls far short of the goal. More realistic goals may be set with more successful outcomes if the precise nature of the patient's paralysis is evaluated.

Disturbances of body image, spatial judgment, and integration of all sensory stimuli occur following stroke in the parietal area of the nondominant hemisphere. These deficits will have a significant effect on the patient's progress in rehabilitation, since he may be unable to interpret which limbs to move or how to move them or how to relate one object to another. Before initiating therapy for his motor defects, it is necessary to help the patient with perceptual problems to reorient himself to space and to develop an awareness of his own body image. The following procedures are suggested.

Neglect

When the patient demonstrates a *neglect of one side of his body* and/or the surrounding space, this area beyond the midline of his body must somehow be brought into his awareness. Initially the therapist strokes the affected arm while the patient watches. If sensation is present, various materials may be used to bring the stimulus (e.g., a piece of cotton or a coin) into the patient's awareness. The patient is then encouraged to stimulate his affected extremities in the same manner. The patient is then taught to move his affected arm in half circles on a table so that he crosses the midline of his body. He may assist this motion by his unaffected arm or a skateboard [2].

If there is a *loss of space perception,* attempts will be made to reestablish awareness through observation of the limbs while placing them in various positions. The therapist helps the patient to move a cane in horizontal, vertical, diagonal, and circular directions from the affected side to the unaffected side. Then the patient repeats these movements unassisted. The patient is then asked to point with his affected hand to an object held by the therapist and to follow the direction of that object with his finger as the therapist moves the object in various directions, encouraging the patient to move his arm across the midline of his body. The patient may also be helped to stand in the parallel bars and place his affected foot in various designated spots on the floor [2].

Disturbance of body image

With disturbances of body image, the patient is encouraged to be aware of his body by naming the various parts of it (first the therapist touches the part, then the patient). Patients are asked to imitate motions of the therapist such as placing hand(s) on different parts of the body, elevating arms above the head. The patient is often requested to perform some of the motions without cues from the therapist. The therapist will gear his motions to the patient's degree of motor paralysis and will encourage him to cross the midline of the body [2].

It is important to note that patients with parietal lobe lesions in the nondominant hemisphere may have perceptual disorders without an accompanying hemiplegia. However, if they neglect the left side of the body, muscle weakness may develop on that side, if no attempt is made to increase their awareness and establish an exercise program for them [2]. Should such weakness occur, staff caring for the patient must be made aware of the nature of the weakness and an exercise established.

Visual and spatial difficulties

Patients with *constructional apraxia* are given visual-motor coordination exercises with blocks, sticks, and multiple forms in two- and three-dimensional patterns. The complexity of the exercises is gradually increased by the therapist in accordance with the degree of impairment and the patient's progress. For *dressing apraxia,* the therapy directed toward unilateral neglect of the body is used. These procedures for reorientation of the patient with perceptual difficulties should be initiated early on in the course of therapy and coordinated with training in activities of daily living (ADL) [2]. These are discussed in detail in Chapter 13.

Lesions of the parietal lobe in the left "dominant" hemisphere in right hemiplegics are frequently accompanied by a bilateral apraxia or Gerstmann's syndrome (dyscalculia, agraphia, loss of left-right discrimination, and finger agnosia). In working with these patients it is important that instructions be made as simple as possible and that directions be given in brief statements spoken clearly and slowly. All motor activities should be taught by breaking them down into the simplest component parts. After the patient has mastered these singly, he can integrate them gradually. It is important to establish a regular routine for these patients and to guide them through the motions when they are unable to initiate or carry through an activity [2].

Spatial disorientation

Patients with perceptual disorders due to a stroke in the *nondominant hemisphere* have difficulty in judging position, distance, and rate of motion. They may also have trouble telling right from left, identifying a vertical axis, and establishing where the various body parts are in relation to the space around them. At times they may confuse the concepts of up and down, inside and outside. Because of these spatial-visual perceptual problems, such patients may bump into objects and have difficulty following the lines of written material or negotiating their way down a straight corridor in a wheelchair. Unfortunately these patients usually have little insight into their problems and vastly overestimate their capabilities for independent activity. They make poor judgments and may act impulsively; therefore they require close supervision to protect them from falls and other accidents.

It is important to remember that patients who have had a stroke in the non-dominant hemisphere have problems interpreting visual sensations. It is far more effective to give these patients verbal instructions than to demonstrate an activity for them to carry out. All instructions should be clear and concise, and it may help to have the patient repeat aloud each step of the task to be performed. Such patients do much better in an environment that is well lighted and free of obstacles, clutter, and other sources of distraction or confusion, such as bright patterns, noise, and moving objects or persons. The patient's ability to orient himself in space and maintain a normal upright posture will be improved if he has a mirror available in which to check his position [8, 18].

Unilateral neglect

Patients who neglect one side of their bodies present a challenge to the staff caring for them, since this disorder affects all aspects of care. The affected limbs must be checked frequently for injuries resulting from improper positioning that go unnoticed by the patient. The meal tray must be prepared so that the patient is aware of all items on it. Bed placement is particularly important, since it has a direct effect on the patient's interaction with his environment. The bed should be positioned so that he can see the activities going on around him and not be unnecessarily isolated with perhaps only a wall to look at. His limited field of vision should be directed toward the door of the room, so that he will not be startled by visitors and staff coming in and will be alert to the activities in his environment. Unilateral neglect is usually associated with limited sensory input, which can lead to consequent isolation and possible disorientation. If the patient is placed with his uninvolved side facing toward activity at regular intervals, this will increase his orientation and allow him to interact with the environment. Since he can easily become distracted by what is happening on the uninvolved side, and thus continue to neglect his involved side, there should also be sessions planned to encourage interaction with the neglected side. This can be accomplished, for example, by placing a television set to the patient's neglected side. The sound will stimulate him to explore that area of space. Families and staff should be encouraged to carry on conversations periodically from the neglected side in order to encourage awareness of that side. The patient may also be placed in a chair with his uninvolved side facing a wall or a place where there is less activity for brief periods. These activities must be planned as a part of the patient's treatment, because initially he may not be alert enough to scan his environment independently [8].

The patient's environment must be arranged so that important items, such as the call bell and drinking water, are placed within his reach on the unaffected side. At the same time he must be taught to care for his affected side. The nurse must remind him continuously of the neglected side of his body, drawing attention to an improperly positioned limb or neglected food or beverage on one half of his meal tray. He should be encouraged to scan his surrounding environment. Since he may perceive only half of what he looks at, the nurse should help by explaining what is going on around him, remembering that such patients will grasp the meaning of verbal stimuli much more readily than visual stimuli [8].

Difficulties with dressing can be handled by placing markers or colored tapes inside the clothing to help the patient identify top and bottom, right and left, and the order in which to put on the various articles of clothing. Written steps in dressing can also help. Some patients must begin by reciting the steps aloud when dressing [8].

The keys to helping patients with perceptual problems reorient themselves to space and compensate for their visual and motor defects are (1) a simplified, structured environment; (2) a well-established routine of activities that reinforces learning through repetition; and (3) sensory stimulation to activate awareness. To provide these elements of care, the staff must have a sound understanding of the perceptual problems involved, an awareness of the appropriate therapeutic techniques, and the patience and creativity to tailor them to each patient's losses and abilities [8].

When establishing a plan for teaching the perceptually handicapped person to compensate for his deficits, one must not lose sight of the effect of brain damage from the stroke on the patient's thought process. Patients with brain damage have difficulty with abstract thinking. They will respond to whatever they are actually experiencing at the moment, without being able to reflect on all aspects of the situation and to make a rational judgment about the most appropriate course of action. These patients will have difficulty integrating facts into new concepts and will interpret situations in accordance with their own concrete thinking. This must be recognized as a pathological result of the stroke [40].

Table 6-1 outlines the more commonly encountered perceptual problems and gives a brief description of the problem, an example, and a suggested therapeutic approach.

REFERENCES

1. Anderson, E. K. The significance of the parietal lobes in hemiplegia. *Hawaii Med. J.* 27:141–146, 1967.
2. Anderson, E. K., and Chay, E. Parietal lobe syndromes in hemiplegia. *Am. J. Occup. Ther.* 24:13–18, 1970.
3. Benson, D., and Geschwind, N. Psychiatric Conditions Associated with Focal Lesions of the Central Nervous System. In S. Arieli (Ed.), *American Handbook of Psychiatry* (2nd ed.). 4, Organic Disorders and Psychosomatic Medicine. New York: Basic Books, 1975. Pp. 208–243.
4. Benton, A. The fiction of the "Gerstmann Syndrome." *J. Neurol. Neurosurg. Psychiatr.* 24:176–181, 1961.
5. Benton A. Disorders of Spatial Orientation. In P. Vinken and G. Bruyn (Eds.), *Handbook of Clinical Neurology. Disorders of Higher Nervous Activity.* New York: Wiley, 1969. Pp. 212–228.
6. Birch, H., Proctor, F., Bortner, M., and Lowenthal, M. Perception in hemiplegia: I. Judgment of vertical and horizontal by hemiplegic patients. *Arch. Phys. Med. Rehabil.* 41:19–26, 1960.
7. Boone, D., and Landes, A. Left-right discrimination in hemiplegic patients. *Arch. Phys. Med. Rehabil.* 49:533–537, 1968.

8. Burt, M. Perceptual deficits in hemiplegia. *Am. J. Nurs.* 70:1026–1029, 1970.
9. Casella, C. Perception of time by hemiplegic patients. *Arch. Phys. Med. Rehabil.* 48:369–372, 1967.
10. Critchley, M. *The Parietal Lobes.* London: Arnold, 1955. Pp. 156–355.
11. Critchley, M. The engima of Gerstmann's syndrome. *Brain* 89:183–197, 1960.
12. DeCencio, D., Leshner, M., and Voron, D. Verticality perception and ambulation in hemiplegia. *Arch. Phys. Med. Rehabil.* 51:105–110, 1970.
13. Denny-Brown, D. *Handbook of Neurological Examination and Case Recording.* Cambridge: Harvard University Press, 1957. Pp. 59–67.
14. Denny-Brown, D. The nature of apraxia. *J. Nerv. Ment. Dis.* 126:9–32, 1958.
15. Diller, L., and Weinberg, J. Evidence for accident prone behavior in hemiplegia patients. *Arch. Phys. Med. Rehabil.* 51:358–363, 1970.
16. Diller, L., and Weinberg, J. Hemi-Inattention in Rehabilitation: The Evolution of a Rational Remediation Program. In E. A. Weinstein and R. P. Friedland (Eds.), *Advances in Neurology* 18. New York: Raven, 1977. Pp. 63–82.
17. Elliot, F. A. *Clinical Neurology.* Philadelphia: Saunders, 1964. Pp. 50–72.
18. Fowler, R. S., and Fordyce, W. E. Adapting care for the brain-damaged patient. *Am. J. Nurs.* 72:1832–1835, 1972.
19. Friedlander, W. Anosognosia and perception. *Am. J. Phys. Med.* 44:1294–1407, 1967.
20. Geschwind, N. The apraxias: Neural mechanisms of disorders of learned movement. *Am. Sci.* 63:188–195, 1975.
21. Goody, W., and Rheinhold, M. Some aspects of human orientation in space. *Brain* 75:472–509, 1975.
22. Lizak, M. D. *Neuropsychological Assessment.* New York: Oxford University Press, 1976. Pp. 10–31; 42–68.
23. Lorenze, E., and Cancro, R. Dysfunction in visual perception with hemiplegia; its relation to activities of daily living. *Arch. Phys. Med. Rehabil.* 43:514–517, 1962.
24. Lucas, M. Perceptual disorders of adults with hemiparesis. *Phys. Ther.* 49:1078–1083, 1969.
25. Luria, A. *Restoration of Function After Brain Injury.* New York: Pergamon, 1963.
26. Luria, A. *Higher Cortical Functions in Man.* New York: Basic Books, 1966. Pp. 123–164.
27. Luria, A. *The Man With a Shattered World.* New York: Basic Books, 1972. Pp. 3–165.
28. Luria, A. *The Working Brain.* New York: Basic Books, 1973. Pp. 1–344.
29. MacDonald, J. An investigation of body scheme in adults with cerebral vascular accidents. *Am. J. Occup. Ther.* 14:75–79, 1960.
30. McFie, J., Piercy, M., and Zangwill, O. Visual-spatial agnosia associated with lesions of the right cerebral hemisphere. *Brain* 73:167–190, 1950.
31. McFie, J., and Zangwill, O. Visual constructive disabilities associated with lesions of the left cerebral hemisphere. *Brain* 83:243–260, 1960.
32. Mossman, P. *A Problem-Oriented Approach to Stroke Rehabilitation.* Springfield, Ill.: Thomas, 1976. Pp. 133–139; 186–228.
33. Nielson, J. M. *Agnosia, Apraxia, Aphasia.* New York: Hafner, 1965. Pp. 24–26; 49–58; 59–62; 76–85; 86–92; 250–254.
34. Paterson, A., and Zangwill, O. Disorders of visual space perception associated with lesions of the right cerebral hemisphere. *Brain* 67:331–358, 1944.
35. Piercy, M., and DeAjuriaguerra, J. Construction apraxia associated with unilateral cerebral lesions – Left and right sided cases compared. *Brain* 83:225–242, 1960.

36. Sawtell, R., and Martin, J. M. Perceptual problems of the hemiplegic patient. *Lancet* 87:193—196, 1967.
37. Strub, R., and Black. F. *The Mental Status Examination in Neurology.* Philadelphia: Davis, 1977. Pp. 85—106; 119—132.
38. Strub, R., and Geschwind, N. Gertmann syndrome without aphasia. *Cortex* 10:378, 1974.
39. Taylor, M. M. Analysis of dysfunction in left hemisphere following stroke. *Am. J. Occup. Ther.* 22:512—518, 1968.
40. Ullman, M. Disorders of body image after stroke. *Am. J. Nurs.* 64:89—91, 1964.
41. Weinstein, E., and Friedland, R. Behavioral Disorders Associated with Hemi-Inattention. In E. A. Weinstein and R. P. Friedland (Eds.), *Advances in Neurology,* Vol. 18. New York: Raven, 1977.
42. Williams, N. Correlation between copying ability and dressing activities in hemiplegia. *Am. J. Phys. Med.* 45:1332—1340, 1967.

7. Assessment of respiratory status and respiratory care for the patient with stroke

ANATOMY AND PHYSIOLOGY OF THE RESPIRATORY SYSTEM

Respiration is the exchange of gaseous substances between the air and the bloodstream. Oxygen (O_2), one of the major substances from which all body cells derive their energy, is taken from the air we breathe in a continuous exchange for carbon dioxide (CO_2), a by-product of cell metabolism [12, 13].

The most immediate concern in the acute phase of stroke is to maintain or restore the patient's vital functions. The first task at hand is to establish a patent airway and assure respiration. Emergency measures are often required to prevent aspiration of secretions and maintain adequate ventilation. An understanding of the respiratory system and its functions is essential to the nurse who will be responsible for monitoring the patient's respiratory status and may be required to institute measures for restoring and maintaining respiratory function.

Upper Respiratory Tract

The respiratory tract is divided into an upper and a lower portion. The *upper respiratory tract* consists of the nose, nasopharynx, and oropharynx. Its function is to warm, filter, and humidify inspired air. The nasopharynx consists of the pharyngeal tonsils and the auditory tube, which connects the nasopharynx to the middle ear and opens during swallowing to allow for regulation of pressure within the middle ear. Irritation to the auditory tube, which may result from placement of a nasotracheal tube to maintain an adequate airway, can result in blockage of the middle ear. The oropharynx is in effect the posterior wall of the mouth, where the digestive and respiratory tracts cross. The swallowing reflex, which serves to propel food into the esophagus, is initiated here. This reflex simultaneously causes the epiglottis to close over the larynx, preventing passage of food or aspiration of fluids and secretions into the trachea [7, 12].

Lower Respiratory Tract

The lower respiratory tract consists of the larynx, trachea, bronchi, bronchioles, lungs, and pleura. It is in this portion of the respiratory system that gas exchange occurs.

The *larynx* contains nine cartilages, the three most important being the thyroid, epiglottis, and cricoid. The largest of these is the thyroid cartilage, which projects into the midline of the neck and is commonly referred to as the "Adam's apple." The epiglottis is attached to it, and the vocal cords lie inside it. The best-known function of the larynx is the production of voice, however. It serves two more important functions, prevention of aspiration and an important role in the cough reflex. The vocal cords close during coughing, thus allowing a buildup of pressure in the tracheobronchial tree with contraction of the thoracic and abdominal muscles. When the vocal cords reopen, the high expiratory rate resulting from this buildup of pressure helps to expel secretions. Since the mucosa of the larynx is supplied with sensory fibers from the vagus nerve, any foreign material coming in contact with the larynx will initiate coughing. It is important to remember that this defense mechanism may not function for the patient with stroke, since it may be suppressed or eliminated by unconsciousness or neurological impairment [7, 22].

The *trachea* is approximately 5 inches (11 cm) in length and extends from the cricoid cartilage of the larynx into the thorax, where it bifurcates to form the right and left bronchi. It consists of C-shaped rings of cartilage open posteriorly and fibroelastic membrane that is shared posteriorly with the esophagus. Elective tracheotomy is performed through the second tracheal ring [7, 12].

There are two main stem *bronchi*. The right is shorter, wider, and more nearly in line with the trachea than the left, which extends out from the trachea at a much narrower angle. This anatomical difference is particularly significant in caring for the patient with stroke who requires intubation. The endotracheal tube may be inadvertently passed too far and positioned in the right main bronchus, thus allowing for aeration of only one lung. Furthermore, aspiration, with resultant danger of pneumonia, usually occurs in the right lung. The two main bronchi subdivide into five branches to serve the upper middle and lower lobes of the right lung and the upper and lower lobes of the left lung. These five branches then subdivide into eighteen segmental bronchi, ten on the right and eight on the left. Further subdivisions of the bronchial tree include the terminal bronchioles and finally the respiratory bronchioles, alveolar ducts, and alveoli, which together make up the gas-exchanging units of the lung [7, 12, 20].

Alveoli are the most important structures involved in gas exchange. Each individual alveolus consists of an alveolar wall and a surfactant, which serve as a gas—liquid interface. The alveolar wall contains the alveolar membrane, a network of capillaries, and interstitial fluid. Alveolar lining fluid, on the surface of the alveolar wall, surrounds alveolar gas. The alveolar surface has the property of surface tension, which allows for shrinking or contracting of the surface area. The surfactant present at the liquid surface has the property of *progressively* lowering the surface tension as the surface becomes smaller. The pulmonary surfactant thus serves to equalize the pressure within each alveolus during the expansion and contraction that occur with inspiration and expiration. During inspiration, surface tension increases. High surface tension at the beginning of expiration reduces lung volume. With the decreased alveolar surface area toward the end of expiration, surface tension is lowered [7, 12].

Groups of alveoli distal to a respiratory bronchiole, together with the bronchiole and blood vessels supplying them, are referred to as *lobules*. The lobule is the primary functional unit of the lung. Large numbers of lobules form the eighteen bronchial segments of the lung — the right lung, which is the larger, possessing ten and the left, eight. The right lung is divided into three lobes: (1) the upper, which consists of an apical, anterior, and posterior segment; (2) the middle, consisting of a lateral and medial segment; and (3) the lower, which includes the superior lateral and anterior segments. The left lung is divided into two lobes: (1) the upper, consisting of the anterior, apical posterior, superior, and inferior segments; and (2) the lower, which includes the superior, anterior medial, and lateral segments [7, 12].

The movement of gases for alveolar ventilation is supplied via the respiratory bronchiole and the alveolar duct. A branch of the pulmonary artery, which brings unoxygenated venous blood from the right ventricle, and a branch of the bronchial artery, which carries arterial blood from the aorta to nourish the lower respiratory tract, enter the lobule with the respiratory bronchiole. The pulmonary vein then takes oxygenated blood from the capillaries at the periphery of the lobule to the left atrium, where it is pumped by the left ventricle into the peripheral circulation [20].

Each lung is enclosed in a serous membrane, the *pleura,* which has two layers. The parietal layer lines the thoracic cavity, and the visceral layer adheres to the lung. A potential space, the *pleural space,* exists between these two layers, which are separated by a thin film of pleural fluid. This allows the lung to have an easy gliding movement along the chest wall. It also creates a negative pressure that means considerable force is required to pull the pleura away from the chest wall. The pleural space is defined by the diaphragm, the chest wall, and the mediastinum [7].

One of the chief *muscles of respiration* is the diaphragm, which is attached to the ribs, sternum, and spine and separates the thorax from the abdominal cavity. When relaxed, it is dome-shaped. The contraction that occurs with *inspiration* causes it to flatten, thereby expanding the thoracic cavity downward. Contraction of the external intercostal muscles simultaneously elevates the ribs, resulting in lateral expansion of the chest wall as well. Each half of the diaphragm receives its own innervation from one of two phrenic nerves. Damage to a phrenic nerve will result in paralysis of the diaphragm on the affected side, thus restricting movement of that lung [7, 20].

Under normal conditions, *expiration* is a passive act. It results from the elastic recoil of the lungs and from the surface tension in the film of fluid that lines the alveoli. Passive elastic recoil of the chest and abdominal muscles also contributes to expiration. With forced or labored breathing, the internal costal muscles draw the ribs and sternum downward, and contraction of the abdominal muscles results in an elevation of the diaphragm further into the thoracic cavity [20].

Ventilation

In order for respiration, which is the exchange of oxygen and carbon dioxide across the alveolar wall, to occur, *ventilation,* or the movement of these gases, must take place. An understanding of this physiological process is most important in planning care for the patient with stroke, who may have inadequate ventilation secondary to pooled or aspirated secretions. The patient may require mechanical ventilation because of damage to the respiratory center or paralysis of the respiratory muscles.

For ventilation to be effective, the volume of air brought into the lungs (*tidal volume*) must (1) actually reach the alveoli, (2) be sufficient for metabolic needs, and (3) be distributed effectively throughout the alveoli [20]. Average normal values for tidal volume vary significantly, but a range of 400–600 ml is usually considered normal. The mechanical properties of the lungs and thorax serve to regulate ventilation, which pumps air into and out of the lungs with each inspiration and expiration [7, 20].

The mechanics of breathing are affected by compliance, nature of the airflow, resistance to airflow, and pressure changes outside and within the pulmonary system. *Compliance* is the relationship between airway pressure and tidal volume. Changes in the elastic properties of the lung and thorax will alter compliance. Decreased compliance requires increased muscular activity in order to create sufficient pressure to deliver an adequate volume for alveolar ventilation [20]. This will occur with pneumonia, atelectasis, pleural effusion, and pulmonary edema. *Airway resistance* refers to the relationship between pressure and flow and is defined as the ratio of pressure drop across the airway to the airflow rate. A high airway resistance increases the work of breathing. This is seen in chronic obstructive lung disease, in which peripheral resistance in the small bronchiole is greatly increased, and it can also occur when the patient has retained secretions [7].

Only part of the tidal volume brought into the lungs with each inspiration actually reaches the alveoli to take part in gas exchange. This volume is called *alveolar ventilation*. The balance, approximately one third of the air inspired, remains in a part of the bronchial tree and is referred to as the *anatomical dead space*. This volume is called *dead space ventilation* [7]. The average anatomic dead space in the adult is approximately 150 ml but is most frequently expressed as the ratio of dead space to tidal volume. This is based on the determination of the partial pressure of carbon dioxide in the arterial blood (Pa_{CO_2}) and of the partial pressure of carbon dioxide in expired gas ($P\bar{E}_{CO_2}$) rather than on measurements of actual volume [7]. The rate at which carbon dioxide is removed from the alveoli, and therefore the arterial carbon dioxide pressure (Pa_{CO_2}), depends on the amount of alveolar ventilation. Normal alveolar ventilation is the level that results in a normal arterial carbon dioxide pressure of 40 mm Hg. Alveolar *hypoventilation* occurs when ventilation is below that required to maintain a normal arterial carbon dioxide pressure. The decreased alveolar level of oxygen is inadequate to cellular metabolic needs, and hypoxia results. In addition, inadequate ventilation makes levels of carbon dioxide build up, producing hypercapnea. Alveolar *hyperventilation* occurs when there is an increase in ventilation above that required to maintain normal arterial carbon dioxide pressure [7].

Blood flow and transport of oxygen

The main function of the pulmonary circulation is to oxygenate venous blood. For this to occur, oxygen must be transported to the capillaries and carbon dioxide must be removed. Blood flow and alveolar ventilation are therefore closely related. The heart must pump the blood through two circulations, the systemic and the pulmonary. Venous blood returns from the systemic circulation to the right atrium through the inferior vena cava and the superior vena cava. The contraction of the right ventricle pumps the blood through the pulmonary artery into the pulmonary circulation to permit gas exchange. The main pulmonary artery carries mixed venous blood. Oxygenated blood from the pulmonary circulation is brought to the left atrium by the pulmonary veins and pumped by the left ventricle through the aorta back into the systemic circulation [12, 20].

Oxygen is carried in the blood in two forms, dissolved in plasma and in chemical combination with hemoglobin. The total amount of oxygen carried in the blood in these two forms is referred to as the *oxygen content* and is expressed in milliliters of oxygen per 100 milliliters of blood. The largest proportion of oxygen is carried within erythrocytes in chemical combination with hemoglobin. When blood is exposed to a partial pressure of oxygen (PO_2) of 150 mm Hg or more, the hemoglobin becomes 100% saturated. Under normal conditions the hemoglobin concentration of blood is approximately 15 gm per 100 ml. At full saturation, 100 ml of blood contains about 20 ml of oxygen. Hemoglobin is about ninety-seven percent oxygenated when the arterial oxygen tension is within the normal range of 90—95 mm Hg. The degree of oxygen saturation of the hemoglobin molecule, therefore, is dependent on the partial pressure of oxygen. The relationship between the two is expressed graphically as the *hemoglobin dissociation curve* (Fig. 7-1) [7].

Each minute approximately one liter of oxygen is pumped into the circulatory system via the aorta by the left ventricle. The amount of oxygen delivered to the tissues depends on total blood flow (cardiac output) as well as on the oxygen

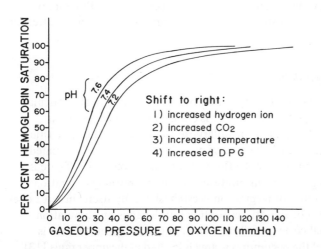

Figure 7-1
The hemoglobin dissociation curve and oxygen transport (From A. G. Guyton, Textbook of Medical Physiology *[5th ed.]. Philadelphia: Saunders, 1976.)*

content of arterial blood [7]. Oxygen supply to a particular site depends upon the adequacy of the blood flow to that area. This is determined by the relationship between blood flow, blood pressure, and resistance to blood flow within the vascular bed. Oxygen content is increased with an increase in blood pressure and a decrease in resistance to blood flow. Smooth muscles of the arterioles contract, thereby increasing resistance, in response to nervous system stimulation by sympathomimetic drugs, hypoxia, acidosis, and elevation of body temperature [7].

The exchange of oxygen and carbon dioxide across the alveolar membrane takes place through *diffusion,* the process by which gases spread from one place to another. This diffusion is passive due to the pressure gradient between the gases within the alveoli on one side of the membrane and those in the blood on the opposite side. The PO_2 within the alveoli is higher than the PO_2 in the mixed venous blood within the capillaries. Under normal conditions diffusion occurs rapidly, with oxygen entering the red blood cells in less than one second and carbon dioxide leaving the plasma in less than half a second [20]. For diffusion to occur, the following conditions are necessary: (1) ventilation must be adequate to maintain the pressure gradient between the gases on both sides of the alveolar membrane, (2) there must be an adequate flow of blood that contains sufficient hemoglobin for chemical combination with the oxygen, and (3) the alveolar capillary membranes must be permeable to both oxygen and carbon dioxide molecules. During diffusion, oxygen molecules entering the respiratory system must traverse the alveolar liquid lining and the alveolar membrane, pass into the interstitial fluid, and from there pass through the capillary membrane into the plasma, where they enter the red blood cells to combine with hemoglobin. Any pathological condition that interferes with this pathway will affect respiration adversely. Pulmonary edema, which increases interstitial fluid, will slow down the diffusion of oxygen. Inadequate ventilation of the lung as well as inadequate blood flow will decrease the rate of gas exchange. Pulmonary emboli will completely prevent transfer of oxygen and carbon dioxide in the affected alveoli [7, 20].

Neurological regulation of ventilation

Ventilation is controlled by the respiratory center, which is located in the reticular substance of the medulla and pons. This center is composed of neurons and is divided into three areas: (1) the area of medullary rhythmicity, (2) the apneustic area, and (3) the pneumotaxic area. The area of medullary rhythmicity is located in the medial half of the medulla below the floor of the fourth ventricle. There is an intermingling of neurons governing inspiration and those governing expiration in this area, where the basic rhythm of respiration is established. By itself this area does not establish a normal pattern of smooth respiration but depends on stimulation from the spinal cord, cerebral cortex, midbrain, and pons. The apneustic area is located in the lower pons, and the pneumotaxic area is located in the upper pons [13].

The brainstem chemoreceptors, two areas located on either side of the medulla, are particularly sensitive to changes in the hydrogen ion concentration of cerebrospinal fluid, which are brought about by changes in the level of carbon dioxide in the blood. An increase in hydrogen ion concentration will cause an increase in respiratory activity, and a decrease in hydrogen ion concentration will result in decreased respiratory activity under regulation of acid-base balance (see Chapter 9) [13].

The respiratory center also receives stimuli from chemoreceptors located outside the central nervous system, which help in regulating respirations. These are the carotid bodies, located in the bifurcations of the common carotid arteries, and the aortic bodies, located along the arch of the aorta. They respond to changes in levels of oxygen, carbon dioxide, and hydrogen ion concentration. When the oxygen tension of arterial blood falls below normal, these peripheral chemoreceptors stimulate the respiratory center to increase alveolar ventilation [13].

Stretch receptors in the lungs send impulses to the respiratory center to inhibit inspiration when the lungs are fully inflated. This effect is called the *Hering-Breuer inflation reflex*. A Hering-Breuer *deflation* reflex inhibits expiration as the lungs empty. In addition to altering respiratory rhythmicity the Hering-Breuer reflexes help to maintain the respiratory rhythm [13].

Blood gases, pH, and regulation of acid-base balance

Arterial blood gases refer to the partial pressures of oxygen (PO_2) and carbon dioxide (PCO_2) in the blood and are used to measure the effectiveness of ventilation, blood flow, and diffusion. When arterial blood gases are analyzed, determinations of the hydrogen ion concentration in the plasma (pH), the bicarbonate level (HCO_3), and the oxygen saturation of the blood (SO_2) are usually performed as well [1, 2, 20].

The partial pressure of oxygen is an indicator of the lung's efficiency in transmitting oxygen to the blood. The normal range of arterial PO_2 is 95–100 mm Hg. It is a direct reflection of the amount of oxygen that has diffused from the alveoli via the capillaries into the arterial circulation. A low PO_2 indicates that the patient is not receiving an adequate supply of oxygen. The condition may be corrected by increasing the concentration of oxygen being administered via mask, nasal prongs, or respirator. The patient's decreased arterial PO_2 may also be secondary to physiological shunting. This can result when the patient is kept in the same position, thereby preventing full ventilation of the lung and allowing unoxygenated blood to return to the left atrium. This is particularly important to keep in mind when positioning the patient with stroke. Physiological shunting can be decreased by changing the patient's position frequently. Venous PO_2 is normally 35–40 mm Hg. This is a measure of peripheral perfusion and reflects the patient's cardiac output, blood volume and gaseous exchange in the lungs. A low venous PO_2 may be the result of a low circulating volume, which will require blood replacement. It may also be due to low cardiac output secondary to myocardial damage. Stroke patients who are having difficulties handling secretions may have retained secretions which are preventing adequate gas exchange. Suctioning the secretions can correct the situation [1, 2, 6].

The partial pressure of carbon dioxide shows the adequacy of ventilation. The arterial PCO_2 level is normally 40 mm Hg and the venous PCO_2 is 45 mm Hg [1].

A low P_{CO_2} is referred to as *hypocarbia,* which means that the patient is blowing off carbon dioxide too rapidly. This may be caused by hyperventilation, atelectasis, or injury to the respiratory center. An elevated P_{CO_2}, or hypercapnea, indicates that the patient is accumulating carbon dioxide. This may be caused by inadequate ventilation due to acute airway obstruction or central nervous system depression [2].

The *pH or concentration of free hydrogen ions in body fluids* determines whether they are acidic or alkaline. Differences in the pH of the blood reflect the rate at which carbon dioxide from cellular metabolism is entering the blood. The pH serves as an index of the patient's acid-base balance [1, 2, 8, 18, 21]. Acid-base balance is essential to normal cellular functioning, since the cell, which is the basic living unit of the body, requires a slightly alkaline environment for maintenance of life.

There are four major disturbances in acid-base balance: metabolic acidosis, respiratory acidosis, metabolic alkalosis and respiratory alkalosis. These disturbances, which frequently occur in varying combinations, and the body's three defense mechanisms, which regulate hydrogen ion concentration — (1) the buffer systems, (2) the respiratory system, and (3) the kidney — are discussed in detail in Chapter 9.

RESPIRATORY FAILURE

Patients with stroke may develop respiratory problems either as a result of the stroke or as a result of preexisting pulmonary disease. Disturbances of ventilation, blood flow, or diffusion of oxygen and carbon dioxide will lead to impairment of gas exchange. This in turn may result in respiratory failure. Respiratory failure is defined by Wade as "the inability of the respiratory apparatus to maintain adequate oxygenation of the blood, with or without carbon dioxide retention [20, p. 140]. An arterial P_{O_2} of less than 60 mm Hg or a P_{CO_2} of more than 50 mm Hg is indicative of respiratory failure. The impaired gas exchange may result in *hypoxemic failure,* with a low arterial P_{O_2} and a normal or slightly lowered P_{CO_2}, or in *hypoventilatory failure,* with a decreased P_{O_2} and an elevated P_{CO_2}, as judged by blood gas determinations [20].

When respiratory failure results from acute upper airway obstruction, in stroke the manifestations are most obvious and require immediate institution of emergency measures to establish a patent airway and restore adequate ventilation. The less dramatic signs and symptoms of impending respiratory failure are often not readily discerned by the nurse, however. These are hypercapnea, hypoxemia, and hypoxia [20].

Hypercapnea

Hypercapnea is an excess of carbon dioxide in the body fluids, which builds up when alveolar ventilation is not able to remove the amount produced by cell metabolism. The nurse should recognize the clinical manifestations of an elevated P_{CO_2}, which acts principally as a central nervous system depressant. These include drowsiness, confusion, and irritability. Patients with carbon dioxide retention frequently have altered sleep patterns, with daytime drowsiness and wakeful nights. Tranquilizers or sedatives will only compound the problem by depressing the respiratory center further and increasing an already elevated PCO_2 level. Uncontrolled administration of oxygen can be lethal. With extreme hypercapnea the increased PCO_2 fails to serve as a stimulus to the respiratory center to increase ventilation, and the resulting hypoxia becomes the primary stimulus for respiratory activity. If the extremely hypercapnic patient is treated with a high concentration of oxygen, he is deprived of his last effective stimulus for respiration [21]. The patient may become comatose rapidly and die. Therefore, administration of oxygen to such patients must be monitored carefully [16, 20, 22].

Hypoxemia

Hypoxemia, a deficiency of oxygen in the blood, is always present with acute respiratory failure. *Acute hypoxemia* may arise from acute airway obstruction, circulatory failure, or pulmonary edema. The immediate response is an elevation in blood pressure, with a rapid pulse and increased cardiac output. If the condition is not reversed, the blood pressure falls and the patient becomes cyanotic. Acute hypoxemia results from hypoventilation *and* impaired ventilation–perfusion ratio and is corrected by ventilatory support. *Chronic hypoxemia* is seen most often in patients who have chronic obstructive lung disease and in these cases result mainly from altered ventilation–perfusion ratios. Hypoventilation is rarely the cause. Patients with hypoxemia may complain of headache, show signs of air hunger, become euphoric, or develop impaired motor function. With prolonged hypoxemia the patient will lapse into unconsciousness [20].

Hypoxia

Hypoxia means a low oxygen pressure anywhere in the body. It signals a much more serious situation than hypoxemia alone, since it indicates decreased oxygen in the tissues and possibly an inadequate supply of oxygen to the vital organs. Hypoxia is also much more difficult to recognize than hypoxemia. The most useful determination of oxygen perfusion to the tissues is a central venous PO_2 [16].

Hypoxia may be the result of acute airway obstruction or circulatory failure, in which case acute changes in the patient's condition will be readily apparent. It may also occur more gradually as the result of reduced arterial PO_2 due to hypoventilation, anemia, reduction in cardiac output, or an increased requirement for oxygen as with fever. Malfunctioning oxygen or mechanical ventilatory equipment can also contribute to hypoxia by reducing the concentration of inspired oxygen. When hypoxia develops slowly, the changes in the patient's condition will be subtler and the clinical manifestations less specific. They can include headache, confusion, tachycardia, an elevated blood pressure, and a sudden drop in blood pressure. Cyanosis develops to a degree that depends on the amount of unsaturated hemoglobin in the blood. Unfortunately it does not become apparent until arterial saturation drops to about seventy-eight percent. Therefore, administration of oxygen is indicated whenever cyanosis is evident. It should be noted, however, that oxygen therapy is not without significant risks. The nurse should familiarize herself with its action, and side effects and with the principles of safe administration. The same thoughtful attention must be given to the concentration and flow rate of oxygen as is given during administration of any other potentially lethal drug [16, 20].

The body attempts to adjust ventilation, hematocrit, and cardiac output to assure that its available oxygen will be supplied to the brain, heart, kidneys, and lungs to avoid jeopardizing the functioning of these vital systems. When hypoxia is present or suspected, the nurse should be most attentive for signs of dyspnea, oliguria, and changes in cerebral function. The body is capable of storing oxygen sufficient to maintain vital functions for only about four minutes. With respiratory arrest, death from hypoxia will result if oxygen perfusion to the heart and brain is not restored within this brief period of time [16, 20].

Management of patients in respiratory failure

Management of patients with respiratory failure will depend on whether failure is hypoventilatory or hypoxemic. If it is hypoventilatory, efforts should be directed primarily toward restoring adequate ventilation. If it is hypoxemic, supplemental oxygen must be given to provide adequate tissue oxygenation. Regardless of the cause, the following principles of patient management should be followed when respiratory failure threatens or occurs: (1) assure airway patency, (2) provide sufficient oxygen, (3) provide adequate ventilation, (4) control hydrogen ion concentration, (5) provide adequate hydration, (6) maintain cardiac output, and (7) prevent infection [16, 20].

AIRWAY PATENCY
Restoring and maintaining an adequate airway is the most immediate concern in the care of the patient in acute respiratory failure. Maintaining airway patency is also vital for unconscious patients or those with problems handling secretions, such as the stroke patient with facial paralysis, depressed or absent protective airway reflexes, or — in brainstem stroke — pharyngeal paralysis. Obstruction of the airway by a foreign body, such as a food particle, dentures, or mucous plug, can result in sudden death if the obstruction is not moved immediately [16]. Artificial airways may be required. These come in three types: (1) oropharyngeal tubes, which provide for an airway down to the larynx; (2) endotracheal tubes, which are inserted via the nose or mouth and passed through the larynx into the trachea; and (3) tracheostomy tubes, which are inserted directly into the trachea below the level of the larynx [16].

OROPHARYNGEAL AIRWAYS
Oropharyngeal airways are used for unconscious patients who have spontaneous respirations and no ventilatory problems. Such an airway provides a route for aspiration of oropharyngeal secretions and prevents the tongue from falling back and occluding the patient's upper airway. It conforms to the curvature of the palate and extends from the lips to the pharynx. If properly placed, it displaces the tongue anteriorly and allows the patient to breath both through and around it. In placing

an oral airway, see that the patient is supine with his head tilted back, or positioned on his side if there is danger of aspiration. Open his mouth with a tongue depressor and insert the airway sidewise, then rotate it carefully into position. The airway is held in place with a band that goes around the outside of the jaw and ties. A bite block around the tube will keep the patient from clamping down on the tube and obstructing the airway and also will help prevent movement of the tube during suctioning. Bite blocks are available commercially. In hospitals where they are not provided, use rolled gauze secured with tape. Gauze or foam pads should be placed between the tape and the jaw to prevent pressure necrosis. Check the skin frequently for pressure. See that the tube is kept in the center of the mouth and avoid moving it unnecessarily, since this may cause coughing or gagging. It is very important that oral hygiene be provided frequently [7].

NASOPHARYNGEAL AIRWAYS
Nasopharyngeal airways are inserted through the nares and extend to just above the epiglottis. They are for short-term use in the semiconscious patient, when an oral airway would stimulate the gag reflex. The nasopharyngeal airway should be replaced by an endotracheal tube if the patient continues to require an artificial airway. These tubes should be checked frequently and changed whenever they become coated with mucus or occluded. A hand or a wisp of tissue over the outer end of the airway will test the flow of air. Bushnell recommends changing the airway every 8 hours, alternating nares [7].

ENDOTRACHEAL AIRWAYS
Oral or nasal endotracheal intubation is often required to secure airway patency. In addition to providing a route for suctioning pulmonary secretions and preventing the tongue from occluding the upper airway, an endotracheal tube protects against aspiration of stomach contents or secretions. It can also provide a route for short-term mechanical ventilation, but if this is required for more than a few days, a tracheostomy is ordinarily performed.

Orotracheal tubes are inserted through the mouth into the trachea. They are held in place with a bite block, which is tied around the tube and secured with a tape that passes along the patient's jawline and around the head to hold the tube in place. The bite block should be changed daily or more often by the nurse or respiratory therapist. When the tube is inserted, it is marked at the point where it emerges from the mouth. This mark acts as an indicator of any movement or displacement of the tube. Bushnell recommends that the position of the tube be changed from one side of the mouth to the other once every 8 hours by an experienced nurse or physician [7]. *Nasotracheal* tubes are inserted through the nose into the trachea. These are usually preferred for long-term intubation, since fixation and retention of the tube are better assured than with the orotracheal tube and this type of intubation is usually more easily tolerated by the patient [7].

In a *cuffed* tube an inflatable attachment is added to an endotracheal or tracheostomy tube to provide a snug fit. The cuffed tube isolates the trachea from the digestive tract, thereby preventing aspiration of gastric contents, and is required whenever controlled or assisted ventilators are used. It also prevents leakage of air and secretions outside the tube as well as aspiration of secretions. The cuff should be deflated at least every one to two hours for approximately five minutes to allow for return of circulation to tracheal mucosa and prevent damage due to continued pressure over one area of the trachea. Before the cuff is deflated, suction should always be applied to the oropharynx and nasopharynx to remove any secretions that may have settled above the inflated cuff and around the exterior of the tube. To prevent secretions and feedings from seeping into the lung, the cuff should always be inflated while tube feedings are being given. Prolonged intubation frequently causes laryngeal damage and also may lead to subglottic stenosis from the continued pressure of the tube. Because of the seriousness of this complication, an elective tracheostomy may be performed [7, 16].

TRACHEOSTOMY

A tracheostomy is rarely required as an emergency procedure in patients with stroke but is most commonly the elected method of maintaining airway patency in a patient who requires prolonged mechanical ventilation or deep and frequent suctioning to remove excessive and/or tenacious secretions. A tracheostomy may also be performed when a patient cannot tolerate an endotracheal tube. If the patient is conscious, the nurse should prepare him for this frightening procedure by explaining why it is necessary. He must understand that he will not be able to speak while the tube is in place, but he must also realize that this will not be a permanent loss. It is particularly important to reassure him that he will never be left unattended and that every effort will be made to anticipate his needs. A system of wordless communication should be set up if at all possible. The nurse should also take the time to explain the tracheostomy to the patient's family, stressing its importance for his well-being. The family should understand that it is a temporary measure and that the patient will not be able to talk while the tube is in place [7, 14, 16, 20].

Three types of tracheostomy tubes are customarily used: (1) the three-part silver tube, consisting of an inner cannula, outer cannula, and obturator, to which an inflatable rubber cuff can be attached; (2) the plastic tube with built-in inflatable cuff; and (3) the controlled pressure cuff tube, with an external control balloon, designed to prevent ischemia of the mucosa. The tracheostomy tube should be tied securely around the patient's neck by tape tied through slots on the side of the tube and fastened with a knot at side of the neck. Strict aseptic technique should be maintained in care of the tracheostomy. Dressings should be gauze flats rather than cotton-filled sponges because of the risk of cotton fiber aspiration. The area around the tracheostomy should be cleansed with gauze dampened with normal saline whenever application of a new dressing is necessary. There should be an extra sterile tracheostomy tube of the same size and an intubation set at the patient's bedside at all times. If a three-part silver tube is in place, an obturator of the same size should also be kept at the bedside [16, 20].

Since secretions accumulated on the tube's surface will support bacterial growth, the tubes should be changed frequently. Aseptic technique must always be used when caring for the tracheostomy wound or stoma. Tubing connected to the tracheostomy tube should be changed daily [16, 20].

CARING FOR THE PATIENT WITH AN ARTIFICIAL AIRWAY
The following principles should be adhered to in caring for patients with artificial
airways: (1) make certain that room air or oxygen is adequately humidified; (2) control secretions; (3) prevent infection; (4) maintain sufficient pressure in cuff of
endotracheal tube to support adequate ventilation, and deflate properly to assure
integrity of the mucosa; and (5) provide a safe means of communication.

Humidity.   The normal means of humidifying inspired air is bypassed. Room air
may contain some humidity, but pressurized oxygen has none. Moisture must be
added to prevent thickening of bronchial secretions, which can contribute to atelectasis, and drying of the tracheal mucosa. This can be accomplished by means of
nebulizers and humidifiers, which provide warmed, moistened air and oxygen mix-
tures to the patient through a mask, or by means of attachments to the ventilator.
Excessive condensation within the tubing can be prevented by using wide-bore
tubing of less than four-foot lengths.

Control of secretions and prevention of infection.   In order to keep the patient's
airway patent it is important to prevent accumulation of respiratory tract secretions.
Moistening the inspired air and oxygen and maintaining adequate hydration will
help keep secretions thin and fluid and prevent formation of thick, tenacious sputum.
Encouraging the patient to cough and breathe deeply and changing his position frequently will help prevent pooling and stagnation of secretions. If the patient does
not have an adequate cough reflex, however, suctioning must be used to remove
secretions.
   The nurse who accepts responsibility for the care of critically ill patients must be
thoroughly competent in the proper technique for inserting airways and applying
suction to maintain a patent airway. She or he must also understand the possible
untoward effects, both long- and short-term, of improper technique. The structures
involved are exceedingly delicate and should be handled in the gentlest manner
possible. Damage to the trachea, larynx, or epiglottis may be irreversible and most
certainly will be painful. Repair of these structures will be costly as well as painful.
Deep and frequent suctioning may be required to maintain pulmonary toilet, and
vigorous suctioning can mean the difference between life and death or the end result
of prolonged cerebral anoxia. To be thorough, however, one need not be rough.
   Even the patient who appears to be unconscious should have the procedure
explained to him and be informed each time he is to be suctioned. He should be
told why suctioning is required, that he will feel short of breath for a few minutes,
and that he will be allowed to rest in a short time. Shouting will not necessarily
help the uncommunicative patient acknowledge your explanation, but a gentle
manner and an adequate warning concerning this exceedingly unpleasant invasion
can do much to alleviate his anxiety.
   Suctioning should be carried out whenever there is any question as to the patency
of the airway or whenever there are audible or visible secretions. It serves to remove
secretions effectively, prevent aspiration, and initiate the cough reflex. It is always
a sterile procedure. Introduce the suction catheter through the nose, mouth, or, if

the patient is intubated, the tube. Suction should never be applied while the catheter is being advanced. Once the catheter has been introduced, apply suction by placing the thumb over the end of the Y connecting tube while gently rotating the catheter and withdrawing it from the orifice. To clear both lungs, the patient's head should be turned first to one side and then to the other. Oxygen should be administered prior to and after suctioning, as both secretions and oxygen are withdrawn during the process. If the patient is on a mechanical ventilator, a self-inflating manual ventilator bag should be used before and after suctioning. Always provide adequate humidity, and observe the stoma site for bleeding if the patient has a tracheostomy. Allow the patient to rest for about three minutes between suctioning, and do not apply suction for more than 6–10 seconds, as hypoxia or ventricular irritability can occur due to anoxia [7].

Unfortunately, the introduction of suction catheters can lead to infection, which in turn will produce excessive secretions. Frequent culturing of sputum will be required to monitor the growth of bacterial organisms in the lung. Every effort must be made to maintain the normal flora of the lung and to prevent introduction of pathogenic organisms during suctioning or tracheostomy stoma care or through careless maintenance of oxygen and ventilatory assistance equipment. Strict sterile technique must be maintained for suction and for care of the tracheostomy stoma [16].

Pneumonia.   Perhaps one of the most common respiratory problems affecting the stroke patient is *pneumonia* since any condition that promotes retention of secretions in the bronchi predisposes the lungs to pneumonia. Pneumonia may be classified according to the location of the disease process — for example, *bronchopneumonia,* in which infection is located in the bronchioles, and *lobar pneumonia,* in which a substantial portion of one or more lobes is involved [4] — or according to the causative organisms, such as streptococcal, staphylococcal, Friedländer's (*Klebsiella pneumoniae*), and viral pneumonia. *Aspiration* of a foreign body into the lungs can cause pneumonia, and *hypostatic pneumonia* occurs when immobility prevents normal clearing of lungs [4].

Patients are most susceptible to developing pneumonia when there is interference with the normal protective mechanisms of the respiratory system, such as inability of the cilia to clear airways of microorganisms that are normally present, impaired swallowing and gag reflexes, and depressed cough reflex. Chronic disease, exposure to pollution or infection, excessive mucus that provides a medium for bacterial growth, and any factor that puts stress on mucous membranes of the respiratory system increase susceptibility to pneumonia.

Symptoms vary depending upon the organism and extent of lung involvement. *Lobar pneumonia* can involve extensive amounts of lung tissue. The patient may experience chills, fever, pallor, and pain that may be sharp and increased in intensity on cough or exertion. Although initially cough may be nonproductive, with progression of the inflammatory process, rust-colored sputum will be produced. Pleurisy with pleural friction may be present. Mononuclear lymphocytes, plasma cells, and macrophages are usually found if the pneumonia is viral, while presence of leukocytosis with polymorphonuclear leukocytes is diagnostic for bacterial pneumonia [4].

In *bronchopneumonia* the initial infection usually is less severe. However, the lesions can cause serious lung impairment because of airway obstruction similar to that seen in acute bronchitis. This condition is frequently associated with preexisting bronchitis. The sputum may be purulent and difficult to raise. The treatment is symptomatic when the causative agent is viral. Therapy with antibiotics will be instituted depending on the culture and sensitivity findings.

In hospitalized patients with stroke, aspiration pneumonia and hypostatic pneumonia are seen most often. *Aspiration pneumonia* is associated with inhalation of foreign material such as fluid, food, or gastric contents, into the lung. The patient who is obtunded, lethargic, or has depressed gag and swallowing reflexes is most susceptible to this type of pneumonia. Patients receiving nasogastric tube feedings are prime candidates for aspiration, unless precautionary measures are taken to prevent it. Dyspnea, cyanosis, tachycardia, hypotension, hypoxia, and even circulatory collapse can occur with aspiration. Aspiration of gastric contents can cause acute inflammation, and obstructive atelectasis from inhaled solid materials and the pneumonia can progress to necrosis and suppuration [5]. Treatment may include chest physical therapy with percussion, vibration, and postural drainage. Tracheobronchial suctioning may be necessary. Steroid therapy may be started to abort an inflammatory process. Antibiotics are usually prescribed [7]. Patients who are susceptible to aspiration require vigilant nursing care, identification of potential problems, and institution of preventive measures. These are described in detail in Chapter 9.

Hypostatic pneumonia can result from any condition that restricts mobility, since with immobility, secretions are retained in the dependent areas of the lung and bacterial growth in the stagnant secretions results in infection. Nursing measures can prevent hypostatic pneumonia. Stroke patients who are incapacitated or restricted to bed rest should have a program directed toward prevention of this complication. Their positions should be changed frequently to facilitate drainage of dependent lung areas, and as soon as he is able the patient should be instructed to cough and breathe deeply to stimulate clearing of secretion. Pulmonary therapy should be provided for those patients who cannot perform these exercises independently or who need additional treatment. Careful monitoring of respiratory status is essential for all patients who are physically restricted. Chapter 12 outlines in detail the program for positioning the comatose and/or paralyzed patient.

Oral hygiene is most important for the comfort and well-being of all patients. It is particularly important for the unconscious patient who is intubated. When strict attention is not paid to this area, the mouth may become a focus of infection. The normal flora of the mouth may be altered by medications and by changes in pH. Accumulated secretions and debris provide an excellent culture medium for organisms. Irritation from artificial airways and suction catheters can lead to tissue breakdown, which will foster bacterial growth. An occasional swipe with a swab saturated in glycerine and lemon juice simply will not do. The mouth must be meticulously cleansed on a regular basis. The procedure best suited to the needs of the particular patient should be spelled out in the care plan and followed religiously. Several preparations and procedures for mouth care, which are geared to certain conditions and adaptable to individual cases, are outlined in Chapter 11.

INFLATION AND DEFLATION OF CUFFED TUBES
As described earlier, endotracheal and tracheostomy tubes can be provided with an inflatable attachment that allows the tube to fit snugly within the trachea. When a cuffed tube is in place, it must be deflated regularly to prevent tissue necrosis. This should be done at least every two hours for approximately five minutes. Prior to deflation suction should be applied to remove secretions that will have accumulated above the cuff. The cuff must be reinflated to prevent aspiration and leakage of air. The pressure gauge should be monitored closely and extreme caution must be used to maintain correct pressure within the cuff. Underinflation defeats its purpose and overinflation can cause tissue damage or burst the cuff and thereby also defeat its purpose. Many tubes are now available with pressure-controlled inflation valves. This prevents cuff pressure from exceeding 25 cm H_2O which is the suggested minimal occluding volume (MOV). The MOV represents the amount of air required to inflate the cuff to provide an airtight seal during mechanical ventilation. This pressure should be measured at the end of exhalation and should be checked and recorded each time the cuff is inflated. An increased MOV indicates a faulty cuff, a slow leak, or tracheal wall damage. When the patient requires tube feedings, the cuff on the endotracheal tube must be inflated during feeding to avoid the dangers of aspiration [20].

PROVIDING A MEANS OF COMMUNICATION
The patient who is intubated cannot speak to make his needs known. He is completely dependent on the nurse to anticipate his needs, interpret his behavior, and establish a safe means of communication. He must be reassured that he will never be left unattended, but every effort must be made to'set up some means for him to communicate with the staff caring for him as well as with his loved ones. The patient with stroke may be unresponsive; often his stroke will have resulted in aphasia or left him with perceptual disabilities or paralysis. All these factors may reduce his ability both to express himself and to comprehend what has happened to him and what is going on around him. Establishing communication with such a patient is indeed a challenge. Even if he is apparently unconscious, the nurse must continue to explain to him whatever she is about to do and why. The particular problems of the aphasic patient who requires intubation are most complex, whether the aphasia be expressive or receptive, and are dealt with in more detail in Chapter 5. It is important to note here that the extent of the patient's neurological deficits must be thoroughly understood before any aids to communication can be devised.

The simplest communication aid for the nurse is a pad and pencil or a magic slate. Needless to say, this will work only if the patient can read and write. Distortions due to visual or perceptual impairment and inability to hold a pencil because of hemiplegia will also preclude this form of communication. When a tracheostomy tube is in place, the nurse can read the patient's lips in order to interpret his needs, as long as the patient is not aphasic, is able to comprehend instructions, and does not have his facial musculature severely impaired by the stroke. In many nursing units flash cards or visual aids have been devised that indicate patients' most common needs, such as "bedpan," "pain relief," "suction," or "change of position." Frequently one must resort to phrasing questions so that they can be answered by a nod for "yes" or a shake of the head for "no." This is certainly at least as frustrating to the patient as it is to the nurse. The means of communication must be tailored to the needs and limitations of each patient. These limitations may include a limited mental capacity and visual problems before the stroke, any of a variety of deficits resulting from the stroke, and an overwhelming sense of isolation, frustration, and helplessness because of inability to communicate. Family and friends must be encouraged to attempt to communicate with the patient to help keep up his morale and to provide him with mental stimulation [14, 16].

COMPLICATIONS OF ARTIFICIAL AIRWAYS

The most common complications of artificial airways result from injury to the respiratory tract, occlusion of the airway, and infection. Laryngeal edema from injury to the vocal cords may result in severe stridor. Although this complication is reversible, it is nevertheless life-threatening. When placement of the airway is difficult, there is always the danger that the mucous membranes or the delicate structures of the upper respiratory tract will be lacerated and that hemorrhage will ensue. Hemorrhage is also a risk in the immediate postoperative period following tracheostomy. When an oropharyngeal or nasopharyngeal tube is used, there is always the danger of aspiration of secretions or gastric contents. Aspiration pneumonia is particularly difficult to treat. It rapidly brings about acute toxemia with high fever, tachycardia, and extreme dyspnea; and, in spite of vigorous treatment by suctioning, ventilatory assistance, and parenteral antibiotics and steroids, often results in multiple lung abscesses.

The major complications of endotracheal intubation are related to trauma or laryngeal edema secondary to insertion, obstruction due to mucous plugs, improper placement of the tube, or prolonged or improper cuff inflation. Improper cuff inflation is also a problem with cuffed tracheostomy tubes. Overinflation or herniation of the cuff will occlude the lumen of the tube, and irritation and eventually necrosis of the tracheal mucosa will result if the cuff is not deflated regularly to allow for proper blood flow. Tracheostomy tubes may slip out of the trachea and become embedded in the subcutaneous tissues. Patients who have had a tube in for a long time usually develop tracheal stenosis. Stenosis may also result if the cuff has not been deflated regularly, since erosion of the tracheal wall will be followed by formation of granulation tissue. Prolonged intubation may lead eventually to the formation of a tracheoesophageal fistula from erosion of the tube through the trachea, and this may cause a fatal hemorrhage. Intubated patients may develop local infection of the tracheostomy site as well as pneumonia [16, 20].

In caring for the acutely ill patient, the highest priority must always be given to maintaining vital functions, but the long-term effects of complications must not be ignored. Any of the complications just described can result in prolonged hospitalization, costly and potentially dangerous therapeutic measures, and, most important, often unnecessary debilitation, pain, and suffering for the patient. The serious long-term consequences of improper mouth care must also be stressed. Patients intubated for prolonged periods of time often require extensive and costly dental work to repair the effects of improper mouth care — a complication that the nurse responsible for care of the acutely ill patient will rarely, if ever, be made aware of.

It is not within the scope of this book to provide an exhaustive coverage of respiratory nursing for critically ill patients. The reference list at the end of this chapter includes several excellent texts.

Oxygen therapy

The most important indication for oxygen therapy is hypoxia. Hypoxia may result from inadequate tissue perfusion or a decrease in the oxygen content of arterial blood. The central nervous system is particularly sensitive to hypoxia. Availability of oxygen to the tissue depends on blood flow as well as on the amount of oxygen carried in the hemoglobin. Inadequate blood flow makes it more likely that arterial hypoxemia will result in hypoxia. Supplemental oxygen should be administered whenever oxygen transport to the tissues is compromised. The optimal inspired oxygen concentration is one that results in an arterial oxygen tension of 70—100 mm Hg. The goal in providing supplemental oxygen is to provide a concentration which will allow for effective use of the oxygen-carrying capacity of arterial blood and provide adequate oxygenation of the tissues [7].

If the patient does not require intubation, and unless otherwise prescribed, oxygen may be administered with nasal prongs at 4—6 liters per minute to provide 30—40% oxygen concentration. The prongs should be removed from the nares every 4—6 hours to check for patency. Face masks are available for delivery of 24%, 28%, 35%, and 40% oxygen. Oxygen flow rate is adjusted to that indicated on each mask to deliver the accurate concentrations. When a mask is used, it must fit snugly, and areas around bony prominences should be padded. The patient must be watched for pressure over bony prominences and for skin irritation. The oxygen should be humidified, since it is a drying agent and can have an irritating effect upon the mucous membranes [7].

COMPLICATIONS
Administration of oxygen must be supervised carefully to avoid potential physiological dangers. The complications that most often arise with stroke patients receiving oxygen therapy are (1) respiratory depression, (2) atelectasis, (3) circulatory depression, and (4) oxygen toxicity. *Respiratory depression* with somnolence and even coma can occur during oxygen therapy when hypercapnia results from decreased alveolar ventilation. This most often happens to patients who have been sedated or who have an underlying obstructive lung disease. Ventilatory assistance must be provided, blood gases carefully monitored, and sufficient oxygen supplied. *Atelectasis* can result when the oxygen concentration is too high. The increased oxygen content in the lungs will wash nitrogen away, diminishing the surfactant in the alveolar lining

fluid and increasing surface tension. This leaves the alveoli with only water, oxygen, and carbon dioxide. Because of the increased surface tension, if the alveoli are not hyperinflated, the oxygen will be absorbed by the pulmonary blood flow, and the alveoli will collapse. *Circulatory depression* can occur when oxygen is given to a hypoxic patient. The oxygen can cause dilation of the blood vessels, which previously had been constricted due to loss of interstitial plasma resulting from the hypoxic state, and this vasodilation can lead to circulatory collapse. Central venous pressure and blood pressure must be monitored carefully during administration of oxygen to the hypoxic patient in order to assure that intravascular volume is maintained. *Oxygen toxicity* results in damage to the lungs themselves and is related to the concentration of oxygen provided and the length of time over which it is given. The goal in oxygen therapy should always be to provide sufficient oxygen to keep arterial oxygen pressure as close to normal as possible, but to reduce the concentration as soon as it is safe to do so. This can be ascertained through monitoring of blood gases. The nurse should always be aware of the concentration of oxygen that is being administered and should check the flow meter regularly to be certain it has not been accidentally set too high [7, 20].

METHOD OF ADMINISTRATION
Oxygen can be administered via (1) nasal catheter, (2) nasal prongs, or (3) mask. The conscious patient should always be told that he is to receive oxygen before the equipment arrives at the bedside. Most elderly patients and their families view the administration of oxygen as a last resort. They should be told why oxygen is needed and what relief of symptoms is expected from it. They should also be instructed as to the rules in force while oxygen is being administered, such as the prohibition against smoking in the room and against disconnecting or otherwise obstructing the flow of oxygen through the tubing.

Nasal catheters are used for short-term therapy. They are made of soft rubber or plastic and are inserted via the nares. The humidified oxygen flow should be adjusted to equal the patient's normal ventilation. A flow of 6–8 liters per minute provides an oxygen concentration of 30–50%. As these catheters are themselves irritating to the mucosa, however, the higher flow rate should be avoided, as it adds to the irritation. A fresh nasal catheter should be placed in the alternate nostril every 6–8 hours. *Nasal prongs* provide oxygen through both nares via two 5/8-inch soft plastic tips. A flow of 4–6 liters per minute will provide an oxygen concentration of 30–40%. The prongs are more comfortable than nasal catheters, but patients experience frontal sinus pain from high flow rates, and the flow is more easily obstructed than with a nasal catheter. *Oxygen masks* are designed to cover both the nose and the mouth and come in a variety of shapes and sizes. The tight fit of a mask allows up to 100% concentration of oxygen, if needed. A face mask must be removed for short periods of time to dry the face and check for pressure areas. An artificial airway must be in place when an oxygen mask is used on an unconscious or obtunded patient. The types generally used for stroke patients requiring oxygen therapy are (1) disposable face masks, (2) partial rebreathing masks, and (3) Venturi masks [7].

The *disposable face mask* allows expired air to be vented through holes on either side. The concentration of oxygen inspired will vary, since it is related to the fit of the mask, the flow rate at which the oxygen meter is set, and the patient's inspiratory rate. A rough approximation of the oxygen concentration that can be provided with a simple disposable face mask is as follows [7]:

OXYGEN CONCENTRATION (%)	FLOW RATE (LITERS/MINUTE)
35—45	6— 8
45—55	8—10
55—65	10—12

Partial rebreathing masks conserve oxygen with reservoir bags, from which one third of the exhaled oxygen is rebreathed. The carbon dioxide reinhaled in the process can be kept to a negligible amount by adjusting the flow rate of the oxygen meter to provide about 4 liters of oxygen per minute and prevent collapse of the reservoir bag during inspiration. With a snug-fitting mask and a flow rate set at 6—10 liters per minute, an oxygen concentration of 35—65% can be achieved [7].

Venturi masks, so called because their function is based on the Venturi high airflow—oxygen enrichment principle, contain a device that will maintain a fixed oxygen—air ratio. This control of oxygen concentration is particularly helpful for patients with chronic obstructive lung disease, who are vulnerable to respiratory depression and carbon dioxide retention from high concentrations of oxygen. The mask must be selected according to the oxygen concentration prescribed (they will deliver 24, 28, 35, or 40% oxygen concentration), and the flow rate must be adjusted according to instructions on the mask [7, 16].

OXYGEN CONCENTRATION (%)	FLOW RATE (LITERS/MINUTE)
24	4
28	4
35	8
40	8

Mechanical ventilation

Mechanical ventilation or use of a respirator is indicated whenever a patient is unable to maintain safe levels of oxygen (PO_2) and carbon dioxide (PCO_2) in his arterial blood through his own spontaneous breathing. The variety of machines available are all designed to provide adequate alveolar ventilation and thereby guarantee a sufficient supply of oxygen to the tissues. The basic differences between these ventilators are related to (1) how the machine is "triggered," that is, how the mechanism starts and stops to assure a complete cycle of inspiration and expiration for each respiration, and (2) how the flow of oxygen and air is delivered to the lungs. The three basic *triggering mechanisms* for respirators are (1) pressure within the airway, (2) a time cycle device, and (3) an electrical device. The *delivery of air and oxygen* may be accomplished by a generator, which can provide: (1) a constant pressure of gas, (2) a constant flow of gas, or (3) a pattern of variable gas flow. When a patient is placed on a ventilator, the nurse is responsible for understanding the principles of mechanical ventilation, recognizing deviations in blood gas patterns or mechanical failure of the ventilator, and knowing what to do should the machine fail [7, 19].

Once the decision has been made to institute mechanical ventilation, the following steps must be taken to assure proper functioning: (1) the machine should be turned on and checked to be certain that it is producing a flow of gas; (2) appropriate settings must be selected for the particular tidal volume, respiratory rate, and oxygen concentration that are required for the patient; and (3) within 30 minutes of placing the patient on the ventilator, arterial blood gases should be measured to assess the effectiveness of ventilation [7, 19].

Lung ventilators are connected to the patient's airway via an endotracheal or tracheostomy tube to either assist or control ventilation. *Assisted ventilation* works only if the patient has sufficient spontaneous inspiratory effort and as long as his spontaneous respiratory rate does not exceed 25 breaths per minute. In this case the ventilator is used to increase the patient's tidal volume. Inspiration is triggered by the patient's spontaneous effort, which is boosted by the respirator. *Controlled ventilation* is used when there is no respiratory stimulus or drive. The ventilator is preset at a specific tidal volume and respiratory rate and does not depend on any inspiratory effort by the patient. Inspiration is initiated and the work of breathing is accomplished by the ventilator at a predetermined frequency. *Assist-controlled ventilation* allows the ventilator to control the respiratory pattern or assist respiration if the patient makes an inspiratory effort that is out of phase with the ventilator, or if the patient becomes apneic [7].

With *volume-cycled ventilators* the changeover from the expiratory phase of respiration to the inspiratory occurs when a preset volume of gas passes a specified point. *Time-cycled ventilators* will cause this changeover to occur when a preset time interval has elapsed. *Pressure-cycled ventilators* permit this changeover when a preset pressure similar to that of the lung pressure has been attained. *Patient-cycled ventilators* allow the changeover to take place with the patient's spontaneous inspiratory effort. *Mixed-cycle ventilators* are designed to allow the changeover to occur with any combination of events listed above [7].

TYPES OF MECHANICAL LUNG VENTILATORS
Pressure preset ventilators are run by gas, usually a mixture of air and oxygen, under pressure. The ventilator delivers the gas directly into the airway until a preset pressure is reached, at which time the inspiratory valve of the respirator will close and the expiratory valve will open to allow passive exhalation of gas from the lungs. This happens regardless of the actual volume of gas delivered to the lungs. The inspired tidal volume will depend upon lung compliance, airway resistance, rate of gas flow from the respirator, and the preset peak pressure. If there is a decreased lung compliance, as is the case with pulmonary edema or pneumonia, or an increased airway resistance, as with chronic obstructive lung disease, the pressure preset ventilator may not necessarily provide an effective tidal volume. Therefore inspiratory pressure, ventilator rate, and expired tidal volume must be measured hourly and any deviation from the physician's written orders reported immediately. The *Bird Mark 7*

is an example of a pressure preset ventilator that can function to assist or control ventilation. The *Bennett PR II* is a positive-pressure-cycled, time-cycled, flow-sensitive ventilator that can function to assist or control ventilation [7, 16, 19].

Volume preset ventilators, usually run by electricity, deliver a preset volume of gas into the patient's lungs at a fixed rate. They are less affected by changes in pulmonary mechanics than are pressure preset ventilators, and they allow oxygen concentration to be varied according to the patient's need. Sufficient pressure is built up to allow delivery of the preset tidal volume. Expired tidal volume and airway pressure must be monitored so that any increased resistance, obstruction, or gas leakage will be detected promptly. The *Emerson* ventilator is volume-limited, allows inspiratory and expiratory rates to be set independently, and permits ventilator rate, expired tidal volume, and inspired oxygen concentration to be preset. The *Engstrom* is a volume-controlled and time-cycled ventilator. The *Bennett MA-1* can provide either assisted, controlled, or assist-controlled ventilation. Inspiratory pressure can be controlled, and exhalation is time-controlled. Oxygen and humidity concentrations are easily controlled with this machine as well. The *Ohio 560* is a volume preset ventilator that can be used to assist or control ventilation. The inspiratory phase is volume-controlled, and inspiratory pressure may be limited. The volume preset ventilators have the advantage of providing an effective tidal volume in spite of changes in compliance or airway resistance, as long as there is no leakage of gas in the system [7, 16, 19, 20].

NURSING MEASURES FOR PATIENTS ON VENTILATORS
All patients receiving mechanical ventilation will have artificial airways and will be receiving oxygen. The principles of care, nursing measures, and complications related to artificial airways and administration of oxygen have already been covered in detail in this chapter. Patients on ventilators require, in addition, being turned, coughed, and suctioned as well as intermittently deep-breathed with a self-inflating manual ventilator bag every 1–2 hours. Auscultation of breath sounds should be performed regularly and aeration of all parts of both lungs assessed periodically in any patient with potential or actual respiratory or pulmonary problems. Proper inflation and deflation of endotracheal and tracheostomy tube cuffs is critical, since leakage of air can interfere with the triggering mechanism of the ventilator. A nurse who has a demonstrated competence in caring for patients receiving mechanical ventilation should be in constant attendance, and a self-inflating manual pressure bag must be kept at the bedside at all times.

WEANING THE PATIENT FROM THE MECHANICAL VENTILATOR
Mechanical ventilatory support is used for patients with a marked inability to provide the necessary exchange of oxygen and carbon dioxide in the lungs. Once the patient's ventilatory status has improved sufficiently, he is gradually weaned from dependence on the respirator. Before the weaning process can be started, blood gas determinations should be within a safe range, the patient must be capable of spontaneously ventilating his lungs and have regained sufficient strength to keep it up. The weaning process must be carried out gradually, starting with brief trial periods

of two or three minutes of unassisted respiration in an oxygen-enriched atmosphere [7]. Prior to initiating the weaning process, physiologic tests are carried out to determine if the patient is capable of adequate spontaneous ventilation. The most common of these tests are vital capacity, tidal volume, inspiratory force, physiologic dead space/tidal volume ratio, and arterial blood gas determinations [7, 20].

Vital capacity (VC) is the measurement of the maximum volume of gas that can be expired from the lungs after a maximum inspiration. It is a critical measure of pulmonary function. The normal vital capacity is approximately 70 ml per kilogram of body weight. It decreases with age at a rate of about 300 ml per decade. Measurements of vital capacity can be made at the bedside with a portable respirometer. Tidal volume (VT) is the amount of air moved into and out of the lungs with each inspiration and expiration. Only a portion of this volume takes part in the exchange of gases at the level of the alveoli, however. The rest remains within the airways, which are referred to as deadspace (VD). The ratio of tidal volume to physiologic dead space is that portion of the tidal volume actually taking part in effective gas exchange and alveolar ventilation. This is commonly expressed as VD/VT. Thus a patient with a tidal volume of 600 ml and a physiological dead space of 180 ml would have a VD/VT ratio of 0.3. The normal VD/VT ratio is 0.3 [7, 20]. The significance of blood gas determinations has already been discussed with respect to the measurement of the effectiveness of ventilation.

When weaning is attempted, the nurse should be in constant attendance to provide reassurance and monitor the patient's progress. She should be especially vigilant to note any signs of fatigue, distress, or emotional stress. The patient should be in a sitting position to decrease pressure of the abdominal contents on the diaphragm. Serial blood gas levels and vital capacity measurements will be performed to ensure adequate ventilation. Blood pressure, pulse, and respirations should be checked every 5 minutes. The patient should be placed back on mechanical ventilation if the blood pressure rises more than 20 mm Hg, the pulse goes above 120, respirations increase to 30, or the patient becomes anxious and agitated. While off the ventilator, the patient should be encouraged to take deep breaths. If he is unable to do so, a self-inflating bag can be used to supplement his tidal volume and expand the alveoli.

Patients who have required mechanical ventilation for a period of time often are extremely frightened by the prospect of being deprived even momentarily of their life support mechanism. The nurse can be a great help to the patient through the period of transition to complete independence from the ventilator. This can be accomplished through reassurance, making him aware of his respiratory movements, making certain that he understands the process of weaning and precisely how long he will be off the ventilator at each trial period. Periods off the ventilator should never be prolonged, and a nurse must be in constant attendance during them. If the patient becomes anxious and exhausted because he has been left off the machine for a longer period than was ordered, he may be apprehensive and reluctant to come off the ventilator at the next weaning session. If there are no setbacks, progressively longer sessions will be allowed until the patient is able to support his own ventilation adequately [7, 16, 20].

Pulmonary physical therapy

Chest physical therapy is directed toward prevention of respiratory complications and improvement of function in acute pulmonary disease. The methods employed include coughing and deep breathing exercises, vibration, percussion, and postural drainage.

COUGHING AND DEEP BREATHING

Coughing and deep breathing exercises are aimed at full expansion of the chest. The patient should be supported in bed by pillows with the knees and arms slightly flexed to help relax the abdominal muscles and allow maximum movement of the diaphragm. He is instructed to breathe as follows: (1) inhale deeply through the nose, (2) exhale completely through the mouth, and (3) inhale deeply and produce a deep abdominal cough by a short, sharp expiration. He should use the abdominal muscles, intercostal muscles, and the diaphragm to facilitate deep inhalation and prolonged expiration. The abdominal muscles may be splinted by the nurse's hands or by a temporary abdominal binder. The nurse may elevate both of patient's arms with inspiration to permit use of all accessory muscles available for chest stretching [7, 20].

PERCUSSION AND VIBRATION

Percussion and vibration are manual techniques used by the nurse or the pulmonary physical therapist to promote drainage of mucus and secretions from the lungs, to dislodge mucus adhering to bronchioles and bronchi, and to help mobilize secretions. Percussion involves striking the chest wall in a rhythmical fashion with cupped hands over the chest segments to be drained. Vibration is the manual compression and tremor to the chest wall during the exhalation phase of respiration. The nurse places her hands on the patient's chest at the level of secretions and applies pressure followed by continued vibration, which is transmitted through the chest wall to the underlying pulmonary tissue [20].

POSTURAL DRAINAGE

Postural drainage uses gravity and positioning of the body to achieve drainage of each segment of the lung. This technique can affect secretions lodged in the distal airways, whereas a suction catheter can only reach the major airways. Postural drainage is an important therapeutic measure when the patient is unable to initiate a voluntary cough, as is true of comatose patients or those who have neurological abnormalities. It can also be used prophylactically to prevent retention of secretions in unconscious patients or those who require mechanical ventilation [7, 16, 20].

Specific positions are employed to drain the lower lobes, the right middle lobe, the left lingula, and both upper lobes. These positions assure that the segmental bronchi are vertical, so that gravity can assist in drainage of secretions from the pulmonary segment into the major bronchi or trachea, where they can be suctioned or coughed up. Some or all of the specific postural drainage positions are chosen for each patient according to the specific lobe or segment involved.

The patient's overall condition must also be considered when setting up a program of postural drainage. If the patient is unable to tolerate the prone position, he may be changed from side to side instead. Patients with tracheostomy tubes may not be able to tolerate certain positions. Postural drainage is contraindicated for patients who have unstable vital signs or cerebral edema. The program should be coordinated with administration of bronchodilators and nebulizer or aerosol treatments, if these are prescribed, to assure maximum benefit from both modalities. Postural drainage should never be performed right after meals, tube feedings, or administration of oral medications.

The patient should always have a pillow under his head, and his knees and hips should be flexed to provide relaxation of the abdominal muscles. Coughing and deep breathing exercises should be carried out in each position used. If percussion and vibratory motion have been prescribed, these should also be carried out in each position, to promote maximum drainage from each area. Each position should be maintained for approximately 20–30 minutes, three or four times daily. The character and amount of material expectorated or aspirated should be noted, and the patient should always receive mouth care following postural drainage.

IPPB

Intermittent positive pressure breathing (IPPB) increases alveolar ventilation by administration of oxygen or air under pressure during inspiration. This may be done with a self-inflating bag, a positive pressure ventilator, or a simple positive pressure device such as the Hand-E-Vent. It can be used as a therapeutic or prophylactic measure [7] to

1. prevent atelectasis by deep inflation of the lung
2. administer bronchodilator aerosols to aid in expectoration
3. decrease the work of breathing
4. help mobilize secretions
5. augment labored or inadequate spontaneous ventilation

RESPIRATORY ASSESSMENT

The observation skills of the nurse are vital to the identification of respiratory problems. Many aspects of respiratory dysfunction can be observed at the bedside, independently of the more sophisticated testing and equipment available. The value of direct patient observation cannot be overrated. It is unfortunate when nurses rely heavily on technology to the exclusion of bedside observation.

Respiratory assessment includes observation of skin color, chest movement on inspiration and expiration, rate and rhythm of respirations, ease or difficulty of breathing, presence or absence of cough, and mental status. *Cyanosis* may indicate poor oxygenation. *The chest* should be examined for symmetry; asymmetry may be noted with certain types of respiratory dysfunction or cardiac disease. *Chest movement* should be observed in relation to rate and rhythm of respirations. The ratio of respirations to the pulse is normally 1 : 4, while the ratio of inspiration to expiration should be fairly equal. Prolonged expiration may be an indication of obstructive lung disease, while short, panting breaths on inspiration may indicate hypoxia. Shallow and frequent respirations indicate restrictive pulmonary disease. Chest movement may be compromised in the presence of respiratory dysfunction. Retraction of the intercostal spaces on inspiration indicates airway obstruction, while pleural effusion or emphysema may cause bulging of the intercostal spaces. Normally the *accessory muscles* are used only in heavy exercise; their use at rest or on only moderate exercise indicates respiratory dysfunction [4]. Any *cough* should be noted for frequency, pattern, and the presence or absence of sputum. *Sputum* should be inspected for color, consistency, and amount. The characteristics, predisposing factors, and location of *pain* are significant. Pleuritic pain is usually produced when the thorax moves, is usually unilateral, and is accentuated when the patient breathes deeply. Generalized thoracic pain can be caused by cardiac disease, hiatus hernia, or costal chondritis. Dyspnea or shortness of breath may occur at rest or with exertion [4].

The nurse may use auscultation with a stethoscope to identify the presence or absence of normal or abnormal breath sounds. Breath sounds are produced by movement of air in the tracheobronchial tree and alveoli throughout the respiratory tract. They have distinctive characteristics of intensity, pitch, quality, and duration that can be related to certain disease processes. The patient is asked to take deep breaths through the mouth while the examiner listens to the chest. The examination is begun by first listening anteriorly at the apices, then working downward and listening to the posterior chest, then starting again at the apices and working downward, comparing symmetrical points sequentially. *Vesicular breath sounds* are normally heard over the lung surfaces. They are soft, low-pitched, and present mainly on inspiration. *Bronchovesicular breath sounds,* normally heard over the area of the trachea, are loud and higher pitched than vesicular sounds. The presence of these sounds over other areas of the chest indicates consolidation of the lungs. *Bronchial breath sounds* are heard when there is obstruction of air in the alveoli and indicate consolidation or compression of lung tissue. These sounds are high-pitched and have a hollow quality. *Adventitious sounds* are abnormal breath sounds superimposed upon normal ones, and are the result of secretions, exudates or other obstructions in the alveoli and tracheobronchial tree. Rales, rhonchi, wheezes, and pleural friction rub are adventitious sounds. *Rales* are produced by air flow through fluid in the alveoli and are more evident on inspiration. Rales may be fine, medium, or coarse. Fine rales are sharp, crackling sounds that are sometimes referred to as crepitation. Medium rales are heard over bronchioles, are more coarse, and make a loud clicking sound. Coarse rales have a loud, gurgling sound and are heard over the bronchi. *Rhonchi and wheezes* are usually heard as musical sounds that result from air passing through an obstruction in the bronchus or bronchioles. Mucus plugs, spasm, and edema are frequently their cause. *Rhonchi* are low-pitched and probably originate in large bronchial tubes, whereas *wheezes* are high-pitched and originate in smaller radicles. *Pleural friction rub* is a rough sound produced by the rubbing together of two inflamed surfaces and is heard with inflammation of the pleura when there is insufficient lubricating fluid between the opposing pleural surfaces. The absence of all breath sounds indicates that no air is being moved in the area [4, 9, 11].

REFERENCES

1. Beland, I., and Passos, J. *Clinical Nursing* (3rd ed.). New York: Macmillan, 1975. Pp. 401–472.
2. Betson, C. Blood gases. *Am. J. Nurs.* 68:1010, 1968.
3. Betson, C. The nurse's role in blood gas monitoring. *Cardiovasc. Nurs.* 7:83, 1971.
4. Beyers, M., and Dudas, S. *The Clinical Practice of Medical-Surgical Nursing.* Boston: Little, Brown, 1977. Pp. 197–310.
5. Bouhuys, A., and Gee, J. B. Environmental Lung Disease. In G. W. Thorn et al. (Eds.), *Harrison's Principles of Internal Medicine* (8th ed.). New York: McGraw-Hill, 1977. Pp. 1378–1388.
6. Broughton, J. O. Understanding blood gases. *Ohio Medical Products Reprint Library* No. 456, 1971.
7. Bushnell, S. S. *Respiratory Intensive Care Nursing.* Boston: Little, Brown, 1973. Pp. 1–14; 15–32; 45–69; 83–98; 111–133; 135–138.
8. Cohen, S. Blood gas and acid base concepts in respiratory care. *Am. J. Nurs.* 76:1, 1976.
9. DeGowin, E., and DeGowin, R. *Bedside Diagnostic Examination.* New York: Macmillan, 1969. Pp. 25–314.
10. Foss, G. Postural drainage. *Am. J. Nurs.* 73:666, 1976.
11. Fowkes, W. C., and Hunn, V. *Clinical Assessment for the Nurse Practitioner.* St. Louis: Mosby, 1973. Pp. 55–63.
12. Goss, C. M. *Gray's Anatomy* (29th ed.). Philadelphia: Lea & Febiger, 1974. Pp. 1111–1153.
13. Guyton, A. C. *Textbook of Medical Physiology* (5th ed.). Philadelphia: Saunders, 1976. Pp. 516–529; 557–571.
14. Lawless, C. A. Helping patients with endotracheal and tracheostomy tubes communicate. *Am. J. Nurs.* 75:2151, 1975.
15. Lee, C. A., Stroot, V. R., and Schaper, C. A. What to do when acid base problems hang in the balance. *Nurs.* 75:32, 1975. Pp. 32–37.
16. Petty, T. L. *Intensive and Rehabilitative Respiratory Care* (2nd ed.). Philadelphia: Lea & Febiger, 1974. Pp. 14–33; 34–47; 136–157; 354–364.
17. Reed, G. M., and Sheppard, V. F. *Regulation of Fluid and Electrolyte Balance.* Philadelphia: Saunders, 1971. Pp. 186–188.
18. Sharer, J. E. Reviewing acid base balance. *Am. J. Nurs.* 75:980, 1975.
19. Tinker, J. H., and Wehner, R. The nurse and the ventilator. *Am. J. Nurs.* 74:1276, 1974.
20. Wade, J. F. *Respiratory Nursing Care* (2nd ed.). St. Louis: Mosby, 1977. Pp. 1–13; 39–53; 54–76; 125–139; 140–168; 170–188; 191–203.
21. Welt, L. J. Acidosis and Alkalosis. In M. M. Wintrobe, et al. (Eds.), *Harrison's Principles of Internal Medicine* (7th ed.). New York: McGraw-Hill, 1977. Pp. 1356–1367.
22. West, J. B. Disturbances of Respiratory Function. In G. W. Thorn et al. (Eds.), *Harrison's Principles of Internal Medicine* (8th ed.). New York: McGraw-Hill, 1977. Pp. 1332–1341.

8. The cardiovascular system and its relationship to stroke

The cerebral circulation is a subsystem of the cardiovascular system. Its function is dependent upon the effective pump action of the heart, the integrity of the systemic vasculature, and the components of the blood for a constant supply of blood and oxygen. The brain requires about twenty percent more oxygen than any other organ of the body [15]. When brain tissue is deprived of blood and oxygen, it will undergo ischemic changes that can progress quite rapidly to irreversible necrosis or infarction [17]. Stroke almost always occurs in conjunction with other illnesses, and because of the close association between the cerebrovascular and cardiovascular systems, conditions such as hypertension, atherosclerosis, myocardial infarction, cardiac dysrhythmias, and valvular heart disease are often cited as etiological factors. Stokes-Adams syndrome, polycythemia, profound anemias, idiopathic thrombocytosis, and complications of anticoagulation therapy may also be implicated [17]. The course of stroke and the stages of recovery can be complicated by these same conditions as well as by the presence of peripheral vascular disease and the development of thrombophlebitis and pulmonary embolism. Underlying cardiovascular problems that remain undetected during the initial examination in the acute stage of stroke can be exacerbated by treatment.

The purpose of this chapter is to provide (1) a brief description of the anatomical and physiological relationship of the cardiovascular system to the cerebral blood supply, (2) a description of the major cardiovascular conditions associated with stroke, (3) the elements of a nursing assessment of the cardiovascular function of patients with stroke, and (4) an overview of the major drugs that may be used in management of the patient with cardiovascular problems. An anatomy and physiology text should be consulted for a more detailed description of the cardiovascular system and its functions, and a cardiovascular nursing or medical text for more complete consideration of the care and management of patients with cardiovascular disorders.

RELATIONSHIP OF THE CEREBRAL BLOOD SUPPLY TO THE CARDIOVASCULAR SYSTEM

The basic physiological function of the circulatory system is to deliver oxygen and metabolites to the tissues and remove the end products of metabolism from them. This is accomplished by means of the blood, which is propelled through the vascular system by the pumping heart. Figure 8-1 is a schematic representation of the right and left heart, showing the route of blood flow from the peripheral venous circulation through the pulmonary circulation and back into the arterial peripheral circulation [3].

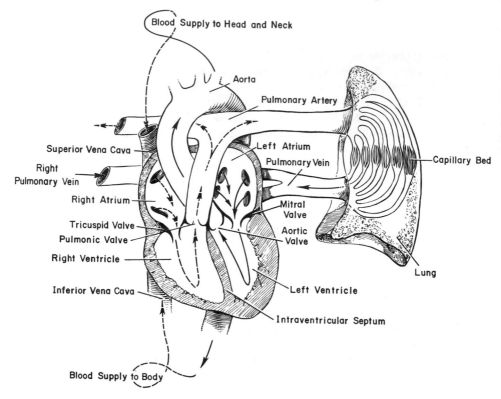

Figure 8-1
Morphological and functional anatomy of the heart in relation to the great vessels and lungs. (From Gerald H. Whipple, Mary Ann Peterson, Virginia Haines, Edward Learner, and Elizabeth L. McKinnon, Acute Coronary Care. *Boston: Little, Brown, 1972.)*

The right heart receives venous blood and pumps it to the lungs for exchange of oxygen and carbon dioxide. The left heart receives oxygenated blood from the lungs and returns it to the systemic arterial circulation. The right atrium receives blood from the venous circulation via the superior and inferior vena cavae and from the coronary sinus. The inferior vena cava returns venous blood from the trunk and the legs, while the superior vena cava carries venous blood back from the head and arms. The coronary sinus drains venous blood from the coronary circulation of the heart muscle. Venous blood is pumped from the right atrium through the tricuspid valve into the right ventricle. With each contraction of the ventricles, blood is pumped from the right ventricle through the pulmonic valve into the pulmonary artery. The pulmonary artery bifurcates to carry venous blood via its branches into both lungs for oxygenation. The relationship between pulmonary circulation and the function of the lungs in oxygen transport has been discussed in Chapter 7. Oxygenated blood is returned to the left atrium by the four pulmonary veins and passes through the mitral or bicuspid valve into the left ventricle. From the left ventricle oxygenated blood is pumped through the aortic valve into the aorta for circulation to the entire body [3].

The two main coronary arteries, which supply the musculature of the heart, originate from the aorta just above the aortic valve [3]. The aorta arches after it arises from the heart, then courses downward following the contour of the spinal column. Three main arteries emerge from the arch of the aorta: (1) the brachiocephalic artery, which gives rise to the right common carotid artery and the right subclavian artery; (2) the left common carotid artery; and (3) the left subclavian artery. The blood supply to the brain is derived from the two internal carotid arteries, which arise from the first bifurcation of the common carotids, and from the two vertebral arteries, which arise from the first branch of the subclavian arteries. The vessels of the head and neck are usually considered as a unit in discussions of cerebrovascular function [26].

When the body is at rest, approximately 5,000 ml of blood per minute normally pass through a given point in the circulatory system. This is called the *cardiac output,* since it represents the amount of blood pumped by the left ventricle into the aorta during that unit of time. *Venous return* is the quantity of blood per minute flowing into the right atrium from the veins. Blood flow throughout the circulatory system is caused by the pumping action of the heart. There is relatively little resistance to blood flow in the large blood vessels but considerable resistance in the arterioles and capillaries. In order to assure blood flow through these smaller vessels, the heart must pump the blood into the arteries under high pressure. *Blood pressure* refers to the force exerted by the blood against the vessel wall. The standard unit of blood pressure is stated in millimeters of mercury (mm Hg) [13]. The arterial pressure fluctuates with the intermittent pumping action of the heart. The pressure at the height of the pulse is called the *systolic pressure,* and the pressure at its lowest point is called the *diastolic pressure.* The difference between the systolic and diastolic pressure is called the *pulse pressure.* Pulse pressure is affected by the *stroke volume output* of the heart, that is, the amount of blood pumped by each ventricle with each heart beat. Pulse pressure is also affected by the compliance or distensibility of the arteries [13].

Thus stroke volume output can be influenced by many factors, including an increased heart rate, a decrease in peripheral resistance, and an increase in mean circulatory pressure. Only two major factors alter arterial compliance, however; a change in mean arterial pressure and pathological changes in the arterial walls that affect their distensibility. Arterial pressure is the product of cardiac output times the total peripheral resistance. An increase in either one of these two factors can cause *hypertension,* which is an elevated arterial pressure. Loss of elasticity of the vessel walls, which usually occurs with old age, is called *arteriosclerosis.* With arteriosclerosis, the arteries become fibrous and sometimes calcified. This condition reduces arterial compliance greatly [13].

The cardiovascular system has three basic controls that regulate the circulation of blood: (1) the ability of the heart to respond automatically to an increased input of blood, or the *Frank-Starling Mechanism*; (2) the ability of blood vessels to adjust their blood flow to the needs of the surrounding tissues, or the *local blood flow regulation*; and (3) the ability of the circulation to regulate extracellular fluid volume and blood volume in conjunction with the kidneys and interstitial fluid system, or the *fluid volume feedback mechanism* [13]. Under normal conditions cardiac output is controlled by the venous return. The tissues in various parts of the body control their own blood flow in accordance with their specific needs. The quantity of blood that flows through the peripheral tissues is returned by the veins to the right atrium. Because of the enormous differences in need between different organ systems and the fluctuations of need within various systems, the heart must adapt itself constantly to widely varying amounts of incoming blood. It does so according to the *Frank-Starling law.* This law states that the more the heart is filled during diastole, the greater the quantity of blood pumped into the aorta. This is possible because, when cardiac muscle is stretched by an increased amount of blood entering the heart, the muscle will contract with greater force, thereby pumping more blood into the arteries. Local blood flow through the tissues is regulated so that each tissue's needs are met exactly. This is brought about by specific factors within the various tissues, acting upon the smooth muscle of the arterioles that supply the tissues and causing these vessels to contract or dilate in response to the metabolic needs of the tissues [13].

These two mechanisms for control of cardiac output presuppose an adequate blood volume and an arterial pressure sufficient to force the blood through the peripheral tissues as it is needed. Both of these conditions are met by the fluid volume feedback mechanism. Ingestion of water and salt increases both extracellular fluid volume and blood volume. Increased blood volume increases the amount of blood available to be pumped by the heart, thereby increasing cardiac output and arterial pressure. The increased arterial pressure will cause the kidneys to excrete both salt and water. When the arterial pressure is high enough to cause excretion of salt and water at the same rate as they are taken in, the extracellular fluid volume, the blood volume, and the arterial pressure will be stabilized, thereby allowing an adequate peripheral blood flow [13]. (Regulation of fluid and electrolyte balance is discussed in detail in Chapter 9.) Diseases of the heart, blood vessels, lungs, and kidneys can disrupt the normal balance and adversely affect arterial pressure, cardiac output, and the blood supply to the brain.

THE MAJOR CARDIOVASCULAR CONDITIONS ASSOCIATED WITH STROKE

The major cause of death in the United States is arterial degeneration [11]. The most prevalent cardiovascular disorder is hypertension, and the second most prevalent is ischemic heart disease [11]. Cerebral thrombosis, which accounts for one third of all strokes, can result from atherosclerotic stenosis or occlusion occurring in the carotid and vertebral arteries of the neck as well as in the intracranial vessels. Cerebral embolism, the cause of about thirty percent of all strokes, is in the majority of cases associated with mitral stenosis, myocardial infarction, and atrial fibrillation. Intracerebral hemorrhage due to hypertension accounts for about eleven percent of all strokes. These figures for frequency of each type of stroke have been reported by the Harvard Cooperative Stroke Registry [17].

Hypertension

Hypertension is usually asymptomatic until it results in secondary organ damage. Therefore, unless noted on a routine examination, it can go undetected until it involves the cardiac, renal, or central nervous system. Damage to the heart from hypertension is the result of increased blood pressure exerted against the left ventricle, which can cause ischemia and angina pectoris. In the coronary arteries the high pressure can cause rapid development of arteriosclerosis with subsequent occlusion of these vessels and myocardial infarction. A similar effect can occur in vessels throughout the body, resulting in clots, weakening of the arteriosclerotic areas, rupture, and hemorrhage. The most significant areas of arterial damage due to hypertension are found in the cerebral and renal arteries.

Hypertension can be caused by (1) a number of conditions affecting the kidneys; (2) endocrine disorders, including pheochromocytoma, which is an adrenal tumor that secretes a vasoconstrictor; (3) any one of the heart disorders that cause an increased stroke volume or an increased cardiac output; and (4) coarctation or arteriosclerosis of the aorta. In addition there is *idiopathic* or *essential hypertension,* for which no specific cause has been identified and which accounts for approximately ninety percent of all cases of hypertension [13]. Heredity and racial factors seem to play a significant role in its development, and studies suggest that excessive salt intake is an important etiological factor [10].

Treatment of hypertension is usually directed toward lowering systemic vascular resistance and may include the use of antihypertensive drugs to inhibit the vasoconstrictor impulses of the sympathetic nervous system. Hypertension is also treated by reduction of intravascular volume and cardiac output through diuretics and peripheral vasodilators, which relax smooth muscle. Therapy must be maintained throughout the patient's lifetime [10].

Atherosclerosis

Atherosclerosis is a patchy form of arteriosclerosis that consists of fatty streaks or raised plaques in the intimal lining of the arteries [11]. These atheromatous plaques are lipid deposits containing large amounts of cholesterol. They are associated with degeneration of the arterial wall and affect the larger vessels. Fibroblasts gradually infiltrate the degenerated areas, and calcium often precipitates with the lipids, causing sclerosis of the arteries (arteriosclerosis). Arteriosclerotic arteries have lost their distensibility and are likely to rupture because of their areas of degeneration. They also become thrombosed easily because of the atheromatous plaques that protrude into the lumen of the vessels [13]. Atherosclerotic lesions, which are irregularly distributed throughout the circulatory system, are found predominantly in the arch of the aorta, the femoral and popliteal arteries of the legs, and the coronary, precerebral, and cerebral arteries. There are many theories concerning the causes of atherosclerosis. The two major factors appear to be hypertension and hyperlipidemia. Other risk factors associated with premature development of atherosclerosis are cigarette smoking, diabetes mellitus, physical inactivity, obesity, emotional stress, and a family history of premature atherosclerosis [11].

Hyperlipidemia refers to elevated triglyceride and cholesterol concentrations in the plasma. Triglycerides are chemical compounds, composed predominantly of fatty acids, that are derived from foods and also synthesized by the body. Their main function is to provide energy for various metabolic processes [13]. Cholesterol is a chemical compound synthesized from the products of fatty acid metabolism. It is derived from food but is also formed to some degree by all cells in the body, predominantly by the liver. The membranous structures of all body cells contain cholesterol, which, together with the triglycerides and phospholipids, serves to maintain the physical integrity of the cells. Cholesterol is also converted by the liver into cholic acid to form bile salts used in the digestion of fats. It is involved in formation of hormones and in the prevention of water evaporation from the skin [13].

No specific plasma concentrations have been defined as absolutely constituting hyperlipidemia. Research on the incidence of premature ischemic heart disease indicates that an increased risk can be detected when the cholesterol level is higher than 220 mg per 100 ml of blood. The Seattle study showed that about one third of cases of hyperlipidemia associated with premature ischemic heart disease are due to genetic disorders [11]. The remainder is felt to be due to dietary habits.

Cholesterol levels are related to consumption of animal fats, while triglyceride levels are related to carbohydrate intake, caloric balance, and alcohol consumption. In adults under fifty-five years of age a cholesterol level of 250 mg per 100 ml or a triglyceride level greater than 200 mg per 100 ml is considered to warrant medical attention. It has not been proved conclusively that reducing hyperlipidemia will halt the progression of atherosclerosis. However, several studies have shown that lowering of cholesterol levels by diet decreases the incidence of complications from ischemic heart disease [11]. To decrease plasma levels of cholesterol it is important to maintain a diet low in both saturated fats and cholesterol composition and also to increase the intake of polyunsaturated fats. When increased quantities of cholesterol are ingested, the liver compensates by synthesizing smaller amounts; but ingestion of saturated fats will stimulate the liver to produce more cholesterol while ingestion of fats containing polyunsaturated fatty acids will actually lower the blood cholesterol level [13]. The diet usually prescribed to prevent or reduce hyperlipidemia emphasizes a decrease in saturated fats and foods high in cholesterol, elimination of alcohol, and balanced caloric intake to maintain a normal weight for age, sex, and body build. A reduction in intake of refined sugars and an increase in intake of fresh fruits and vegetables and use of polyunsaturated fats is encouraged [4, 13].

Ischemic heart disease

As atherosclerotic plaques build up within the arteries, the involved vessels gradually become occluded, diminishing the blood supply to the surrounding tissues. With complete obstruction, lack of tissue perfusion results in necrosis. The clinical picture of cerebral infarction resulting from occlusion of the cerebral and precerebral arteries has been described in Chapter 1. Atherosclerosis that causes occlusion of the coronary arteries with myocardial anoxia is called *ischemic heart disease.*

ANGINA PECTORIS

The diminished perfusion of the myocardium causes *angina pectoris,* the characteristic pain associated with transient myocardial ischemia. It is most often related to physical exertion or to emotional stress, generally subsides with rest, and is relieved by nitroglycerine. There is no noninvasive technique for demonstrating the presence of atherosclerosis. Consequently it is not usually diagnosed until one of its complications occurs. Since myocardial ischemia is not necessarily detected on an electrocardiogram taken with the patient at rest, a stress test or exercise tolerance test may be carried out in which the cardiac workload is increased, thereby increasing myocardial oxygen consumption and inducing a myocardial ischemia that will be reflected in the electrocardiogram [4]. If a patient has established angina pectoris refractory to medical management and is a candidate for coronary artery bypass surgery, coronary angiography may be performed to provide a definitive diagnosis of atherosclerosis of the coronary arteries and an estimate of the severity of the lesions. There is, however, a significant risk of morbidity and mortality associated with this procedure [15].

MYOCARDIAL INFARCTION

Acute myocardial infarction usually results from a complete occlusion of one of the coronary vessels or its branches due to thrombus or embolus or from rupture of an atherosclerotic vessel [4, 11]. Lack of oxygen supply to the surrounding area of the myocardium will result in cessation of cell metabolism, failure of the cell transport system with accumulation of lactic acid, disintegration of the cellular membrane, and release of cellular components into the extracellular fluid [4]. The buildup of lactic acid stimulates the autonomic nerves, producing the crushing chest pain characteristic of an acute myocardial infarction. The cessation of cellular function contributes to cardiac dysrhythmias, congestive heart failure, and shock [4]. It is important to note that, while acute chest pain is the most common symptom associated with myocardial infarction, in at least 15–20% of all cases there is no pain. In such cases, more common among the elderly and in patients with diabetes mellitus, the presenting complaint may be a sudden onset of dyspnea, loss of consciousness, or confusion [21].

The diagnosis of myocardial infarction is confirmed by the electrocardiogram and by elevated serum enzyme levels. Acute myocardial infarction constitutes a medical emergency requiring immediate intervention. The primary objectives of management are prevention of death from arrhythmia and prevention of extension of the infarction. Ideally the patient is placed in a coronary care unit where emergency drugs and equipment are readily available, continuous electrocardiogram monitoring is provided, and a highly trained nursing staff can recognize arrhythmias and is authorized to regulate antiarrhythmic drugs, initiate resuscitation procedures, and apply countershock in an emergency [21]. Immediate therapy for the patient with acute myocardial infarction includes alleviation of pain, administration of supplemental oxygen, and control of complications [4].

The two major complications of myocardial infarction are arrhythmias and pump failure. *Ventricular fibrillation* is the most common cause of death from arrhythmia [21]. Unless ventricular fibrillation is recognized and treated immediately, death will ensue almost instantly, since the chaotic contractions of the ventricles prevent development of sufficient pressure to propel the blood forward, and circulation thereby stops. Consequently all ventricular ectopic activity in patients with myocardial infarction is treated prophylactically by suppression with lidocaine [21]. These patients may also be treated by *cardioversion,* or delivery of an electrical discharge to the patient's chest by means of a synchronized capacitor, to restore normal rhythm to the heart. This technique can be used for various arrhythmias that are refractory to treatment with antiarrhythmic agents [16]. With ventricular fibrillation cardioversion must be applied promptly, since cessation of circulation for more than 2–4 minutes will result in irreversible damage to the heart and brain [23].

Pump failure is the major cause of death in hospitalized patients with acute myocardial infarction [21]. This syndrome, often referred to as cardiogenic shock, is caused by a marked reduction in the quantity of contracting myocardium. The following signs are present: (1) systolic intraarterial pressure of less than 90 mm Hg that has dropped 30 mm Hg from the previous reading; (2) cold, moist skin with cyanosis; (3) dulled sensorium; (4) oliguria of less than 20 ml per hour; and (5) lack of improvement in condition after pain has been relieved and oxygen administered. Cardiogenic shock, which carries a mortality rate of more than 95% and occurs in approximately twenty percent of all patients with myocardial infarction, is a severe form of left ventricular failure [21].

Heart failure

Heart failure is the failure of the heart to pump blood adequately to meet the metabolic needs of the body. Since the right and left sides of the heart constitute two separate pumping systems, the failure may be left- or right-sided. Heart failure may also be described as high- or low-output and as acute or chronic [5].

CONGESTIVE HEART FAILURE
Congestive heart failure is a chronic state of combined left- and right-sided failure [4]. Patients with coronary artery disease, hypertension, myocardial infarction, and valvular disease usually have a low cardiac output failure as opposed to patients with metabolic disease, pulmonary emphysema, and anemias, who generally have a high cardiac output failure [5].

The three mechanisms available to the heart for maintaining adequate cardiac output are tachycardia, cardiac dilatation, and cardiac hypertrophy. With heart disease these three adaptive mechanisms eventually become ineffective [4]. Factors leading to impairment of cardiac output are (1) myocardial disease, including coronary atherosclerosis, myocardial infarction, and metabolic or inflammatory conditions affecting the myocardium; (2) overloading of the heart volume in the presence of aortic stenosis, arterial or pulmonary hypertension, pulmonic stenosis, and mitral or aortic insufficiency; (3) interference with filling of the chambers of the heart during diastole because of mitral stenosis, constrictive pericarditis, cardiac tamponade, blood loss, or shock; and (4) disturbances of heart rate or rhythm such as tachycardia, atrial flutter, or fibrillation, with rapid ventricular rate, ventricular tachycardia, sinus bradycardia, and second-degree and complete heart block [4].

LEFT VENTRICULAR FAILURE
Heart failure usually results in a buildup of fluid behind one or both ventricles. An accumulation of fluid behind the left ventricle results in pulmonary congestion, or *left-sided* or *left ventricular failure*, the classic symptom of which is dyspnea. In its severest form left-sided failure becomes pulmonary edema. Fluid from the capillaries seeps into the alveoli, causing hypoxia, hypercapnea, severe dyspnea, and intense anxiety. This is a life-threatening situation requiring immediate attention. Treatment includes rotating tourniquets to the extremities, placing the patient in a sitting position, and administering morphine, 100% concentration of oxygen under positive pressure, aminophylline, and digitalis [4, 5].

RIGHT VENTRICULAR FAILURE
Right ventricular failure occurs when venous blood returning to the right heart meets resistance because of residual blood in the ventricle or atrium. It is usually a result of left-sided failure but may also be due to chronic obstructive lung disease, in which case it is referred to as *cor pulmonale*. The classic symptom in either case is edema, which may be accompanied by hepatomegaly, ascites, jugular vein distention, oliguria, and pleural and pericardial effusions [4].

When failure is severe or prolonged, both sides of the heart become involved [5]. Because, in left-sided failure, blood remains in the left ventricle at the end of systole, the left atrium, pulmonary veins, capillaries, and arteries as well as the right ventricle are unable to empty completely. This will result in dilation of the right ventricle, eventual loss of contractility, and consequent right-sided failure. In like manner, a decrease in left ventricular function can result from right ventricular failure. The stroke volume of the left ventricle is determined by the amount of blood received from the right heart. If the right heart does not empty completely, the left ventricular stroke volume is diminished, thereby decreasing cardiac output [4]. With chronic congestive heart failure, manifestations of both right and left ventricular failure are revealed by chest x-ray, electrocardiogram, venous pressure, and blood gas determinations.

Therapy for heart failure is directed toward (1) elimination or treatment of the underlying or precipitating factors; (2) control of the failure; (3) reduction of the cardiac work load by rest and weight reduction, if necessary; (4) improvement of myocardial contractility with pharmacological agents such as digitalis, epinephrine, isoproterenol, and dopamine; and (5) control of extracellular fluid by means of dietary sodium restriction, diuretic therapy, and mechanical removal such as thoracentesis, paracentesis or dialysis, if necessary [5]. It should be noted that with congestive failure secondary to myocardial infarction, digitalis cannot be expected to improve the contractility of the infarcted tissue [21].

PUMP FAILURE

Ross et al. have stated that with *pump failure* or cardiogenic shock syndrome following myocardial infarction, left ventricular function may be impaired in the absence of the usual manifestations of left-sided heart failure [21]. When a major coronary artery is obstructed, the resultant infarction greatly reduces the amount of contracting myocardium. This impaired myocardial function causes the arterial pressure to drop, thereby reducing perfusion of blood through the coronary arteries and cutting down nourishment to the myocardium. The diminished coronary blood flow will contribute to extension of the infarction. Thus a vicious cycle is set up in which the complications of arrhythmias and acidosis that result from inadequate tissue perfusion serve to perpetuate the cycle with progressive deterioration of left ventricular function.

Therapy for this state is directed toward raising arterial pressure to maintain coronary perfusion and ensure left ventricular filling pressure. Patients with shock syndrome require continuous monitoring of arterial pressure and frequent monitoring of cardiac output. Control of pain and administration of a 100% concentration of oxygen are also necessary. Hypovolemia is corrected to assure that vascular volume is sufficient to maintain cardiac output, and norepinephrine (Levophed) is administered to maintain systolic pressure around 90 mm Hg so that the vital organs are perfused. An intraaortic balloon pump may be used. The balloon is inserted via the femoral artery and inflates in diastole to enhance coronary artery as well as peripheral blood flow and deflates in systole to reduce the afterload that the left ventricle must contract against [21].

Endocardial and valvular heart disease

Cerebral infarction may result from hypotension complicating myocardial infarction, since the lowered arterial pressure will reduce perfusion of the brain [26]. Embolic stroke can occur with myocardial infarction, which is due to thrombosis of a coronary artery, if embolic material becomes dislodged from a clot that has formed over an infarcted area of the left ventricular endocardium. Vegetation on the heart valves resulting from endocarditis is another source of cerebral emboli: it may be dislodged by dysrhythmias.

Cardiac dysrhythmias

Chronic atrial fibrillation is a common cause of cerebral embolism, and dysrhythmias complicating acute myocardial infarction can precipitate cerebral ischemia and infarction when a clot becomes dislodged from the left atrium [2].

Dysrhythmias include disturbances of heart rhythm, rate, and conduction [23]. Some occur without evidence of organic heart disease. Others are related to specific forms of heart disease, electrolyte imbalance, circulatory disturbance, or drug toxicity [23]. Frequently the nurse is in a position to detect a newly arising dysrhythmia in the acutely ill patient. Therefore it is important that she be able to recognize these abnormalities and understand what action is necessary. There are a number of different dysrhythmias. The following six are life-threatening and require immediate intervention: (1) ventricular tachycardia, (2) ventricular fibrillation, (3) ventricular flutter, (4) ventricular standstill or arrest, (5) severe sinus bradycardia, and (6) complete atrioventricular heart block. The first four have already been discussed briefly as complications of acute myocardial infarction.

SINUS BRADYCARDIA
Sinus bradycardia is characterized by a slow heart rate. It may indicate dysfunction of the sinus node or of atrioventricular (AV) conduction as well as increased intracerebral pressure [23]. Contraction of the heart is regulated by a cardiac system that generates electrical impulses to initiate contractions of the heart muscle and conducts these impulses throughout the heart. The *sinoatrial (S-A) node*, located in the right atrium, is the normal pacemaker of the heart [13]. Impulses arriving here are conducted through the atria, forcing them to contract, and on to the *atrioventricular (A-V) node* and its fibers, which delay further conduction of the impulse to the ventricles until the atria have emptied completely. Specialized fibers from the AV node, which conduct cardiac impulses to the ventricles, divide into two branches, referred to as the left and right *bundle branches* [13].

HEART BLOCK
Heart block is a pathological delay in conduction of the excitation impulses from the sinus node to the ventricles. It is classified according to severity as first-, second-, or third-degree atrioventricular (AV) block. First-degree heart block by electrocardiographic evidence but without other manifestation of disease is not treated. Second-degree heart block is further classified as Mobitz type I, also called Wenckebach, and Mobitz type II. Type I is usually transitory and requires no treatment unless hemodynamic disturbances result [23]. Type II is more serious and may progress suddenly to complete heart block. *Stokes-Adams syncopal attacks* may also occur without warning [23]. These attacks, which may be intermittent or persistent, are caused by a sudden reduction in cardiac output and cerebral blood flow. When conduction of cardiac impulses is disturbed by a complete atrioventricular block, the pacemaker below the block ceases to function, and syncope occurs. Usually the attacks involve a momentary weakness, cardiac standstill, and loss of consciousness due to impairment of cerebral circulation. Longer periods of asystole may occur, however, with prolonged cerebral ischemia and sometimes permanent neurological impairment [1]. Third-degree block is the most severe form and usually is referred to as complete heart block. With this condition the conduction of impulses for contraction of the heart muscle is so disorganized that the atria and ventricles maintain separate and independent rhythms [23]. Myocardial infarction is the most common cause of complete heart block. The patient with second-degree type II or complete heart block is always at risk of a Stokes-Adams attack, which can be fatal or result in cerebral infarction. Therefore, treatment is directed toward prevention of this.

Insertion of a temporary transvenous pacemaker or implantation of a permanent pacemaker is usually the therapy [23].

ATRIAL FIBRILLATION
Atrial fibrillation may develop in patients with digitalis intoxication or valvular, atherosclerotic, or hypertensive heart disease. In atrial fibrillation, the sinoatrial node has lost control of heart rhythm. There is no effective contraction of the atria, so the AV node and ventricles continue to receive very rapid and irregular stimuli simultaneously. Some of these stimuli are blocked by the AV node, while other impulses are conducted to the ventricles, causing rapid irregular ventricular contraction. The ventricles do not have time to fill adequately between successive beats, and cardiac output therefore decreases. Because the atria do not empty, blood stagnates, leading to thrombus formation. Embolic material that breaks away can then reach both the pulmonary and the systemic circulation. Atrial fibrillation can be persistent or paroxysmal. It may be treated by (1) allowing rhythms to remain irregular and controlling ventricular rate with digitalis, (2) using antiarrhythmic agents such as quinidine, or (3) using cardioversion to restore sinus rhythm. The choice of therapy will depend upon the patient's underlying problem and its duration as well as whether or not failure is present. When this dysrhythmia is chronic, and particularly when it accompanies mitral stenosis, anticoagulation therapy may be initiated to prevent thromboembolism. Thromboembolism is a common complication and accounts for 20% of deaths in patients with mitral stenosis [23]. Mitral stenosis is generally the result of one or more acute attacks of rheumatic fever. The diseased mitral valve becomes calcified with time, and thrombus formation takes place on the valve leaflets and in the left atrium. With long-standing mitral stenosis atrial arrhythmias tend to occur. Atrial fibrillation can cause clots in the left atrium to break off and enter the systemic circulation, lodging most frequently in the vessels of the brain, kidneys, and extremities [6].

Thromboembolism

Thromboembolism occurs commonly in patients with large myocardial infarctions and congestive failure as well as in patients with mitral stenosis and dysrhythmias. Venous thrombosis does not have a specific etiological factor, but it is well known that common risk factors include (1) prolonged bed rest, (2) severe illness, (3) immobilization, and (4) congestive heart failure [25]. Patients with stroke may be at risk of thromboembolism due to underlying cardiovascular and lung disease, bed rest imposed as treatment in the acute stage of stroke, and lack of exercise because of paralysis or coma.

The function of the venous system is to carry carbon dioxide and other products of cell metabolism in the blood away from the tissues. The veins are constructed with valves that prevent a backward flow of blood. These structures are particularly important in the legs. The valves are assisted by muscular activity that serves to compress the vessels, thereby propelling the venous blood back toward the heart. When these valves are defective, pooling of blood in the extremities can occur; and with lack of exercise, venous pressure in the legs will rise and predispose to edema. Prolonged venous stasis and edema of the lower legs can lead to skin ulcer formation.

Thrombophlebitis

It is known that thrombophlebitis can occur whenever there is trauma, infection, or chemical irritation of a vein. Prolonged intravenous therapy or administration of irritating substances via the intravenous route will certainly contribute to the development of phlebitis. A thrombus forms in the sinus of the venous valve and attaches to the wall of the vein, most often in the legs. As the thrombus increases in size, it can obstruct the lumen. The greatest danger with thrombophlebitis is that the material obstructing blood flow through the affected vessel will become detached and will be propelled into the pulmonary circulation.

Thrombophlebitis is generally classified as deep or superficial. Superficial thrombophlebitis involves the saphenous vein, while deep thrombophlebitis involves the iliofemoral, femoropopliteal, and small veins of the calf. The iliac and femoral veins most often give rise to large emboli, which may become lodged in the pulmonary artery. Superficial thrombophlebitis is manifested by local pain, swelling, tenderness, and erythema. Deep thrombophlebitis often has no apparent symptoms or signs and may not be detected until a pulmonary embolism has occurred [25]. Mild calf pain and swelling, however, may be found upon pressing the calf from side to side, and Homan's sign may be elicited by forced dorsiflexion of the ankle, which will result in pain in the calf muscles.

Treatment usually involves bed rest, elevation of the affected extremity, and administration of an analgesic. Anticoagulants are generally prescribed for deep vessel involvement. Sometimes elastic hose or bandages are used. It is most important that the nurse check frequently to be certain these are in place smoothly and properly, as often one finds they are actually serving as a tourniquet rather than enhancing blood flow. Moist heat must be applied with *extreme* caution to assure that the tissues are not damaged by the heat or macerated by the moisture. If anticoagulant therapy has been instituted, the patient must be observed carefully for signs of bleeding and protected from injury.

Pulmonary thromboembolism

Pulmonary thromboembolism carries a very high incidence of mortality. According to Moser, this complication is responsible for more than 50,000 deaths in the United States each year [18] ; 60% of all cases coming to autopsy show evidence of thromboembolism. He cites stasis of the blood, vessel wall abnormalities, and alterations in the coagulation system as the three factors involved in the development of thromboembolism.

The immediate effect of a pulmonary embolism is a partial or complete obstruction of the arterial blood flow to the lung. The consequences depend upon the size of the embolism. Unlike cerebral and myocardial tissue, the lung has three avenues for obtaining oxygen for tissue perfusion: the arterial circulation, the bronchial circulation, and the airways. Therefore pulmonary embolism rarely results in infarction of surrounding lung tissue [18]. The involved area of the lung will be ventilated but not perfused, and atelectasis will be noted within approximately 24—48 hours. Because the vascular capacity of the lung is reduced, the resistance to pulmonary blood flow will be increased, thereby causing pulmonary hypertension, acute right ventricular failure, and a decreased cardiac output. The most common symptom is a sudden onset of unexplained dyspnea [18].

Most pulmonary emboli result from deep venous thrombosis. The larger ones are usually from the iliofemoral veins. Activities that cause a sudden increase in venous return are contributing factors to dislodgment of a thrombus, such as movement of extremities that have been immobilized for some time; the Valsalva maneuver, which creates an increase in intrathoracic pressure, causing sudden distention of the large pelvic veins. Embolic material dislodged from a thrombus will travel through the great veins into the right heart and into the pulmonary artery. Depending on the size of the embolism, it can become lodged within the pulmonary artery itself or in any of its smaller branches [4].

When a major artery is occluded, dyspnea may be accompanied by cyanosis, shock, signs of right heart failure, tachypnea, tachycardia, and fever. When small vessels are affected, no symptoms may be present. Pleuritic chest pain and hemoptysis will be found with pulmonary infarction. Chest x-ray, lung scan, or angiography may be used to confirm the diagnosis. Since most pulmonary emboli resolve in time, therapy is most often supportive and includes bed rest, oxygen, and anticoagulant agents. In severe cases, plication or ligation of the inferior vena cava or insertion of a vena cava umbrella may be undertaken to prevent emboli from reaching the lungs. In rare instances pulmonary embolectomy is performed [4, 21].

In caring for the patient with stroke, the nurse must be alert to signs of pulmonary embolism and take measures to prevent it. Turning, positioning, and range of motion exercises (outlined in Chapter 12) are all effective in preventing venous stasis. When carrying out these procedures, however, the nurse must be careful not to dislodge thrombotic material in patients with vascular disease. Since straining at stool can precipitate dislodgment of a clot, the nurse should note whether the patient is constipated or not. When adequate fluids and roughage in the diet are not sufficient to correct this problem, the physician should be contacted concerning the possibility of using fecal softeners or cathartics [4].

Peripheral artery occlusion

Sudden occlusion of a peripheral artery can result from a thrombus, embolism or injury and is usually due to the same disease that underlies the stroke. The most common source of embolism is the heart. Rheumatic heart disease involving the mitral and aortic valves may give rise to emboli, particularly if there is atrial fibrillation. Prosthetic valves may also be the source of emboli. Trauma due to intra-arterial needles or catheters can dislodge atheromatous plaques. When an artery becomes occluded, the blood supply to the surrounding tissue can be completely cut off if there is not adequate collateral circulation. Arterial spasm will cause severe pain, numbness, and paresthesia. The peripheral pulses distal to the occlusion will be absent and the affected extremity pale and cold, with a sharp demarcation between the normally perfused tissue and the ischemic tissue. Loss of sensation and of motor function will follow. When sudden arterial occlusion occurs, the affected extremity should be placed in a dependent position [4, 25]. When collateral circulation is inadequate, immediate surgical intervention is necessary to remove the clot. Otherwise irreversible tissue damage requiring amputation will occur within six hours [25].

CARDIOVASCULAR ASSESSMENT

The nurse's skill as an observer is vital to identification of all the cardiovascular problems outlined in the chapter. An alert and oriented patient can usually express his problems and describe his symptoms when he is in pain or aware of a somatic dysfunction. The patient who has suffered a stroke may be lethargic, confused, or in a coma and be prevented by language and speech difficulties or perceptual disorders from communicating in the usual manner. A patient who is aphasic or has a diminished sensorium will be unable to express symptoms of chest pain or headache. The astute nurse can identify such symptoms by observing the patient's facial expression, restlessness, or other signs of discomfort and distress. It is most important that any change in vital signs or behavior be investigated. One must not assume that all symptoms and behavior are directly related to the stroke. If the patient appears to have leg discomfort, he may have thrombophlebitis. If he is constantly rubbing his chest, he may have chest pain due to a pulmonary embolism or myocardial infarction.

The components of a cardiovascular assessment are familiar to all nurses. They include monitoring of vital signs and apical pulses, observation of skin color and temperature, observation of respiratory pattern, and checking of peripheral pulses. The condition of the extremities is of particular significance, especially for a patient on bed rest. The legs should be inspected daily for signs of swelling, tenderness, or temperature change. A change in skin temperature is of particular importance if it involves only one extremity or a localized area, as this may indicate thrombophlebitis or arterial occlusion. A sudden increase in coldness may indicate a peripheral embolism.

Checking of peripheral pulses is a vital part of the cardiovascular assessment. Absence or the diminished quality of a peripheral pulse may be the first indication that blood flow has been impaired. Pulses should be palpated where arteries lie close to the body surface over a bone or other firm surface that will provide support when pressure is exerted on the artery. The most common sites are the brachial, radial, femoral, popliteal, dorsalis pedis and posterior tibialis arteries. *The radial pulse* on the flexor surface of the wrist is generally used in checking vital signs. The *brachial pulse* is found on the medial aspect of the arm in the groove between the biceps and triceps muscles. The *femoral* pulse is palpated where the artery passes through the groin in the femoral triangle. The *popliteal* pulse is felt in the back of the knee. The femoral artery becomes the popliteal as it enters the knee in the popliteal fossa. The *dorsalis pedis* pulse is located on the dorsum of the foot and is usually felt between the first and second metatarsal bones. It should be noted, however, that this pulse is absent in about 10% of the population. The *posterior tibialis* pulse can be felt just posterior to the ankle bone on the inner aspect of the ankle.

Under normal conditions the pulse is felt immediately. The artery is pressed gently against the bone or underlying structure to occlude the vessel, then gradually and gently released. As blood flow resumes, the pulsation is palpable. Both rate and rhythm of the pulse should be noted. The strength of the beat may be typified as full, bounding, weak, or faint. The strength of the pulsation should be compared to the same pulse in the opposite extremity as well as to the next proximal pulse. Color, temperature, and skin condition will also indicate circulatory insufficiency. Numbness and tingling, which may be caused by poor oxygenation of the tissues, can denote ischemic neuropathy. When oxygenation to an extremity is compromised, it will cause increasingly severe pain [24].

Because of the interrelationship between the cardiovascular and cerebrovascular systems, the nurse must be constantly aware of the stroke patient's cardiovascular status. Any signs of deterioration in the patient's condition must be promptly reported to the responsible physician. The drugs used most frequently in the treatment of patients with cardiovascular disorders will be discussed next. The effective therapeutic action of these agents as well as their adverse effects and unpleasant side effects will generally be manifested by an alteration in the signs that the nurse observes in her assessment of cardiovascular function.

OVERVIEW OF THE MAJOR DRUGS USED IN THE MANAGEMENT OF CARDIOVASCULAR DISORDERS

It is important to remember that drugs have the power to harm as well as to help the patient. Epidemiological studies have shown that drug-induced disease is a large and growing problem, with 5–30% of hospitalized patients having adverse reactions to drugs during hospitalization. The probability of experiencing an adverse reaction is related directly to the number of different drugs taken during one time period [9]. Although the physician initiates orders for medications, the nurse who carries out these orders is responsible for her own actions. It is not enough to know the dosage, route of administration, and expected therapeutic response. Before administering any medication the nurse must be familiar with (1) possible side effects, (2) toxicity, (3) rate of absorption, (4) rate and route of excretion, (5) factors that may increase toxicity or decrease therapeutic response, (6) the drug's interaction with other pharmacological agents, and (7) what immediate action should be taken in the event of an adverse reaction. It is her (or his) professional responsibility to keep abreast of the most current information concerning any drugs that are ordered for patients under her care. Since patients vary in the way they absorb, metabolize, and excrete drugs, it is also her responsibility to be aware of differences in response of various patients and of any history of allergy or previous untoward reaction to pharmacological agents.

Pharmacological agents are integral to the management of patients with cardiovascular disorders. Because of the critical nature and instability of the patient's condition during the acute stage of illness, many different drugs in varying dosages may be ordered in rapid succession. Often these preparations carry the risk of potentially fatal complications. Factors such as congestive heart failure and hepatic or renal impairment can have a significant effect on the absorption, metabolism, and excretion of drugs. This is particularly true of drugs that have a cumulative effect. Since most drugs are administered intravenously in the acute phase, the risk of untoward effect is compounded. In most instances patients with cardiovascular problems will have to take some form of medication for the rest of their lives. Often they are discharged on drugs that carry a very high risk of toxicity. It is the nurse's responsibility to see that the patient or a responsible family member knows what the medications are, what they are for, precisely when and how much to take, what side effects may be expected, and when to seek medical attention.

This responsibility, of course, includes making certain that the patient or a responsible family member knows precisely what the arrangements for medical follow-up are and is aware of how to obtain help in an emergency. It is important that this information be provided in writing, include a clear statement of where to go for follow-up care, and give the name of the physician responsible for supervision of the patient's care. This is especially important for the patient who is discharged to follow-up in a clinic setting. To be effective in patient teaching, the nurse must have a thorough knowledge of the drugs prescribed for the patient's continuing care. Patient teaching concerning medications is critical for patients discharged on antihypertensive preparations. Such patients have to be followed carefully and may require frequent change of dosage and preparation. Often antihypertensive drugs are prescribed in varying combinations. Most of these agents have distressing side effects that will be much more apparent and troublesome to the patient than his hypertension, which may have been entirely asymptomatic. Since the drugs will actually make them feel worse rather than better, without continued encouragement and reinforcement of the principles of therapy, most patients will not adhere to the treatment plan.

It is outside the scope of this book to discuss all pharmacological agents the nurse may be called upon to administer to patients with cardiovascular conditions. This section is intended only as an overview of most frequently used drugs with which the nurse should be familiar. Research in pharmacology provides a continuing source of new therapeutic agents. At the same time the effects of existing drugs continue to be evaluated. As experience is gained through clinical trials, therapeutic regimens may be changed, with new drugs introduced and existing agents discontinued or their use modified.

Most hospitals subscribe to the Hospital Formulary System (provided by the American Society of Hospital Pharmacists). The Formulary includes a description of each drug, its chemistry, pharmacological action, use, absorption, metabolism and excretion, side effects, cautions, any known drug interactions and interference with laboratory tests, dosage, and the preparations available. Several times a year the Formulary is updated to reflect the most current knowledge about drugs. The reader is referred to this source for the most up-to-date information about drugs. Most medical centers and large hospitals have drug information centers staffed by clinical pharmacologists who can provide information to health care practitioners within the area they serve. Because therapeutic regimens change so frequently, and because of the growing problem of iatrogenic illness induced by drugs, the professional nurse should avail herself of these resources.

Drugs used in treatment of cardiovascular disease may be classified as having either a direct or an indirect action on the heart. Drugs having *direct cardiac action* include those that (1) affect the contractility of the myocardium (*positive inotropic agents*), (2) have an effect on the heart rate by altering cardiac rhythm (*antiarrhythmic agents*), (3) affect *conductivity* of impulses through the heart muscle, and (4) affect the *irritability* of the heart. Drugs may *act on the heart indirectly* to achieve any of these four effects by altering either the autonomic influences on the heart or the relationship between oxygen supply to the myocardium and oxygen needs [7]. Many drugs have more than one of these actions. *Antihypertensive drugs* include those that (1) act on the sympathetic nervous system to reduce vasomotor tone, (2) block ganglionic transmission in the autonomic nervous system, (3) inhibit storage of norepinephrine, (4) block release of norepinephrine from the sympathetic nerve endings, (5) block the action of circulating levels of norepinephrine at alpha-adrenergic receptor sites, and (6) relax vascular smooth muscle directly [14]. *Diuretics* are used in the treatment of heart failure to control excessive fluid retention [5]. They are also used in hypertension because of their action on the renal tubules, which affects arterial pressure through sodium diuresis and volume depletion [14]. *Anticoagulant drugs* include coumarin derivatives, which antagonize the action of vitamin K, and heparin, which inactivates thrombin [19]. Anticoagulant therapy is used commonly in the treatment of patients with thromboembolism to prevent further thrombus formation and extension of a thrombus that has already formed.

The major pharmacological agents used in treatment of patients with cardiovascular disease are described briefly in the following tables.

DIGITALIS GLYCOSIDES

ACTION
Augment contractility and irritability of heart muscle
Slow atrioventricular conduction and heart rate
Stimulate vagus nerve to increase strength of contraction while decreasing heart rate
Increase myocardial uptake of calcium

CLINICAL USE
Treatment of congestive heart failure and supraventricular rhythms

PREPARATIONS	ROUTE	ONSET OF ACTION	ELIMINATION
Digitalis leaf	Oral	25 min–2 hr	Kidney excretion up to 2 wks
Digoxin	IV	5–30 min	Kidney/stool excretion,
	Oral	1 hr	2–6 days
Digitoxin	Oral	2–4 hr	Liver metabolism,
			kidney/stool excretion,
			2–3 weeks
Ouabain	IV	3–10 min	Kidney/stool excretion,
			1–3 days

ADVERSE EFFECTS
Digitalis toxicity
Arrhythmias
Anorexia
Nausea
Vomiting
Bradycardia
Yellow vision
Neuralgia
Headache
Drowsiness
Delirium

FACTORS INFLUENCING THERAPEUTIC RESPONSE/TOXICITY
Absorption of digoxin and digitoxin can be reduced by antidiarrheal agents containing kaolin and pectin, nonabsorbable antacids, and neomycin.
Tolerance to digitalis is reduced by age, myocardial infarction or ischemia, magnesium depletion, renal insufficiency, hypercalcemia, electrical cardioversion, depletion of potassium stores.
Digitalis has a cumulative effect, digitoxin has the greatest.
Effects of quinidine, procainamide, and propranolol may be additive to those of digitalis.
Digitalis preparations are synergistic with adrenergic agents.

NURSING CONSIDERATIONS
Digitalization is the process by which a therapeutic blood level is reached over a 24–48 hour period.
When a patient is being digitalized it is most important that medication be given precisely at the time intervals specified in the doctor's orders.
The patient must be observed closely for signs of toxicity, especially if there are predisposing conditions.
Monitor heart rate and rhythm, observe for changes.
Observe for hypokalemia, which is the most common factor precipitating toxicity.
Give oral preparations with or following meals to decrease irritation of gastric mucosa.
Institute patient teaching concerning medication regimen, monitoring of pulse, observation for toxicity, and precise instructions for seeking medical attention.

CATECHOLAMINES AND SYMPATHOMIMETIC DRUGS

1. Alphamimetic drugs

ACTION
Stimulation of alpha-adrenergic receptors in smooth muscle of the blood vessels, causing vasoconstriction, increased arterial resistance, reduced venous return, and increase in blood pressure

CLINICAL USE
To induce hypertension and increase vagal tone reflexly with supraventricular tachycardia
To treat shock due to loss of vasoconstrictor tone when cardiac output is high or normal
These agents are *not* used in treatment of shock due to myocardial infarction.

PREPARATIONS	ROUTE	ONSET OF ACTION
Methoxamine (Vasoxyl)	IM or IV	Immediate, lasting 1 hr
Phenylephrine (Neo-Synephrine)	IM, IV, or SC	15–90 min

ADVERSE EFFECTS
Methoxamine: headache, projectile vomiting
Phenylephrine: marked reflex bradycardia

FACTORS INFLUENCING THERAPEUTIC RESPONSE/TOXICITY
Prolonged administration of methoxamine can reduce plasma volume.
Marked reflex bradycardia caused by phenylephrine may be blocked by atropine.

NURSING CONSIDERATIONS
Observe patients on methoxamine for signs of hypovolemia.
Observe patients with hyperthyroidism, slow heart rate, heart block, or myocardial infarction very carefully when phenylephrine is administered.
Monitor vital signs.

2. Betamimetic drugs

ACTION
Stimulation of beta$_1$-adrenergic receptors in the myocardium, blood vessels, and skeletal muscle, resulting in increased contractility, automaticity, conduction, velocity, and irritability of the heart
Stimulation of beta$_2$-adrenergic receptors, resulting in relaxation of smooth muscle in the blood vessels, trachea, and bronchi
Vasodilation, decreased peripheral vascular resistance, increased heart rate and cardiac output

CLINICAL USE
Enhancement of pacemaker automaticity and facilitation of AV conduction in heart block, thereby increasing ventricular rate
Isoproterenol is *not* used in the treatment of cardiogenic shock.

PREPARATIONS	ROUTE	ONSET OF ACTION
Isoproterenol (Isuprel)	IV infusion sublingual	Several minutes 15 min–2 hr
Mephentermine (Wyamine)	IV, IM, SC	Immediate, lasting 30–45 min 15 minutes, lasting 1–2 hrs

ADVERSE EFFECTS
Headache
Flushing
Angina
Nausea
Tremor
Dizziness
Weakness
Sweating
Hypotension due to hypovolemia
Development of ventricular ectopy
Increased myocardial ischemia

FACTORS INFLUENCING THERAPEUTIC RESPONSE/TOXICITY
During Isoproterenol infusion, expansion of circulating volume may be necessary, because vasodilation will reduce central venous pressure.
Enhanced myocardial contractility and increased rate will increase oxygen consumption and can increase ischemia.
Mephenteramine has no cumulative effects.

NURSING CONSIDERATIONS
Monitor vital signs carefully.
Monitor heart rate and rhythm.
Observe for signs of hypovolemia.
Observe for adverse effects.
Regulate rate of intravenous infusion according to electrocardiogram findings.

3. *Drugs that stimulate both alpha- and beta-receptors*

   a. *Norepinephrine (levarterenol, Levophed)*

      ACTION
      Acts on peripheral alpha-receptors to increase systolic, diastolic, and pulse pressures
      Increases peripheral resistance
      Reflex vagal action decreases heart rate
      Increases coronary blood flow and stroke volume
      Decreases blood flow to kidneys, brain, and visceral and skeletal muscles

      CLINICAL USE
      Treatment of hypotension when peripheral vascular resistance is low and cardiac output is normal or increased
      Treatment of cardiogenic shock

ROUTE	*ONSET OF ACTION*
IV	Immediate

      ADVERSE EFFECTS
      Anxiety
      Respiratory distress
      Headache
      Severe hypertension
      Retrosternal and pharyngeal pain
      Sweating
      Vomiting
      Arrhythmias
      Tissue necrosis due to extravasation of fluid

FACTORS INFLUENCING THERAPEUTIC RESPONSE/TOXICITY
Following prolonged administration, dosage may have to be tapered to prevent vascular collapse.
There may be fluid shift from intravascular to extracellular space, causing depletion of intravascular volume.
Vasoconstrictor action can cause pain and sloughing of tissue. Dosage must be administered intravenously.

NURSING CONSIDERATIONS
The patient must never be left unattended when this drug is being given.
Blood pressure must be monitored and intravenous infusion rate regulated to maintain pressure at prescribed levels.
The infusion site should be observed frequently for signs of extravasation.
The area may be infiltrated with phentolamine (Regitine), an adrenergic blocking agent, to prevent tissue necrosis if there is any extravasation.
Urinary output should be monitored carefully, since it is a sensitive indicator of perfusion of the heart, brain, and kidneys.

b. *Epinephrine (Adrenalin)*

ACTION
Acts directly on beta-receptors in the heart to increase rate and force of contractions, cardiac output, stroke volume, and coronary blood flow.
Small doses lower blood pressure by vasodilation in skeletal muscle.
Large doses elevate blood pressure, increase peripheral resistance, and reduce blood flow to the skin and kidneys.

CLINICAL USE
Initiation of cardiac rhythm in cardiac arrest by stimulating pacemaker

ADVERSE EFFECTS
Ventricular arrhythmias
Angina
Headache
Tremor
Weakness
Elevation of blood sugar

FACTORS INFLUENCING THERAPEUTIC RESPONSE/TOXICITY
Fear and anxiety may aggravate symptoms.
Increased heart rate and force of contractions will increase myocardial oxygen requirement. If coronary flow is inadequate myocardial ischemia can result.
Renal blood flow, glomerular filtration rate, and sodium excretion rate are usually reduced.
Acidosis reduces the effectiveness of epinephrine.
Prolonged administration can cause damage of the vessel walls and endocardium.
This drug must be given parenterally, because it is destroyed by the gastrointestinal juices.

NURSING CONSIDERATIONS
Observe carefully for evidence of adverse reactions.
Monitor vital signs carefully.
Epinephrine should not be administered concurrently with isoproterenol, since both are direct cardiac stimulants. When both drugs are ordered, they should be alternated at 4-hour intervals.

c. *Metaraminol (Aramine)*

ACTION
Similar to that of norepinephrine but less potent and longer lasting
Increases systolic and diastolic pressures through vasoconstriction
Increases the force of myocardial contraction

CLINICAL USE
Treatment of hypotension when immediate elevation of blood pressure is
    needed
Termination of supraventricular tachycardias by reflex vagal stimulation

ROUTE	ONSET OF ACTION
SC	5–20 min
IM	10 min
IV	1–2 min

ADVERSE EFFECTS
Reflex bradycardia
Ventricular irritability
Tissue slough
Sustained elevation of blood pressure
Severe headache

FACTORS INFLUENCING THERAPEUTIC RESPONSE/TOXICITY
Vasoconstriction can lead to sloughing of tissues.
Atropine eliminates reflex bradycardia due to metaraminol.

NURSING CONSIDERATIONS
Care should be taken not to inject drug into areas of arterial insufficiency,
    since vasoconstriction can lead to sloughing of tissues at site of subcu-
    taneous injections or extravasation of intravenous infusions.
Vital signs should be monitored carefully to prevent an excessive rise in blood
    pressure.

d. *Dopamine*

This drug is the immediate precursor of norepinephrine in the synthesis of
    norepinephrine.

ACTION
At low doses it stimulates dopaminergic receptors, thereby dilating mesenteric
    and renal blood vessels and decreasing renal vascular resistance, increasing
    renal blood flow, glomerular filtration rate and excretion of sodium.
As the dosage is increased, stimulation of beta receptors in the myocardium
    induces tachycardia. Higher dosages stimulate adrenergic receptors to
    elevate blood pressure.
It causes both relaxation and contraction of vascular smooth muscle.
When doses are administered that elevate blood pressure, baroreceptor-mediated
    bradycardia occurs.

CLINICAL USE
Treatment of heart failure
Treatment of cardiogenic shock when volume expansion therapy and use of
    other catecholamines has been unsuccessful

ROUTE	ONSET OF ACTION	ELIMINATION
IV	5 min	Excreted by the kidneys

ADVERSE EFFECTS
Nausea and vomiting
Dyspnea
Headache
Angina
Tachycardia
Hypotension
Hypertension
Vasoconstriction
Ventricular arrythmias

FACTORS INFLUENCING THERAPEUTIC RESPONSE/TOXICITY
Inactivated by alkaline solutions
Extravasation can cause tissue necrosis due to vasoconstriction in patients
    with vascular occlusive disease.
Antagonized by propranolol and other beta-adrenergic blocking agents
Should not be used when patient has pheochromocytoma, uncorrected tachy-
    arrythmias, or ventricular fibrillation

NURSING CONSIDERATIONS
Careful monitoring of urine output is required.
Vital signs must be monitored frequently.
Infusions must be titrated for individual patients, with extreme care not to
    administer a bolus.
Since the drug is inactivated by alkaline solutions, it should not be mixed with
    sodium bicarbonate.
Extremities should be checked frequently, particularly if patients have vascu-
    lar occlusive disease, for signs of ischemia due to vasoconstriction.
Infusion must be checked frequently to prevent extravasation.

ANTIARRHYTHMIC AGENTS

1. Quinidine

ACTION
Depresses the excitability of cardiac muscle to electrical stimulation
Decreases the velocity of conductivity
Decreases cardiac output and systemic and pulmonary arterial pressure
Prolongs refractory period of atrial and ventricular muscle

CLINICAL USE
Prevention of recurrent atrial fibrillation after sinus rhythm has been restored
    by electrical countershock
Conversion of atrial flutter to normal sinus rhythm when digitalis has been ineffec-
    tive
Prevention of repeated episodes of supraventricular and ventricular tachycardia
    or fibrillation
Treatment of ectopic premature supraventricular and ventricular beats in acute
    myocardial infarction

ROUTE	ONSET OF ACTION	ELIMINATION
Oral	1–2 hr	Metabolized by the liver and excreted
IM	30–90 min	by the kidneys in 24 hours
IV	Onset not instant	

ADVERSE EFFECTS
Tinnitus
Headache
Distorted vision
Gastrointestinal symptoms
Rashes
Thrombocytopenia
Hypotension
Heart block
Ventricular fibrillation

FACTORS INFLUENCING THERAPEUTIC RESPONSE/TOXICITY
Prolongs prothrombin time, may enhance action of anticoagulants
Potentiates hypotensive effect of antihypertensive agents and diuretics
Metabolism and excretion interfered with by liver disease, congestive heart failure, and renal insufficiency
May decrease force of contraction with acute myocardial infarction
May be antagonized by increasing extracellular sodium and decreasing extracellular potassium

NURSING CONSIDERATIONS
The greatest hazard is sudden death due to ventricular fibrillation.
Gastrointestinal effects may be minimized by giving medication with food.
If drug is given more often than every 2 hours, the effect is cumulative.
A test dose is usually given because hypersensitivity is common.

2. *Procainamide (Pronestyl)*

ACTION
Depresses excitability of cardiac muscle to electrical stimulation
Decreases velocity of conductivity
Prolongs refractory period

CLINICAL USE
Treatment of premature ventricular contractions and ventricular tachyarrythmias, particularly when an intravenous preparation must be used and lidocaine has not been successful in suppressing ectopy

ROUTE	ONSET OF ACTION	ELIMINATION
Oral	At maximum concentration, 1 hr	Metabolized by the liver and excreted by the kidneys
IM	15–60 min	
IV	Immediate	

ADVERSE EFFECTS
Bradycardia
Heart block
Ventricular tachycardia/fibrillation

Nausea, vomiting, diarrhea, anorexia with oral preparations
Drug eruptions
Agranulocytosis
Drug fever
Lupus-like syndrome
Bone marrow depression
Central nervous system depression

FACTORS INFLUENCING THERAPEUTIC RESPONSE/TOXICITY
May potentiate hypotensive effects of thiazides and antihypertensive drugs
May be additive with digitalis, quinidine, and propranolol
Anticholinergic action may oppose the ventricular slowing induced by digitalis.
Digitalis may counteract the decrease in atrial conduction induced by drug.
Can induce asthma attacks in patients with bronchial asthma
Can cause hypotension, especially when given intravenously
Renal insufficiency or hepatic damage may predispose to toxicity.
Presence of partial or complete AV block may cause asystole.

NURSING CONSIDERATIONS
Vasopressors should be readily available.
Intravenous administration should not exceed 50–100 mg/1–3 minutes.
Continuous cardiac monitoring is required.
Liver and kidney function should be monitored and blood counts should be
    checked frequently.

3. *Lidocaine*

ACTION
Controls ventricular arrhythmias by suppressing automaticity in the His-Purkinje
    system and elevating the threshold for electrical stimulation of the ventricle
    during diastole
Enhances conduction at the Purkinje fiber myocardial junctions; this may diminish
    reentrant arrhythmias

CLINICAL USE
Control of ventricular arrhythmias complicating acute myocardial infarction or
    following cardiac manipulative procedures such as catheterization

ROUTE	*ONSET OF ACTION*	*ELIMINATION*
IV bolus	10 sec–3 min	Metabolized rapidly by the liver
IV infusion	10–20 min	and excreted by the kidneys

ADVERSE EFFECTS
Drowsiness
Dizziness
Disorientation
Visual disturbances
Paresthesias
Tremors
Stupor
Convulsions
Hypotension
Heart block

Bradycardia
Cardiac and respiratory arrest

FACTORS INFLUENCING THERAPEUTIC RESPONSE/TOXICITY
The drug is a central nervous system depressant with sedative, central analgesic, and anticonvulsant effects. With high doses, convulsions may result from depression of inhibitory influences on motor pathways.
Overdosage can cause medullary depression and respiratory arrest.
Prolonged infusions may cause local thrombophlebitis.
Anoxia or hypoxia will increase cardiovascular toxicity.
Congestive heart failure, shock, kidney and liver disease predispose to toxicity.
Hypokalemia must be eliminated as a potentiating factor.

NURSING CONSIDERATIONS
Continuous cardiac monitoring is required.
Dosage must be adjusted according to individual patient requirements and response.
Vital signs must be monitored frequently.
Mental status should be checked frequently.
Site of intravenous infusion should be checked regularly for signs of phlebitis.

4. *Diphenylhydantoin (Dilantin)*

ACTION
Reduces automaticity in Purkinje fibers
Raises atrial and ventricular fibrillation thresholds
Decreases force of contraction and rate of conductivity

CLINICAL USE
Treatment of supraventricular and ventricular arrhythmias particularly those resulting from digitalis toxicity
Treatment and prevention of ventricular extrasystoles and tachycardia when other antiarrhythmic agents have not been effective

ROUTE	ONSET OF ACTION	ELIMINATION
Oral	Absorbed slowly	Inactivated chiefly by the liver
IV	5–20 min	and excreted by the kidneys in 6–9 days

ADVERSE EFFECTS
Transient hypotension
Bradycardia
Ataxia
Slurring of speech
Nystagmus
Gastric irritation
Nausea
Vomiting
Skin eruption
Hyperplasia of gums
Hepatocellular damage
Pseudolymphoma

FACTORS INFLUENCING THERAPEUTIC RESPONSE/TOXICITY
Neurological reactions may mimic cerebellar disease.
The drug may be additive or potentiate the action of other central nervous
  system depressants.
Intravenous administration may potentiate hypotensive action of diuretics and
  antihypertensive agents. Rapid administration can cause hypotension and
  cardiac arrest.
Effects may be additive to those of digitalis, quinidine, procainamide, propranolol.
Coumarin anticoagulants inhibit metabolism and can predispose to toxicity.
The drug can also potentiate action of coumarin anticoagulants.

NURSING CONSIDERATIONS
Frequent dental hygiene with gum massage is imperative for all patients receiving
  this drug.
The solution is highly alkaline and can cause pain when instilled into small veins.

BETA-ADRENERGIC RECEPTOR BLOCKING AGENTS

Propranolol (Inderal)

ACTION
Blocks the effects of catecholamines and sympathetic nerve stimulation on heart
  rate, contractility, and cardiac output
Reduces resting heart rate and arterial blood pressure
Reduces oxygen consumption by myocardium

CLINICAL USE
Treatment of angina pectoris when nitrates have failed to provide relief
Abolition and prevention of paroxysmal supraventricular and ventricular tachy-
  cardias when other antiarrhythmic agents have been ineffective
Treatment of tachyarrhythmias due to digitalis toxicity when electric countershock
  is contraindicated
Treatment of hypertension

ROUTE	ONSET OF ACTION	ELIMINATION
Oral	30 min	Metabolized by the liver and
IV	10 min	excreted in the urine

ADVERSE EFFECTS
Nausea
Diarrhea
Visual disturbances
Skin eruptions
Weakness
Lethargy
Shock
Cardiac failure

FACTORS INFLUENCING THERAPEUTIC RESPONSE/TOXICITY
Antagonizes responses to circulating epinephrine, norepinephrine, isoproterenol
Potentiates ventricular slowing of digitalis
Absorption of oral agent is decreased when administered with or soon after feedings.
May precipitate or intensify heart failure

Hypoglycemia may occur in insulin-dependent diabetes.
Plasma levels and clinical effectiveness vary widely.
Large doses may cause sodium retention.

NURSING CONSIDERATIONS
Cardiac monitoring is recommended during intravenous administration.
Propranolol may prevent the appearance of the symptoms of acute hypoglycemia
in insulin-dependent diabetics (tachycardia, sweating).

VASODILATORS

ACTION
Relaxation of smooth muscle
Generalized arterial and venous dilation, resulting in a drop in blood pressure and
tachycardia
Reduction of cardiac workload and myocardial oxygen consumption, due to drop
in blood pressure and reduction of heart size by venous dilation
Dilation of coronary vessels, aiding perfusion of ischemic areas of myocardium

CLINICAL USE
Treatment of angina pectoris
Prevention of anginal attacks that are associated with predictable events known to
precipitate pain such as stair climbing, exposure to cold air, sexual intercourse

PREPARATIONS	ROUTE	ONSET OF ACTION
Glyceryl trinitrate	Sublingual	1—2 min, duration 30 min
(nitroglycerine)	transcutaneous	
Amyl nitrite	Inhalation	10—30 sec
Isosorbide dinitrate	Oral	15—30 min, duration 4 hr
(isordil)	Sublingual	2 min

ADVERSE EFFECTS
Flushing
Throbbing of head
Headache
Hypotension
Nausea
Vomiting
Vertigo

FACTORS INFLUENCING THERAPEUTIC RESPONSE/TOXICITY
Causes increased intraocular and cerebrospinal fluid pressure, should be used with
caution in stroke and glaucoma
Deteriorates when exposed to air, light, heat, or moisture
Drop in blood pressure usually occurs within 1—5 minutes after taking.
Tolerance may develop.

NURSING CONSIDERATIONS
Patient should be instructed about the importance of keeping sublingual preparations under the tongue and keeping a supply with him at all times and explicitly
instructed when to use them.

Because of its hypotensive effect, the patient should be instructed to lie down or
   remain seated after taking it.
Since nitroglycerine deteriorates rapidly, the patient should be instructed to keep a
   supply with him and store the remainder in an airtight container protected from
   heat, light, and moisture. A fresh supply should be procured at least every 6
   months.

ANTIHYPERTENSIVE AGENTS

1. Drugs that have central action

a. Clonidine

ACTION
Acts on sympathetic nervous system centers in the brain to reduce vasomotor
   tone and lower arterial pressure
Inhibits renin secretion

CLINICAL USE
Control of mild to moderate hypertension

ROUTE
Oral

ADVERSE EFFECTS
Postural hypotension
Drowsiness
Dry mouth
Rebound hypertension after abrupt withdrawal

FACTORS INFLUENCING THERAPEUTIC RESPONSE/TOXICITY
Antihypertensive effect is antagonized by tricyclic antidepressants.

NURSING CONSIDERATIONS
The patient should be instructed about the action of the drug and the need for
   continuing therapy and monitoring of blood pressure.
Patient teaching should include measures to prevent adverse effects of postural
   hypertension.

b. Methyldopa (Aldomet)

ACTION
Acts on sympathetic nervous system centers in the brain to reduce vasomotor
   tone and lower arterial blood pressure
Blocks sympathetic nerves
Inhibits renin secretion

CLINICAL USE
Treatment of mild to moderate hypertension with renal impairment

ROUTE	ONSET OF ACTION	ELIMINATION
Oral	4–6 hr	Metabolized by the liver and kidneys;
IV	2 hr	excreted by kidneys and in stool

ADVERSE EFFECTS
Postural hypotension
Fatigue
Sedation
Fever
Gynecomastia and impaired ejaculation
Positive Coomb's test

FACTORS INFLUENCING THERAPEUTIC RESPONSE/TOXICITY
Caution should be used in evaluating results of clinical laboratory tests, since
    falsely elevated values may be found.
If blood transfusion is required, prior knowledge of positive Coomb's reaction
    will help in crossmatching.
Tolerance may develop.
Thiazides have a potentiating effect on methyldopa.
Water and sodium retention occur if a diuretic is not given.

NURSING CONSIDERATIONS
Monitoring of vital signs is necessary.
Patient should be taught about medication regimen and possible side effects.
When mobilizing patient, care should be taken to avoid the effects of postural
    hypotension.
Patient should be observed for signs of edema.

2. Ganglionic blocking agents

ACTION
Inhibit transmission of nerve impulses through both sympathetic and parasympa-
    thetic ganglia to cause a decrease of peripheral vascular resistance and a lowering
    of arterial pressure
Reduce cardiac output
Have a histamine-like effect that dilates blood vessels directly

CLINICAL USE
Control of hypertensive crisis
Treatment of pulmonary edema due to hypertension
Use in severe hypertension when rapid lowering of arterial pressure by parenteral
    administration is required

PREPARATION	ROUTE	ONSET OF ACTION	ELIMINATION
Trimethaphan	IV	Almost immediate, lasting 10–20 min	Excreted by the kidneys
Pentolinium	IM, IV	3 min	

ADVERSE EFFECTS
Postural hypotension
Impaired visual accommodation
Dry mouth
Constipation
Urinary retention
Impotence
Paralytic ileus

FACTORS INFLUENCING THERAPEUTIC RESPONSE/THERAPY
Excessive amounts will prolong action rather than increase hypotensive effect.
Blocking of ganglionic transmission in autonomic system has little effect when
   patient is supine but prevents vasoconstriction in the upright position.
Procainamide potentiates action.
Removal of autonomic control enhances sensitivity of vasoconstricting and vaso-
   dilating receptor sites in the cardiovascular system.
These agents are incompatible with alkaline solutions, iodides, and bromides.

NURSING CONSIDERATIONS
Careful monitoring of blood pressure is required.
The patient should be observed carefully for signs of peripheral vascular collapse.
Adequacy of voiding and bowel function should be watched closely.
Care should be taken when patient assumes an upright position because of
   postural hypotension.

3. Drugs that act on postganglionic nerve endings

a. Rauwolfia alkaloids

ACTION
Inhibit storage of norepinephrine within vesicles in adrenergic nerve endings,
   leading to depletion of catecholamine stores
In parenteral preparations, have a direct effect on vascular smooth muscle

CLINICAL USE
Treatment of mild to moderate hypertension in young patients

ROUTE	ONSET OF ACTION
Oral	Several days to 2 weeks
IV	

ADVERSE EFFECTS
Depression
Nasal congestion
Diarrhea
Impotence
Headache
Dizziness
Nightmares

FACTORS INFLUENCING THERAPEUTIC RESPONSE/TOXICITY
Oral administration has a cumulative effect that may persist for up to 4 weeks
   after the drug has been discontinued.
Depression is most likely to affect the elderly. An early sign of depression is
   an altered sleep pattern.
Depletion of body stores of catecholamines may lead to cardiovascular
   collapse under sudden stress.
These alkaloids cause activation of peptic ulcer disease.

NURSING CONSIDERATIONS
Monitor blood pressure carefully.
Observe patient for signs of depression.
Teach the patient about the medication regimen and possible side effects.

b. Reserpine

ACTION
Inhibits storage of norepinephrine within adrenergic nerve endings, leading to
    depletion of catecholamine stores
Inhibits renin secretion
Parenteral preparations affect vascular smooth muscle directly

CLINICAL USE
Treatment of moderate to severe hypertension
Treatment of hypertensive crisis

ROUTE	*ONSET OF ACTION*	*ELIMINATION*
Oral	3–6 days	Excreted by the kidneys
IM		
IV	1 hr	

ADVERSE EFFECTS
Postural hypotension
Miosis
Sedation bradycardia
Nightmares
Nasal congestion
Weight gain
Increased appetite
Depression

FACTORS INFLUENCING THERAPEUTIC RESPONSE/TOXICITY
Can cause postural hypotension and respiratory depression

NURSING CONSIDERATIONS
Monitor vital signs carefully.
Observe patient for signs of depression.

c. Guanethidine

ACTION
Blocks release of norepinephrine from sympathetic nerve endings

CLINICAL USE
Treatment of moderate to severe hypertension

ROUTE	*ONSET OF ACTION*	*ELIMINATION*
Oral	Full therapeutic effect, 2–7 days	Excreted by the kidneys

ADVERSE EFFECTS
Postural hypotension
Bradycardia
Dry mouth
Impaired ejaculation
Fluid retention
Diarrhea
Impotence

FACTORS INFLUENCING THERAPEUTIC RESPONSE/TOXICITY
More effective in lowering blood pressure in patients who are upright than
  supine, because cardiovascular reflexes are reduced or absent
Blood pressure remains at its lowest point 3—4 days after drug is stopped.
Should be administered carefully to patients with impaired renal function,
  because it can further increase blood urea levels
Depletion of catecholamines can lead to acute cardiovascular collapse when
  the patient is subjected to sudden stress.
Antagonized by amphetamines, tricyclic antidepressants
Since it reduces heart rate, should be given cautiously to patients receiving
  digitalis.
May cause explosive diarrhea leading to incontinence

NURSING CONSIDERATIONS
Patients should be cautioned to avoid prolonged standing or exercise, since
  orthostatic hypotension is a frequent side effect.

d. *Pargyline*

ACTION
Monoamine oxidase inhibitor acts both centrally and peripherally by blocking
  the degradation of catecholamines

CLINICAL USE
Treatment of moderate to severe hypertension in depressed patients

ROUTE	*ONSET OF ACTION*
Oral	Several days to weeks

ADVERSE EFFECTS
Postural hypotension
Insomnia
Nightmares
Muscle twitching

FACTORS INFLUENCING THERAPEUTIC RESPONSE/TOXICITY
Action is cumulative.
Acute hypertension can be induced by foods and drugs containing tyramine.

NURSING CONSIDERATIONS
Patients on this drug must be alerted that foods such as aged cheese, wine,
  beer, and pickled herring contain tyramine, which can release stored
  catecholamines and precipitate a hypertensive crisis.

4. *Agents that act at alpha-adrenergic receptor sites*
(Such as phentolamine and phenoxybenzamine)

CLINICAL USE
Used only in the treatment of hypertension due to pheochromocytoma

5. *Agents that act on beta-adrenergic receptor sites*

   Propranolol (Inderal)

   ACTION
   Blocks beta-adrenergic receptors
   Blocks sympathetic effects on heart
   Reduces cardiac output

   This drug has already been discussed as a beta-adrenergic receptor blocking agent
   for use in treatment of angina pectoris and as an antiarrhythmic agent.

6. *Drugs that affect vascular smooth muscle directly*

   a. *Hydralazine (Apresoline)*

      ACTION
      Acts primarily on arterial resistance to increase cardiac output and increase
      renal blood flow
      Interferes with sensory receptors in the myocardium

      CLINICAL USE
      As adjunct in treatment of moderate to severe hypertension
      In parenteral preparations, in malignant hypertension

ROUTE	ONSET OF ACTION
Oral	
IM	
IV	10 min

      ADVERSE EFFECTS
      Lupus erythematosus-like syndrome
      Headache
      Tachycardia
      Angina pectoris
      Nausea
      Vomiting
      Diarrhea

      FACTORS INFLUENCING THERAPEUTIC RESPONSE/TOXICITY
      Effect on peripheral resistance is partly negated by reflex increases in sympa-
      thetic discharges that increase heart rate and cardiac output. This limits
      usefulness in patients with severe coronary artery disease.
      Tolerance may develop.
      In the presence of myocardial ischemia, these drugs should be used cautiously.

      NURSING CONSIDERATIONS
      Vital signs should be monitored carefully.
      Headache and dizziness accompanying use of this drug will usually disappear
      in 7−10 days when the drug is continued. The patient should be informed
      of this.
      When large doses are prescribed, the patient usually experiences headaches,
      palpitations, flushing, and dyspnea on exertion.

b. *Diazoxide*

ACTION
Diazoxide is not a diuretic, but it acts upon arterial resistance to increase
   cardiac output and increase renal blood flow.

CLINICAL USE
In acute situations it is used as an emergency measure for treatment of severe
   or malignant hypertension.

ROUTE   ONSET OF ACTION
Rapid IV   Immediate

ADVERSE EFFECTS
Sodium retention
Hyperglycemia
Hyperuricemia

FACTORS INFLUENCING THERAPEUTIC RESPONSE/TOXICITY
Reduces carbohydrate tolerance

NURSING CONSIDERATIONS
No titration is necessary, but careful monitoring of vital signs and urine output
   is essential.

c. *Nitroprusside*

ACTION
Direct vasodilation

CLINICAL USE
Emergency use for control of acute hypertension

ROUTE   ONSET OF ACTION
IV   Immediate

ADVERSE EFFECTS
Apprehension
Weakness
Diaphoresis
Nausea
Vomiting
Muscle twitching

NURSING CONSIDERATIONS
Vital signs must be carefully monitored.
Administration must be controlled with infusion pump.

7. *Drugs that act on renal tubules*

  a. *Thiazides, hydrochlorothiazide (Hydrodiuril)*

   ACTION
   Act on renal tubules to cause sodium diuresis and volume depletion
   Reduce peripheral vascular resistance

   CLINICAL USE
   Treatment of mild hypertension and as an adjunct in treatment of moderate
     to severe hypertension

ROUTE	*ONSET OF ACTION*	*ELIMINATION*
Oral	2–6 hr	Excreted by the kidneys

   ADVERSE EFFECTS
   Hypokalemia
   Hyperuricemia
   Carbohydrate intolerance
   Dermatitis
   Purpura
   Nausea
   Vomiting
   Diarrhea
   Dizziness
   Paresthesias
   Muscle cramps

   FACTORS INFLUENCING THERAPEUTIC RESPONSE/TOXICITY
   May cause potassium depletion; precipitating cardiac arrhythmias and increas-
     ing sensitivity to digitalis
   Augment action of other antihypertensive agents
   May cause sodium depletion when the patient is on severely restricted sodium
     diet
   May increase insulin requirement in diabetes

   NURSING CONSIDERATIONS
   Watch patients carefully for signs of electrolyte imbalance.
   Monitor rate and rhythm of heart.
   Administer after meals to reduce gastric irritation.
   Provide foods rich in potassium.
   Measure intake and output carefully.
   Monitor vital signs.
   Weigh daily.

  b. *Furosemide (Lasix)*

   ACTION
   Blocks resorption of sodium and water in proximal renal tubule
   Interferes with resorption of sodium in ascending limb of loop of Henle and
     proximal portion of distal tubule

CLINICAL USE
As a potent diuretic for patients who do not respond to thiazides; when a
    rapid-acting potent diuretic is required, as in pulmonary edema
In oral preparation, for treatment of mild hypertension; as an adjunct to other
    preparations, for treatment of more severe hypertension

ROUTE	ONSET OF ACTION	ELIMINATION
Oral	20–30 min	Excreted by the kidneys
IM	Slightly later than IV	
IV	5 min	

ADVERSE EFFECTS
Dermatitis
Pruritis
Nausea
Vomiting
Diarrhea
Blurring of vision
Weakness
Muscle cramps
Spasms of urinary bladder

FACTORS INFLUENCING THERAPEUTIC RESPONSE/TOXICITY
The potent diuretic effect may lead to severe electrolyte imbalance and exces-
    sive fluid loss with dehydration, circulatory collapse, thrombosis, and
    embolism.
In patients receiving digitalis, potassium depletion can precipitate digitalis
    toxicity.
The drug may produce hyperglycemia in patients with latent diabetes.
It potentiates action of antihypertensive drugs.
Salicylate toxicity can occur at lower dosage than usual, since both agents
    have the same renal site of excretion.

NURSING CONSIDERATIONS
Monitor intake and output carefully.
Weigh patient daily, same time, same scale.
Observe closely for signs of dehydration and electrolyte imbalance.
Monitor vital signs carefully.

c. *Ethacrynic acid (Edecrin)*

ACTION
Blocks resorption of sodium within ascending limb of loop of Henle

CLINICAL USE
Treatment of congestive heart failure when potent diuretic is needed
Treatment of mild hypertension or as an adjunct to other forms of therapy in
    more severe hypertension

ROUTE	ONSET OF ACTION	ELIMINATION
Oral	30 min	Excreted in urine and feces
IV	15 min	

ADVERSE EFFECTS
Skin rash
Deafness
Granulocytopenia
Profuse diarrhea
Nausea
Vomiting
Blurred vision
Headache

FACTORS INFLUENCING THERAPEUTIC RESPONSE/TOXICITY
If used with kanamycin sulfate, can cause irreversible deafness
Can precipitate electrolyte depletion because of rapid electrolyte and fluid
    loss. This may result in hypotension.
May precipitate gout
Potentiates action of antihypertensive agents

NURSING CONSIDERATIONS
Monitor intake and output carefully.
Weigh patient daily.
Observe for signs of metabolic acidosis, dehydration, and electrolyte depletion.
Monitor vital signs.

d. *Spironolactone (Aldactone)*

ACTION
Causes renal sodium loss by blocking the effect of endogenous mineralocorti-
    coids
Reduces resorption of sodium and chloride and retention of potassium
Has diuretic activity only in presence of aldosterone

CLINICAL USE
Treatment of hypertension due to hypermineralocorticoidism
As an adjunct to thiazides
Treatment of congestive heart failure

ROUTE	*ONSET OF ACTION*	*ELIMINATION*
Oral	3 days	Excreted in urine and feces

ADVERSE EFFECTS
Hyperkalemia
Diarrhea
Gynecomastia
Menstrual irregularities
Impotence
Skin rash
Ataxia

FACTORS INFLUENCING THERAPEUTIC RESPONSE/TOXICITY
When administered with other diuretics, the drug produces synergistic response
    and decreases potassium secretion caused by other diuretics.
Stupor and coma may occur in patients with severe liver disease.

It may potentiate action of hypotensive agents.
Aspirin may antagonize diuretic effect.

NURSING CONSIDERATIONS
Patients should be instructed to avoid excessive intake of potassium-rich foods
   and potassium salt substitutes.
Serum electrolytes should be monitored.
Patients should be instructed about side effects.
Patients should be instructed not to take aspirin without a physician's order.

e. *Triamterene (Dyrenium)*

   ACTION
   Impedes sodium resorption
   Reduces potassium loss

   CLINICAL USE
   Treatment of hypertension
   As an adjunct to thiazides

ROUTE	*ONSET OF ACTION*	*ELIMINATION*
Oral	2 hr	Detoxified by liver and kidneys; excreted in urine and feces

   SIDE EFFECTS
   Nausea
   Vomiting
   Diarrhea
   Headache
   Skin rash
   Elevated blood urea
   Hyperkalemia
   Leg cramps

   FACTORS INFLUENCING THERAPEUTIC RESPONSE/TOXICITY
   This drug potentiates action of hypotensive drugs.
   Hyperkalemia may cause cardiac irregularities.

REFERENCES

1. Adams, R. D., and Braunwald, E. Faintness, Syncope and Episodic Weakness.
   In G. W. Thorn et al. (Eds.), *Harrison's Principles of Internal Medicine* (8th ed.).
   New York: McGraw-Hill, 1977. Pp. 75–89.
2. *American Neurological Association. Report of the Joint Committee for Stroke
   Facilities,* Vol. VII. Medical and Surgical Management of Stroke. Washington,
   D.C.: U.S. Department of Health, Education and Welfare, March-April 1973.
3. Andreoli, K., Fowkes, V., Zipes, D., and Wallace, A. *Comprehensive Cardiac
   Care* (3d ed.). St. Louis: Mosby, 1975. Pp. 1–7.
4. Beland, I., and Passos, J. *Clinical Nursing Pathophysiological and Psychosocial
   Approaches* (3rd ed.). New York: Macmillan, 1975. Pp. 508–509; 533–686.

5. Braunwald, E. Heart Failure. In G. W. Thorn et al. (Eds.), *Harrison's Principles of Internal Medicine* (8th ed.). New York: McGraw-Hill, 1977. Pp. 1178–1187.

6. Braunwald, E. Valvular Heart Disease. In G. W. Thorn et al. (Eds.), *Harrison's Principles of Internal Medicine* (8th ed.). New York: McGraw-Hill, 1977. Pp. 1243–1248.

7. Braunwald, E., and Pool, P. E. Pharmacologic Treatment of Cardiovascular Disorders. In G. W. Thorn et al. (Eds.), *Harrison's Principles of Internal Medicine* (8th ed.). New York: McGraw-Hill, 1977. Pp. 1206–1216.

8. Carini, E., and Owens, G. *Neurological and Neurosurgical Nursing* (6th ed.). St. Louis: Mosby, 1974. Pp. 11–40.

9. Cluff, L. E., and Caldwell, J. R. Reactions to Drugs. In G. W. Thorn et al. (Eds.), *Harrison's Principles of Internal Medicine* (8th ed.). New York: McGraw-Hill, 1977. Pp. 346–352.

10. Engelman, K., and Braunwald, E. Elevation of Arterial Pressure. In G. W. Thorn et al. (Eds.), *Harrison's Principles of Internal Medicine* (8th ed.). New York: McGraw-Hill, 1977. Pp. 188–192.

11. Fredrickson, D. S. Atherosclerosis and Other Forms of Arteriosclerosis. In G. W. Thorn et al. (Eds.), *Harrison's Principles of Internal Medicine* (8th ed.). New York: McGraw-Hill, 1977. Pp. 1297–1307.

12. Goldberg, L. J. Drug therapy dopamine – clinical uses of endogenous catecholamine. *N. Engl. J. Med.* 29:707, 1974.

13. Guyton, A. C. *Textbook of Medical Physiology* (5th ed.). Philadelphia: Saunders, 1976. Pp. 160–175; 222–236; 250–264; 916–927.

14. Jagger, P. J., and Braunwald, E. Hypertensive Vascular Disease. In G. W. Thorn et al. (Eds.), *Harrison's Principles of Internal Medicine* (8th ed.). New York: McGraw-Hill, 1977. Pp. 1307–1317.

15. Lesch, M., Ross, R., and Braunwald, E. Ischemic Heart Disease. In G. W. Thorn et al. (Eds.), *Harrison's Principles of Internal Medicine* (8th ed.). New York: McGraw-Hill, 1977. Pp. 1261–1270.

16. Lown, B. Electrical Reversion of Cardiac Arrhythmias. In G. W. Thorn et al. (Eds.), *Harrison's Principles of Internal Medicine* (8th ed.). New York: McGraw-Hill, 1977. Pp. 1216–1218.

17. Mohr, J. P., Fischer, C. M., and Adams, P. D. Cerebrovascular Diseases. In G. W. Thorn et al. (Eds.), *Harrison's Principles of Internal Medicine* (8th ed.). New York: McGraw-Hill, 1977. Pp. 1832–1868.

18. Moser, K. Pulmonary Thromboembolism. In G. W. Thorn et al. (Eds.), *Harrison's Principles of Internal Medicine* (8th ed.). New York: McGraw-Hill, 1977. Pp. 1401–1406.

19. Nossel, H. L. Congenital Disorders of Blood Coagulation Factors. In G. W. Thorn et al. (Eds.), *Harrison's Principles of Internal Medicine* (8th ed.). New York: McGraw-Hill, 1977. Pp. 1720–1728.

20. Olsen, E. Hazards of immobility. *Am. J. Nurs.* 67:780–782, 1967.

21. Ross, R., Lesch, M., and Braunwald, E. Acute Myocardial Infarction. In G. W. Thorn et al. (Eds.), *Harrison's Principles of Internal Medicine* (8th ed.). New York: McGraw-Hill, 1977. Pp. 1271–1282.

22. Ryan, R. Thrombophlebitis: Assessment and prevention. *Am. J. Nurs.* 76:1634–1636, 1976.

23. Sobel, B., and Braunwald, E. Cardiac Dysrhythmias. In G. W. Thorn et al. (Eds.), *Harrison's Principles of Internal Medicine* (8th ed.). New York: McGraw-Hill, 1977. Pp. 1187–1206.

24. Sparks, C. Peripheral pulses. *Am. J. Nurs.* 75: 1132–1133, 1975.

25. Strandness, D. E. Vascular Diseases of the Extremities. In G. W. Thorn et al. (Eds.), *Harrison's Principles of Internal Medicine* (8th ed.). New York: McGraw-Hill, 1977. Pp. 1321–1330.
26. Toole, J., and Patel, A. *Cerebrovascular Disorders.* New York: McGraw-Hill, 1974. Pp. 216–226; 375–391.
27. Whipple, G., et al. *Acute Coronary Care.* Boston, Little, Brown, 1972. Pp. 213–243.

9. Fluid and electrolyte balance and nutrition

BASIC PHYSIOLOGY OF FLUID AND ELECTROLYTE BALANCE

The basic living unit of the body is the cell. It is composed mainly of five basic substances: water, electrolytes, proteins, lipids, and carbohydrates. The human body contains 75 trillion cells. Each organ is actually an aggregate of various cells, with all cells requiring nutrition for maintenance of life. While each different type of cell is specifically adapted to perform one particular function within the body, all cells utilize almost identical nutrients, and the mechanisms for converting these nutrients into energy are basically the same for all cells. One of the major substances from which all cells derive energy is oxygen (O_2) which combines with carbohydrates (CHO), fats (F), and proteins (P) to release the energy required for cell function. The end products of these chemical reactions are delivered by the cell into the body fluids which surround each cell [6].

About fifty-six percent of the adult body is fluid. This represents approximately forty liters in a person weighing 70 kg. Fluid within the cells is referred to as *intracellular,* and that which fills the spaces surrounding the cells is called *extracellular.* Plasma, or intravascular fluid, accounts for 25% of the extracellular fluid, while 75% exists as interstitial fluid which immediately surrounds the cells. The cell obtains its essential nutrients and excretes its wastes by means of a constant exchange of materials with the extracellular fluid through the cell membrane. Thus cell activity affects the composition of extracellular fluid [6]. The functions of each organ system in the body are designed to maintain *homeostasis* or a state of constant balance within and between the extracellular and intracellular compartments of the body.

The essential difference between extracellular and intracellular fluid is the distribution of electrolytes within each of them. *Electrolytes* are chemical substances that form electrically charged particles when they are in solution. These particles are called ions. The unit of measure used for ions is milliequivalents (mEq) per liter, while molecules are expressed in milligrams or grams per 100 milliliters of fluid [11]. Positively charged ions are called *cations.* The principal cation in extracellular fluid is sodium (Na^+), and in intracellular fluid, potassium (K^+). Negatively charged ions are *anions.* The principal anion in extracellular fluid is chloride (Cl^-) and in intracellular fluid is the phosphate ion (HPO_4^{--}) [6].

Each of these ions serves an important function in the body. To assure healthy functioning of the cells the volume of body fluid must be maintained at an optimum level, and the level of each electrolyte must be maintained within a certain range, which is referred to as normal. Any deviation above or below this normal range will result in an adverse effect upon the body's physiological processes. Four basic physiological processes that are affected by electrolytes are (1) distribution of water,

(2) osmolality of body fluids, (3) neuromuscular irritability, and (4) acid-base balance [1, 11].

Extracellular fluid is called the internal environment of the body. It contains large quantities of sodium (Na^+) and chloride (Cl^-) ions and fairly large amounts of bicarbonate ions (HCO_3^-) but only small quantities of potassium (K^+), calcium (Ca^{++}), magnesium (Mg^{++}), phosphate (HPO_4^{--}), sulfate (SO_4^{--}), and organic acid ions. The plasma portion of the extracellular fluid contains a large amount of protein as well. The interstitial component contains much less protein. When the body is functioning normally, the constituents of its internal environment, the extracellular fluid, are regulated to assure the cells are surrounded by a fluid containing the electrolytes and nutrients required for cellular functioning [6].

Intracellular fluid, in contrast to the extracellular, contains only small amounts of sodium (Na^+) and chloride (Cl^-) ions and almost no calcium (Ca^{++}) ions. It has large quantities of potassium ions (K^+) and phosphate ions (HPO_4^{--}) and moderate amounts of magnesium (Mg^{++}) and sulfate (SO_4^{--}) ions. The cells also contain approximately four times the protein that is present in the plasma portion of the extracellular fluid (Fig. 9-1).

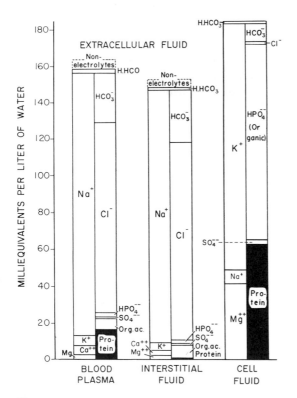

Figure 9-1
The composition of plasma, interstitial fluid and intracellular fluid. (From A. G. Guyton, Textbook of Medical Physiology *[5th ed.]. Philadelphia: Saunders, 1976.)*

The cell membrane that separates these two body fluid compartments into extracellular and intracellular fluid is semipermeable, that is, it allows water to pass through but not some of the dissolved solutes. Through the process of *osmosis,* when the concentration of nondiffusible substances is greater on one side of the cell membrane than the other, water passes through the membrane to the side that has the greater concentration of nondiffusible material. Osmosis results from the kinetic motion of the molecules in solution on both sides of the membrane. The individual molecules are equally active on both sides, but the nondiffusible solute on one side of the membrane displaces water, thereby reducing the concentration of water. The chemical activity of the water molecules on that side becomes less, resulting in a diffusion of water molecules to the solute side. In the healthy body a state of osmotic equilibrium is maintained constantly, since any disequilibrium is instantly corrected through osmotic transfer of water across the cell membrane. The potential pressure of nondiffusible particles is called the *osmotic pressure* of the solution. The amount of osmotic pressure exerted by a solute is proportional to the concentration of the solute in numbers of molecules or ions. This concentration in terms of numbers of particles is referred to as *osmolality.* One osmol is the number of particles in one gram molecular weight of undissociated solute [6].

Approximately four-fifths of the total osmolality of interstitial fluid and plasma is caused by sodium (Na^+) and chloride (Cl^-) ions. Approximately half the intracellular osmolality is caused by potassium (K^+) ions. The volume of both extracellular and intracellular fluids can be changed markedly due to (1) ingestion of water; (2) dehydration; (3) intravenous infusions of different types of solutions; (4) loss of fluid from the gastrointestinal tract, perspiration, or the kidneys [6]; (5) alterations in antidiuretic hormone (ADH) secretion; or (6) shock.

EFFECT OF ADDING WATER TO EXTRACELLULAR FLUID
Water can be added to extracellular fluid through infusion directly into the bloodstream, injection beneath the skin, or oral administration with absorption through the gastrointestinal tract into the blood. Addition of water to the extracellular fluid dilutes it, causing it to become hypotonic with respect to the intracellular fluids. At the cell membrane, osmosis begins immediately, causing large amounts of water to pass into the cells. Within minutes water is almost evenly distributed among both fluid compartments [6].

EFFECT OF DEHYDRATION
When water leaves the body by evaporation from the skin and lungs and/or excretion of very dilute urine, it is removed from the extracellular compartment. Immediately, by osmosis, water from the intracellular compartment passes into the extracellular compartment to maintain equal osmolalities in the two [6].

EFFECT OF ADDING SALINE SOLUTION TO THE EXTRACELLULAR COMPARTMENT
Fluids are classified as isotonic, hypotonic, or hypertonic according to their effect on the cell. An *isotonic* solution is one that causes neither swelling nor shrinkage of the cell. A 0.9% solution of sodium chloride is isotonic. A *hypotonic* solution is

one that causes the cells to swell. A solution of sodium chloride with a concentration of less than 0.9% is hypotonic. A *hypertonic* solution causes the cells to shrink. Any solution of sodium chloride with a concentration of over 0.9% is hypertonic [6].

When an isotonic solution is added to the extracellular compartment, there is no change in the osmolality of the fluid. Only the volume of fluid is increased. If a hypertonic solution is added, osmolality of the extracellular fluid increases, thereby causing osmosis of water out of the cell and into the extracellular compartment. The addition of a hypotonic solution to the extracellular compartment results in decreased osmolality, allowing some of the extracellular fluids to pass into the cells [6].

EFFECTS OF INFUSING HYPERTONIC GLUCOSE, MANNITOL, OR SUCROSE SOLUTIONS INTO THE EXTRACELLULAR COMPARTMENT

The purpose of administering concentrated solutions of glucose (greater than 5%), mannitol, or sucrose is to create an immediate decrease in intracellular fluid volume. Since these three substances are all excreted rapidly by the kidneys, and glucose is metabolized by the cells, the effect lasts only for several hours. However, since the intracellular fluid volume can be decreased by several liters in a matter of minutes, this effect can be used as a life-saving measure to reduce cerebral edema caused by pressure in the cranial vault, which obstructs the cerebral circulation [6].

EFFECT OF SOLUTIONS PROVIDED FOR NUTRITION

When the patient is too ill to take food and fluids by mouth, intravenous infusions are often administered to provide nutrition. In this case an attempt is made to adjust the concentration of the solution to as close to isotonic as possible (a 5% glucose solution is isotonic) or to regulate the rate of infusion slowly enough that osmotic equilibrium of the body fluids is not upset. Once the glucose or other nutrient has been metabolized, the excess water remaining will be excreted in the form of dilute urine, provided kidney function is normal. If kidney function is impaired, the patient will become overhydrated and possibly "water intoxicated." This is manifested by mental irritability and convulsions [6].

MANAGEMENT OF PATIENTS WITH FLUID AND ELECTROLYTE DISTURBANCES

In caring for the acutely ill patient who has suffered a stroke, regulation of fluid and electrolyte balance is a major objective. Such patients are prime candidates for body fluid disturbances. Intelligent management requires a thorough knowledge of the mechanisms that regulate fluid volume and electrolyte balance, the manifestations of their disturbance, and those factors that contribute to such disturbances. The management of patients with such problems is neither simple nor precise. Therefore, the nurse must be aware of the effect of chronic illness and the interrelationship of various organ systems on the causes and treatment of fluid and electrolyte imbalances. She must also be knowledgeable concerning the approximate exchange of water and various ions that occurs in maintaining and restoring body fluids to normal volume and effective osmolarity. The nurse carries a great responsibility for early detection of body fluid disturbances. Maintaining an accurate record of the patient's total intake and elimination with specification of the type of fluid lost will facilitate proper restoration and resolve many of the complex problems concerning disorders of hydration.

Disturbances in body fluids are usually characterized by a change in volume, concentration, osmotic pressure, or hydrogen ion concentration. The most frequently seen disturbances are those resulting from either an excess or a deficit of water, sodium, potassium, calcium, or hydrogen ions. Often these imbalances occur simultaneously in various combinations.

Disturbances in Body Fluids and Electrolyte Balance

As has been previously noted, homeostasis, or the maintenance of an optimum biochemical environment in the fluids surrounding the cells, is a fundamental requirement for cellular function. The concentration of various ions in the body fluids is important in the processes of nerve conduction and muscle contraction. Therefore, electrolyte disturbances usually manifest themselves in abnormalities of conduction and contraction. Conduction of an impulse depends on a change in the nerve cell membrane's permeability to the positively charged sodium ions that are concentrated in the extracellular fluid. Calcium ions serve to render the cell membrane permeable to sodium ions, which diffuse into the nerve cells. This diffusion of positively charged sodium ions into the cell creates a negative charge outside and a positive charge inside the cell. When the positive charge becomes excessive, it causes the concentration of positively charged potassium ions within the cell to move out. As this process spreads through the nerve fiber, the impulse is transmitted. To restore the nerve cell to its original state, the process is reversed [11].

Many factors contribute to disturbances in the equilibrium of fluids and electrolytes. The most important are (1) a simple deficit or excess of water and/or electrolytes provided to the patient; (2) an inability to ingest or absorb water or electrolytes; (3) kidney failure; (4) excessive loss of fluid or electrolytes through the skin, gastrointestinal tract, lungs, or kidneys; (5) loss of fluid resulting from injury to the tissues and/or blood loss; (6) shift of fluid from one compartment to another, as in the development of ascites or edema. The ultimate effect of any of these factors will be determined by how they influence the volume, distribution, osmolality and concentration of fluid and electrolytes in each compartment [1].

WATER DEFICIT
Effect. The most frequent disturbance of fluid and electrolyte imbalance is a deficit of water, caused either by inadequate intake or excessive output. The resulting loss of extracellular fluid leads to an increase in the concentration and osmolality of the extracellular fluid, which will cause osmosis of water out of the cell and into the more concentrated extracellular fluid. The result is an increased concentration of serum sodium and cellular dehydration. The normal response to this is thirst. Failure to drink is the commonest cause of a water deficit and is of particular significance for the patient with stroke. His sensorium may be clouded, or he may be too weak to respond to thirst, unable to drink because of paralysis of the face and upper extremity, or unable to communicate his thirst because of aphasia [1].

Tube feedings may be initiated for stroke patients because of prolonged coma or inability to swallow. If feedings contain large quantities of protein, and the patient is unable to store large amounts of nitrogen, he may develop a water deficit that goes unnoticed because there is a large amount of unconcentrated urine excreted and the patient is unable to communicate his thirst [14].

Fluid lost through the integumentary, respiratory, or urinary systems may be in the form of water alone or water with electrolytes. Sweat usually contains some sodium and chloride. However, normal perspiration as well as diarrhea can cause a loss of water with little or no electrolyte loss, in contrast to profuse diaphoresis, in which large amounts of electrolytes are also lost. Deep, rapid breathing contributes to greater water loss than normal breathing. Thus the lethargic, comatose, or confused patient is more likely to develop a water deficit if strict attention is not paid to his fluid intake and elimination. Whenever a loss of water continues without a comparable loss of electrolytes, the amount of available intracellular fluid may be insufficient to correct the water deficit in the extracellular fluid compartment. This will result in elevated levels of hemaglobin, nonprotein nitrogen, sodium, and other electrolytes in the blood. The hematocrit (Hct), which represents the proportion of red blood cells to blood plasma, will also rise. The kidneys will excrete small volumes of highly concentrated urine. In patients with normal kidney function, a urine output of less than 500–800 ml in a 24-hour period indicates an insufficient intake of water [1]. As dehydration increases, water will continue to be taken from the extracellular spaces. The skin and mucous membranes will become dry, and with severe dehydration the eyeballs will become soft.

Prevention and Correction of Water Deficit.   Adequate fluid intake prevents a water deficit. The adequacy of the intake is evaluated by monitoring the urine output, fluid intake, condition of mucous membranes, and weight. The urine output should be at least 500–800 ml per 24-hour period. The mucous membranes should be clean and moist. Weight loss of more than 1 pound per day or an increased irritability may indicate an insufficient intake of water [1].

If the patient is unable to tolerate oral fluids, intravenous infusions will be required. The nurse must see that the correct amount and solution of parenteral fluid is administered at the rate prescribed. Fluids provided over a 12–24 hour period usually contribute more to the patient's fluid and electrolyte balance than those given within a 6-hour span. However, the rate at which intravenous solutions can be administered safely varies with the condition of the patient and the concentration of the solution [1, 14].

Hypotonic solutions (glucose solutions of less than 5%, electrolyte solutions with a concentration of less than 150 mEq/liter, or saline solutions of less than 0.9%) should not be administered to prevent or correct a water deficit, since addition of the hypotonic solution to the extracellular compartment will cause more extracellular fluids to pass into the cells.

Hypertonic solutions (glucose solutions of greater than 5% or saline solutions of greater than 0.9%) should not be given at a rate of more than 200 ml per hour. The maximum rate of flow for glucose solutions is 0.5 gm per kilogram of body weight per hour, since a faster rate will result in glycosuria and loss of potassium [1].

Isotonic solutions can be given at a higher rate, but always slower for elderly patients because of the reduced compliance of their circulatory systems and impaired cardiac and renal function. If urinary output exceeds 50 ml per hour, the rate should be slowed down in all cases.

WATER EXCESS

Effect. Water excess results from an increased volume of water in one or both body fluid compartments due to an intake of fluid in excess of the total output. It is usually reflected first in the extracellular compartment and may result from an excessive amount of intravenous fluid administered too rapidly. This excess of water dilutes the sodium (hyponatremia) and other osmotically active substances in the extracellular fluid, thereby decreasing its osmolality. Water then passes through the cell membrane, causing the cell to swell. The result of this may be disturbed cerebral function, coma, and even death. It is important to note that the severity of the patient's reaction to the fluid overload is related to the rapidity with which the water passes from the extracellular compartment into the intracellular rather than to the degree of dilution created in the extracellular fluid. Water intoxication can occur if the patient's renal function is impaired and if other mechanisms for elimination of water fail [1, 14].

Prevention and Correction of Water Excess. The flow rate of all intravenous solutions must be monitored carefully and regulated properly. Weight should be taken daily at the same time and under similar conditions (e.g., same scale and clothing) and recorded. The color and amount of urine should be carefully noted and its specific gravity measured to determine the ability of the kidney to concentrate urine. When impairment of renal function is suspected or documented, the urinary output should be measured hourly. The patient should be observed carefully for signs of confusion or dyspnea, and fluid intake should be restricted once it has been determined that there has been an overload of fluid [1, 14].

SODIUM DEFICIT (HYPONATREMIA)

Effect. Hyponatremia, or a deficit of sodium in the extracellular fluid, occurs when the patient's serum sodium level drops to less than 135 mEq per liter. It may be caused by a decreased intake of sodium, an increased output of sodium, an increased intake of water, or an increased output of water. It is seen most commonly when there is dehydration or edema, in which salt is lost in excess of water or water retained in excess of salt [14]. Excessive sweating with an intake of plain water can cause sodium deficit, as can repeated tapwater enemas, intravenous infusions of electrolyte-free solutions, or the use of potent diuretics. The symptoms of hyponatremia include a feeling of apprehension or impending doom, abdominal cramps, oliguria or anuria, or clouded sensorium. If the deficit is severe, hypotension will occur and the pulse will be rapid and thready. The patient may develop cyanosis, cold clammy skin, and even seizures and coma [1, 14].

Treatment. When hyponatremia complicates the course of illness, its treatment requires replacement of both sodium and water. If this cannot be accomplished with oral feedings, intravenous replacement will be necessary. A hypertonic solution is used unless the patient has edema or is known to have impaired renal function or inappropriate secretion of ADH. Administration of sodium increases the osmotic activity of the intracellular fluid by promoting movement of water from the cells into the extracellular compartment as its osmolarity is increased [1, 14]; thus osmotic equality is preserved throughout the body.

Syndrome of inappropriate antidiuretic hormone (SIADH)

The antidiuretic hormone (ADH), or vasopressin, assists in maintaining the constancy of osmolality and volume of body fluids by conserving water and concentrating urine. This hormone is stored in the posterior portion of the pituitary. Its secretion is stimulated by the supraoptic nuclei of the hypothalamus in response to concentration of electrolytes within the neurons of the lateral hypothalamus, activation of carotid and aortic baroreceptors in severe hypotension and neural impulses from the left atrium via the vagus nerve in volume depletion.

When ADH, or vasopressin, is released into the blood, it acts primarily on the collecting ducts of the kidneys to cause massive reabsorption of water [13]. A syndrome of inappropriate ADH secretion (SIADH) occurs in association with many clinical disorders, among them cerebral vascular thrombosis and subarachnoid hemorrhage. SIADH seen in cerebrovascular disorders is felt to be the result of stimulation of the hypothalamic-neurohypophyseal system [13]. The syndrome involves continual release of ADH, unrelated to plasma osmolality, and it is characterized by hyponatremia due to water retention in the presence of a urinary osmolality that is greater than the plasma osmolality. The patient with SIADH is unable to excrete dilute urine, and the fluids that he receives are retained, resulting in expansion of his extracellular fluid volume and development of dilutional hyponatremia. With this syndrome, the amount of ADH released and the elevation of urine osmolality are inappropriate only in relationship to the level of the plasma osmolality or the serum sodium concentration [13].

TREATMENT

SIADH associated with cerebrovascular disorders is transient and clears with the underlying disease. Signs and symptoms are related to acute water intoxication. Patients are usually treated with fluid restriction. However, some patients may also require intravenous saline for treatment of severe hyponatremia. When there is congestive heart failure, careful diuretic therapy may also be prescribed [13].

Excess of sodium (hypernatremia)

EFFECT

Hypernatremia or an excess of sodium in the blood occurs when the serum sodium level exceeds 147 mEq per liter. It is, in effect, a concentration of sodium in the serum, and may be caused by a decreased intake or loss of water or by the administration or ingestion of salt in excess of water. High fever or rapid breathing can contribute to a loss of water [14].

The patient with hypernatremia will have dry sticky mucous membranes and a rough dry tongue and will complain of intense thirst. This may be accompanied by flushed skin, an elevated temperature, excretion of very concentrated urine, and oliguria or anuria. Sometimes there is profuse watery diarrhea and excitement progressing to mania or convulsions.

The sodium excess results in water retention, thereby increasing the extracellular fluid volume. When the body's mechanism for eliminating excess sodium and maintaining homeostasis breaks down, edema develops. The most serious results of hypernatremia are overloading of the circulatory system and pulmonary edema [1].

Hypernatremia poses special problems in the management of patients with (1) renal failure; (2) disorders in which the circulation of blood through the kidneys is inadequate, as congestive heart failure; (3) cirrhosis of the liver; (4) disorders characterized by overproduction of aldosterone by the adrenal cortex; and (5) conditions requiring large doses of adrenal corticoids [1].

PREVENTION AND CORRECTION OF SODIUM EXCESS

Hypernatremia is treated by correcting the situation responsible for the concentration of sodium in the extracellular fluid. This will include restriction of sodium intake, increase of water intake, and correction of underlying causes such as fever, glycosuria, and diarrhea [14]. Because patients with stroke frequently have a history of hypertension, cardiovascular disease, renal impairment, and/or diabetes mellitus, maintaining electrolyte balance is a challenge. If hypernatremia is to be prevented, it is important that the nurse carefully observe and record the patient's intake and elimination and be alert to changes that would indicate an electrolyte or body fluid imbalance.

Potassium deficit (hypokalemia)

EFFECT

Hypokalemia, a deficit of potassium in the extracellular fluid, occurs when the serum potassium level falls below 4 mEq per liter. It may be due to prolonged use of parenteral fluids without the addition of potassium or depletion due to use of diuretics, steroids, or sodium bicarbonate. It may also be due to losses from the gastrointestinal tract because of vomiting, diarrhea, or drastic use of cathartics or enemas [4, 14].

Potassium is important in maintaining intracellular fluid volume and helps to regulate neuromuscular irritability and cardiac function. It is a key factor in maintaining the hydrogen ion concentration in the blood (see Acid-base Balance) [1].

Symptoms of hypokalemia include muscle weakness, irritability, anorexia, nausea, vomiting, paralytic ileus, and diarrhea. As potassium has an effect on the myocardium, a deficiency may lead to a weak pulse, heart block, and hypotension. Definite changes will be noted on the electrocardiogram. The patient with hypokalemia will have shallow respirations and experience thirst [4].

PREVENTION AND TREATMENT OF POTASSIUM DEFICIT
The consequences of a deficit of potassium may be dangerous, but replacement of this ion is not without serious risk. The greatest hazard is the possibility of cardiotoxic effects caused by a too rapidly administered or a too concentrated intravenous replacement. It is safer to replace losses orally because there is a delay in their absorption from the gastrointestinal tract. When intravenous solutions containing potassium are administered, the rate of infusion must be monitored and regulated carefully in accordance with serum level determinations and electrocardiogram patterns. As a safeguard against too rapid infusion, the concentration of potassium may be limited to 50 mEq per liter of intravenous solution. Meat broths, bananas, and citrus fruits are all rich in potassium. If the patient is able to take oral feedings safely, he should be encouraged to have some of these foods daily, especially if he has been on a sodium-restricted diet, is receiving diuretics, or is recovering from diabetic acidosis [1, 14].

With hypokalemia the sensitivity of the heart muscle to digitalis is increased. Doses of digitalis in the usual therapeutic range may cause digitalis toxicity in patients with a deficit of potassium. Early signs of this are anorexia, nausea, and vomiting. The patient may complain of yellow vision and may have disturbances in cardiac rhythm, the most common being premature ventricular contractions (PVC) due to increased irritability of the ventricles. Heart block and even ventricular fibrillation and sinus arrest may occur. The nurse must be alert to the onset of any of these problems in stroke patients who have been receiving digitalis preparations for a preexisting heart condition [1].

Potassium excess (hyperkalemia)

EFFECT
Hyperkalemia, an excess of potassium in the extracellular fluid, occurs when serum levels of potassium exceed 5.6 mEq per liter. It can be caused by an unduly large dose of potassium replacement or by adrenal insufficiency or advanced kidney disease. With hyperkalemia the patient may be irritable and have nausea, intestinal colic, and diarrhea. As the excess of potassium increases, weakness will be noted and this may progress to paralysis. There may be severe renal impairment. Because of the effect of potassium on the heart muscle the patient may develop cardiac arrhythmias and possibly arrest [4].

PREVENTION AND TREATMENT OF EXCESS OF POTASSIUM
It is important to remember that hyperkalemia, like all other fluid and electrolyte disturbances, does not necessarily occur as a distinct and separate condition. Frequently the stroke patient who has less than optimum kidney function and a host of

other complicating illnesses will manifest a combination of disturbances in fluid and electrolyte balance. The nurse must be aware that the correction of one problem may create others.

Potassium excess occurs most commonly with parenteral administration of potassium to correct a deficiency or to meet the daily maintenance needs of a patient who is unable to take sufficient nourishment by mouth. The rate of all intravenous infusions should be regulated with care, but those containing potassium, in particular, require the utmost attention in order to prevent the possibility of the irreversible and catastrophic effects of an overdose.

If the patient's kidneys are functioning properly, hyperkalemia may be treated by avoiding additional intake of potassium. If the patient is able to eat, protein intake will be restricted. When there is impairment of renal function, peritoneal dialysis or even hemodialysis may become necessary [1].

Deficit of calcium (hypocalcemia)

EFFECT
Ninety-nine percent of the body's calcium is found in bone. The remaining 1% exists in the blood in two forms. That which is bound to serum protein and is non-diffusible accounts for 45%. The remainder (55%) of the serum calcium is ionized and diffusible. Hypocalcemia, or a deficit of calcium in the extracellular fluid, occurs when the serum calcium level drops below 4.5 mEq per liter [1, 4]. The level of calcium in the blood is regulated by the parathyroid hormone, which stimulates dissolution and reabsorption of calcium from the bone and increases absorption of calcium via the gastrointestinal tract when serum levels are low. An elevated serum calcium level will inhibit further release of this hormone. The level of serum calcium is regulated in relation to the level of phosphate ions in the extracellular fluid [11].

Calcium is required for bone formation. It also functions in the regulation of neuromuscular irritability, blood coagulation, and irritability of heart muscle [1]. Ionized calcium in the body fluids regulates the permeability of cell membranes. When hypocalcemia occurs, permeability of the cell membrane increases, thereby permitting leakage of both potassium and sodium across the cell membrane. The result of this leakage across nerve fibers can result in rapid, uncontrollable spasms, known as tetany, once the serum calcium level drops 30% below normal. This condition can be lethal when it causes spasm of the respiratory muscles [11].

Hypocalcemia may occur in the stroke patient who is alkalotic, has been treated for acidosis, or has advanced renal disease in which the kidney has lost its ability to conserve calcium. Administration of citrated blood or calcium-free intravenous solutions can also cause a deficiency of calcium in the blood. Sensory manifestations include tingling of the fingers, lips, tongue, and feet. Motor manifestations consist of facial and muscle spasms (tetany), laryngospasm, and convulsions [1, 4].

PREVENTION AND TREATMENT OF HYPOCALCEMIA
In acute calcium deficit a 10% solution of calcium gluconate is administered intravenously. The effect is immediate but of only short duration, and additional calcium

replacement may therefore be required. The flow rate of the infusion must be very carefully regulated for patients receiving digitalis, since rapid infusion of calcium may lead to cardiac arrest [1].

Excess of calcium (hypercalcemia)

EFFECT
Hypercalcemia, or an excess of calcium in the blood, occurs when the serum level of calcium exceeds 5.8 mEq per liter. It has a number of causes, including hyperparathyroidism, overdose of vitamin D, and multiple myeloma. Hyperfunction of the parathyroids, a common complication of advanced kidney disease, may result in retention of calcium. Prolonged immobilization also encourages calcium retention.

The patient with hypercalcemia will have hypotonicity of the muscles. An elevated serum calcium decreases the permeability of the cell membrane and, in contrast to the effect of hypocalcemia, decreases the excitability of the nerve fibers, causing depression of the central nervous system and sluggish, relaxed muscles. Flank and bone pain as well as kidney stones may occur [4, 11].

PREVENTION AND TREATMENT OF HYPERCALCEMIA
Treatment of hypercalcemia is directed toward correction of the underlying condition. Care must be exercised in administering calcium replacements so as not to induce hypercalcemia.

Deficit of Magnesium

EFFECT
Magnesium deficit is not common but may arise with impaired gastrointestinal absorption of magnesium as a result of chronic alcoholism, vomiting, diarrhea, and other gastrointestinal disease. It is also likely to be observed with diabetic acidosis. Magnesium is concentrated within the cells and is necessary to the activation of many enzyme systems such as the phosphatase enzymes. It is the cofactor with thiamine in the intermediate carbohydrate metabolism. It also functions in the metabolism of calcium and phosphorous and is important in the regeneration of protein [1, 4, 14].

Approximately fifty percent of the body's magnesium is in the bone. The concentration in serum is fairly constant, between 1.5 and 2.0 mEq per liter. Approximately one-third of this is bound to protein. A serum level of less than 1.4 mEq per liter is considered hypomagnesemia and is manifested by weakness, agitation, confusion, disorientation, muscle fasciculations, and possibly convulsions and coma [14].

PREVENTION AND TREATMENT OF MAGNESIUM DEFICIT
Since the body's conservation of magnesium is very efficient, there may be no deficiency until the patient is on prolonged parenteral fluid maintenance without magnesium replacement. The condition can be resolved by addition of a magnesium supplement. This deficit is easily mistaken for a potassium deficit. When a magnesium deficiency is suspected, and the serum potassium level is within the normal range, magnesium sulfate is usually administered as a therapeutic test. It is difficult

to evaluate the specific characteristics of the response to magnesium therapy, since the quantitative nature of the deficit cannot be defined. Magnesium sulfate is usually administered in doses containing 10 mEq of magnesium with frequent checks of serum levels. Serum levels as high as 4 mEq per liter have not resulted in untoward effects [14].

Protein deficit in extracellular fluid (hypoproteinemia)

EFFECT

A deficit of protein can result from trauma, blood loss, decreased food intake, or pressure sores. Its symptoms include easy fatigability, loss of muscle mass and tone, weight loss, and depression. A protein deficit leads to a decreased resistance to infection. Under normal conditions the osmotic pressure of plasma is higher than that of interstitial fluid because of the presence of plasma proteins, but in hypoproteinemia the concentration of the plasma, and therefore the level of plasma colloid osmotic pressure, is reduced, creating edema.

PREVENTION AND TREATMENT OF PROTEIN DEFICIT

During the acute phase of stroke the patient's inability to take nutritional foods by mouth because of unconsciousness, swallowing difficulties, or paralysis often results in a protein deficiency. In addition prolonged immobilization may lead to development of pressure necrosis, which will create an even greater protein deficiency. Since hypoproteinemia also leads to edema, special attention should be paid to prevention of skin breakdown. Attempts must be made to guarantee a sufficient protein intake as soon as possible.

ACID-BASE BALANCE

Acid-base balance is one of the most important aspects of homeostasis. The most significant item in acid-base balance is the hydrogen ion (H^+). Various organ systems regulate acid-base balance by regulating hydrogen ion concentration in extracellular and intracellular fluids. *Acid* refers to any substance that can give up a hydrogen ion, and *base* refers to any substance that can accept a hydrogen ion [6, 15].

The symbol pH represents a formula used to express the hydrogen ion concentration. A low pH means a high concentration of hydrogen ions and hence greater acidity; a high pH means a low concentration of hydrogen ions, hence less acidity or greater alkalinity. At a pH of 7 a solution is neutral. A solution with a pH of less than 7 is acid, while one above 7 is alkaline or basic. The pH of arterial blood is approximately 7.4. Any arterial pH above 7.4 is alkalemia and any below 7.4 is acidemia [15]. Alterations in body functions follow any change in the normal range of pH of body fluids. The lowest limit at which a patient can live for more than a few minutes is about 7.0. The uppermost limit is 7.8. As blood levels approach pH 7.0, the central nervous system is depressed, the patient goes into coma, and death may ensue. With an increasing pH, the hyperexcitability of the central nervous system leads to tetany and paralysis of the respiratory muscles [11, 15].

The body has three control systems that regulate acid-base balance and restore it to normal when excess acid or base enters the body: the buffers, the respiratory system, and the kidney. These three systems supplement each other; when one fails, the others attempt to compensate [11, 14].

ACID-BASE BUFFER SYSTEMS

The first line of defense is the buffer systems, which are able to act within a fraction of a second against changes in the pH of body fluids. Buffers are present in all body fluids. They are solutions of two or more chemical compounds that can combine with strong acids to form weak acids or with strong bases to form weak bases by altering the pH. There are three major buffer systems, each of which performs under specific conditions: the bicarbonate, the phosphate, and the protein buffer systems [11, 12].

The *bicarbonate buffer system* is composed of carbonic acid (H_2CO_3), which is very weak, and sodium bicarbonate ($NaHCO_3$), which is a salt of that acid. If a strong acid is added to this buffer, it will react with the sodium bicarbonate to form more carbonic acid, which is a weak acid. If a strong base is added, it will combine with the hydrogen ion in the carbonic acid to form water and more sodium bicarbonate, which is a weak base. In either case a significant alteration in pH has been prevented [11, 15].

The *phosphate buffer system* is composed of disodium phosphate (Na_2HPO_4) and monosodium phosphate (NaH_2PO_4). Strong acid added to the system will convert some disodium phosphate to monosodium phosphate, a weak acid. When a strong base is added, it will react to form disodium phosphate, a weak base [11, 15].

The *protein buffer system* is the most powerful of the three buffer systems and carries out 75% of the body's buffering activity. Both intracellular and extracellular fluid contain proteins, which are composed of various amino acids linked together. Since some amino acids have free acidic radicals and some have free basic radicals, proteins can react as either acids or bases to maintain the pH level [11, 15].

RESPIRATORY REGULATION OF ACID-BASE BALANCE

The body's second line of defense against changes in hydrogen ion concentration is alteration in the depth and rate of respiration. Carbon dioxide (CO_2) is being formed continuously by intracellular metabolic processes in which the carbon in foods is oxidized. Carbon dioxide thus formed diffuses into the interstitial fluids and the blood, by which it is transported to the lungs. There it diffuses into the alveoli and is excreted by pulmonary ventilation. The respiratory system controls the pH of body fluids by varying the rate of carbon dioxide removal. An increase in the depth and rate of respirations increases alveolar ventilation, thereby increasing carbon dioxide removal. This lowers the hydrogen ion concentration, thus shifting the pH of the body fluids toward decreased acidity or increased alkalinity. Conversely, a decrease in the depth and rate of respirations decreases alveolar ventilation and slows down carbon dioxide removal. This increases hydrogen ion concentration and shifts the pH of body fluids toward increased acidity or decreased alkalinity [6, 11, 15].

The respiratory center in the medulla controls breathing and regulates respiratory rate and depth to maintain acid-base balance whenever an accumulation of carbon dioxide in body fluids jeopardizes the normal concentration of hydrogen ions. This mechanism functions within a matter of minutes [11].

The pressure of carbon dioxide in body fluids is expressed as PCO_2. The normal PCO_2 in venous blood is 45, while that for arterial blood is 40. Intracellular fluid has a PCO_2 of 46. Carbon dioxide will diffuse from an area of high concentration to a lower one. An increased metabolic rate will increase PCO_2 in venous blood, increase the hydrogen ion concentration and acidity, and decrease the pH. This acts as a direct stimulus on the respiratory center to increase the depth of inspirations. With a higher level of carbon dioxide the respiratory center is stimulated to accelerate the rate of respirations as well. The increase in ventilation lowers the PCO_2 in alveolar air, facilitates diffusion of CO_2, decreases the hydrogen ion concentration, and restores the body fluid pH to normal. Without further stimulus to the respiratory center the depth and rate of respirations returns to normal [2, 3, 11, 15].

It is important to note that, just as the concentration of hydrogen ions in body fluids can stimulate the respiratory center, variation in respiration will have an effect on the pH of body fluids. Any decrease in alveolar ventilation decreases the effectiveness of the respiratory mechanism in controlling acid-base balance. This is very significant in the care of the stroke patient, whose respiratory function may be severely impaired [11, 15].

RENAL REGULATION OF HYDROGEN ION CONCENTRATION
As a third line of defense the kidneys regulate acid-base balance by increasing or decreasing the rate of four basic processes in response to the body's need for relief from either excess acid or alkali. These processes are (1) tubular secretion of hydrogen ions, (2) reabsorption of sodium ions, (3) conservation of bicarbonate, and (4) ammonia synthesis [11, 15].

When extracellular carbon dioxide levels are high because of an increased metabolic rate and/or respiratory insufficiency, the kidney acts to remove the excess carbon dioxide by accelerating the process of secretion of hydrogen ions by the tubular cells. Each hydrogen ion secreted is exchanged for a sodium ion, which is reabsorbed. A bicarbonate ion is formed in the tubular cells each time a hydrogen ion is formed. These bicarbonate ions diffuse into the peritubular fluid in combination with the reabsorbed sodium ions, thus conserving bicarbonate. In addition, bicarbonate ions combine with the hydrogen ions to form carbonic acid, which dissociates into carbon dioxide and water. The carbon dioxide diffuses into the peritubular fluid, and the water passes into the urine [11, 15].

Hydrogen ions can also be transported from the tubules to the exterior by combining with ammonia, which is continuously synthesized by the proximal and distal tubules. The ammonia reacts with the hydrogen ions to form ammonia ions, which are then excreted in the urine in combination with chloride or other tubular anions [11, 15].

The ammonia-secreting mechanism is particularly important, because it can adapt readily to handle greatly increased loads of acid elimination. Most of the negative ions in tubular fluid are chloride. Very few hydrogen ions could be transported in combination with chloride, since the resulting hydrochloric acid would cause the pH to fall to 4.5, and hydrogen secretion would cease. In combination with ammonia the hydrogen ions form a neutral salt. When tubular fluids remain highly acid for prolonged periods, the formation of ammonia will increase steadily to restore the pH [11, 15].

CLINICAL ABNORMALITIES OF ACID-BASE BALANCE

There are four major disturbances of acid-base equilibrium: (1) respiratory acidosis, (2) metabolic acidosis, (3) respiratory alkalosis, and (4) metabolic alkalosis. (See Table 9-1). These occur frequently in combination.

Respiratory acidosis.   Respiratory acidosis is caused by inadequate elimination of carbon dioxide by the lungs due to hypoventilation or uneven ventilation in relation to blood flow. The decrease in effective pulmonary ventilation leads to an accumulation of carbon dioxide in the extracellular fluid and an increase in hydrogen ion concentration. The retention of carbon dioxide will increase the P_{CO_2}. Respiratory acidosis may arise from damage to the respiratory center, airway obstruction, paralysis of respiratory muscles, pneumonia, pulmonary edema, decreased alveolar surface as in emphysema, or any other condition that interferes with exchange of gases between the blood and alveolar air [13a, 15].

The signs of respiratory acidosis include restlessness, dulled sensorium, disorientation, elevated pulse, increased perspiration, and eventual coma. The pH is decreased and the P_{CO_2} elevated. Both these factors stimulate ventilation. The kidneys also respond to help eliminate acid and alter electrolyte composition. If the underlying condition worsens and hypercapnea continues in response to stimulation of the respiratory center, sensitivity to the repeated stimulation of an elevated P_{CO_2} diminishes until hypercapnea becomes extreme. At this point the ensuing hypoxia serves as the stimulus for respiratory activity since an increased P_{CO_2} is no longer an appropriate stimulus. Correction of the hypoxia with concentrations of oxygen may remove the last effective stimulus for respiratory activity, and the patient will become confused, rapidly lapse into coma, and die. Oxygen therapy should therefore be carried out with the utmost caution, and strict regulation of the oxygen concentration must be maintained. The patient should be watched carefully for any changes in mental status. Frequently a mechanical respirator may be required to provide the necessary ventilatory exchange [15].

Metabolic acidosis.   Metabolic acidosis refers to an acid-base imbalance due to any other cause than respiratory. It results from either a primary loss of bicarbonate or an accumulation of metabolic acids. Loss of bicarbonate is caused most frequently by prolonged or severe diarrhea. Prolonged vomiting may also result in metabolic acidosis when alkaline intestinal fluids are lost along with gastric secretions. Primary loss of bicarbonate is also seen in renal disease. Metabolic acids accumulate in diabetic acidosis and renal insufficiency when the kidneys fail to rid the body of acids formed by the daily metabolic processes. Intravenous administration of metabolic acids, a decreased food intake, and systemic infections may contribute to metabolic acidosis [6, 13a, 15].

Metabolic acidosis is characterized by headaches, lethargy, or coma with deep, rapid breathing. There may be a fruity odor to the breath. With metabolic acidosis, the reduction of bicarbonate and increase in carbonic acid reduces the pH of

Table 9-1
Clinical abnormalities of acid-base balance

Acidosis	Alkalosis
Respiratory (Acute)	*Respiratory* (Acute)
Arterial hypercapnea	Arterial hypocapnia
Blood Gases	*Blood Gases*
Elevated PCO_2	Low PCO_2
Low pH	Elevated pH
Normal HCO_3^-	Normal HCO_3^-
Primary Causative Factor	*Primary Causative Factor*
Hypoventilation	Hyperventilation
Mechanism	*Mechanism*
Reduced alveolar ventilation slows rate of CO_2 excretion from lungs	Increased alveolar ventilation speeds up rate of CO_2 excretion from lungs
Retention of CO_2 in body raises PCO_2	Depletion of CO_2 in body lowers PCO_2
CO_2 reacts with body fluids to form carbonic acid	Reduction of carbonic acid raises the ratio of bicarbonate to carbonic acid
$$CO_2 + H_2O \rightleftharpoons H_2CO_3^- \rightleftharpoons H_2 + HCO_3^-$$	$$CO_2 + H_2O \rightleftharpoons H_2CO_3^- \rightleftharpoons H_2 + HCO_3^-$$
Metabolic	*Metabolic*
Excess of any acid in the body other than CO_2	Excess of base in body fluids
Blood Gases	*Blood Gases*
Low PCO_2	Normal to elevated PCO_2
Low pH	Elevated pH
Low HCO_3^-	Elevated HCO_3^-
Primary Causative Factor	*Primary Causative Factor*
Loss of alkali or retention of metabolic acids	Loss of acidic contents of gastro-intestinal tract
	Depletion of K^+ due to diuretics
	Ingestion of large amounts of alkaline drugs
Mechanism	*Mechanism*
Accumulation of metabolic acid load due to renal insufficiency, circulatory failure, or diabetes	Loss of acid or retention of bases due to vomiting, diarrhea, diuretic therapy, or suction and ingestion of alkaline substances increases the ratio of base to acid and results in an elevated HCO_3^- and pH.
Addition of large amounts of fixed acids to blood or depletion of bicarbonate from prolonged diarrhea results in loss of base (HCO_3^-) and decrease in pH.	

extracellular fluid. This serves as a stimulus to increase pulmonary ventilation, and Kussmaul breathing develops. These deep, rapid respirations compensate for acidosis by rapid removal of carbon dioxide from the body fluids. With accelerated excretion of carbon dioxide, the PCO_2 will drop, and any change in pH will be minimized. The kidneys respond to metabolic acidosis with almost total reabsorption of filtered bicarbonate and an increase in urinary excretion of acid [15].

In diabetes mellitus, lack of insulin secretion by the pancreas prevents normal use of glucose for metabolism, so fats and protein must be used for energy. Metabolism of fats increases the number of ketone bodies, which are acidic, in the blood. Their excretion as sodium salts of ketone in the urine depletes sodium bicarbonate as well. Adequate insulin coverage will promote restoration of acid-base balance [15].

In chronic renal failure, metabolic acidosis may be due to inadequate reabsorption of bicarbonate and may be corrected by administering sodium bicarbonate.

In general, treatment of metabolic acidosis consists in correcting the condition causing the abnormality, if possible. Sodium bicarbonate may be given intravenously but cautiously, since it has possible complications. One is overcorrection of the acidosis and resultant alkalosis. The other is hypocalcemic tetany. Many patients with metabolic acidosis have increased calcium excretion. While acidotic the patient is protected from tetany due to hypocalcemia. With administration of sodium bicarbonate and correction of the pH, tetany can result if there is a severe calcium deficiency. Effective calcium in the extracellular fluid is ionized to a degree proportional to the acidity of the extracellular fluid. With decreased acidity the calcium deficit in the extracellular fluid causes hyperexcitability of the nerve fibers with spasms and convulsions. Therefore calcium gluconate is given prior to administration of sodium bicarbonate. The two solutions must not be mixed, since calcium carbonate will precipitate as a result.

When sodium bicarbonate is administered, there is an increase in excretion of potassium in the urine. If this loss is not replaced, a potassium deficit will occur. Depleted potassium serves to intensify the alkalosis resulting from administration of sodium bicarbonate [15].

Respiratory alkalosis. Respiratory alkalosis is due to hyperventilation, which causes carbon dioxide to be excreted faster than it is produced. Carbonic acid is reduced and bicarbonate is increased. Hydrogen ion concentration decreases, and pH increases. Hyperventilation with resultant alkalosis may be caused by anxiety or induced by hypoxia caused by pulmonary or cardiopulmonary disease. Although uncommon, lesions in the respiratory center of the brain may also cause sustained hyperventilation and alkalosis [11, 13a, 14].

The symptoms of transient respiratory alkalosis include lightheadedness, circumoral and peripheral paresthesias, muscle tremors, and carpopedal spasm. These symptoms usually disappear before renal compensation is necessary. Increasing the P_{CO_2} by breathing into a paper bag will relieve the symptoms. In cases of sustained hyperventilation due to lesions in the medulla, the kidney's response will result in a decreased concentration of bicarbonate in the extracellular fluids, thereby decreasing the pH to normal [15].

Metabolic alkalosis. Metabolic alkalosis occurs when there is an increased concentration of bicarbonate without an equivalent increase in the P_{CO_2}. This results in a loss of acid from the extracellular fluids and an elevation of the pH. There are many possible causes, including excessive ingestion of alkaline preparations, loss of chloride due to vomiting or gastric suction, excessive secretion of acid in the urine, and movement of hydrogen ions from the extracellular fluid into the cells due to a deficit of potassium [13a, 15].

The major effect of uncompensated metabolic alkalosis is overexcitability of the nervous system, usually affecting the peripheral nerves, which go into a state of tonic spasm. The patient becomes nervous, and convulsions and tetany may develop. The respiratory system responds to metabolic alkalosis by slowing down alveolar ventilation, which causes retention of CO_2. Since the resulting hypoxia and hypercapnea will subsequently stimulate respiratory activity, this compensation is limited. The kidney compensates by decreasing its excretion of hydrogen ions and reducing absorption of bicarbonate, thus reducing the concentration of bicarbonate in extracellular fluid [6, 15]. The principal therapy for metabolic alkalosis is correction of the condition that precipitated it [6]. Occasionally ammonium chloride is given, but this must be done with great care so as not to induce a metabolic acidosis.

MEASURES FOR THE MAINTENANCE OF HYDRATION AND NUTRITION

Intravenous therapy

During the initial phase of stroke, fluid and electrolyte needs may have to be maintained by intravenous therapy because of coma, lethargy, or inability to swallow. An understanding of the principles of intravenous therapy is essential, since the nurse is responsible for the safe administration of intravenous fluid and electrolyte replacement prescribed by the physician. Patients receiving intravenous therapy should be observed closely for development of complications. The most commonly occurring complications are (1) local infiltration of the solution, (2) circulatory overload, (3) thrombophlebitis at the site of infusion, and (4) local skin infection.

LOCAL INFILTRATION
Local infiltration of the intravenous solution occurs whenever the needle becomes dislodged, allowing the solution to infuse into the surrounding subcutaneous tissues. The following are indications that this has happened:

1. Edema at the site of the infusion
2. Failure to demonstrate a return of blood in the tubing when the bottle or bag is placed lower than the site of the infusion
3. Discomfort at the site of insertion of the needle or catheter
4. Cessation or significant decrease in the rate of flow of the solution

If there is infiltration, the needle should be removed from the vein and the infusion restarted in another site. In cases of extreme extravasation the physician should be contacted regarding local skin care.

FLUID OVERLOAD
Excessive amounts of intravenous fluid may overload the circulatory system, causing increased venous pressure, venous distention, elevated blood pressure, and pulmonary

edema. Coughing, shortness of breath, an increased respiratory rate, severe dyspnea, and cyanosis may be noted. The infusion should be stopped and the physician alerted immediately. To guard against this complication, the nurse should clarify with the physician the total amount of fluid prescribed within a 24-hour period and the rate of infusion and make frequent checks to ascertain that the flow continues at the recommended rate [1].

THROMBOPHLEBITIS AT THE SITE OF INFUSION
Thrombophlebitis is associated with clot formation in an inflamed vein. It may arise as a consequence of long-term intravenous therapy at one site and is indicated by pain along the course of the vein and redness and edema at the site of insertion. When this is noted, the infusion should be restarted at another site and the responsible physician contacted regarding orders for treatment of this complication.

LOCAL SKIN INFECTION
When intravenous therapy is prolonged, repeated applications of tape to anchor the needle can cause local excoriation of the skin. Failure to provide adequate cleansing and protection of the skin can lead to infection [8].

Prevention of Complications. In most cases complications of intravenous feeding can be prevented by nursing measures. In patients with hemiplegia, muscle action that would normally enhance peripheral circulation is diminished in the affected arm. Therefore the intravenous feeding should not be administered via the paralyzed limb. As the patient receiving intravenous replacement therapy may also require frequent venipunctures for monitoring electrolyte balance, the venous sites available are restricted. For patients with quadriplegia there is little choice as to the site of the infusion. Therefore the nurse must be doubly cautious in her efforts to prevent complications of therapy in these patients. It should be understood that the hemiplegic patient will try to use his one functioning upper extremity in spite of the intravenous infusion, to reach for tissues, call bell, urinal, and other objects necessary to his comfort and well-being, if these needs are not anticipated by the nurse.

The needle or catheter should not be inserted in veins over movable joints. Once it has been inserted into the vein, it is most important that it be properly anchored and the tubing adequately secured. Applying an overabundance of tape will not necessarily solve the problem of maintaining an open intravenous line. It may, however, cause excessive pressure that can lead to compression of the vein with the possibility of puncture or to a decrease in the patency of the vein or intravenous catheter, thereby slowing down the rate of flow considerably [8]. If the restraining tape or gauze acts as a tourniquet, this can severely impair circulation to the extremity. Furthermore this restraint doubles the hemiplegic patient's deficit, rendering him completely helpless and sometimes agitating a confused and frustrated patient to the degree that he is constantly attempting to free his only functioning arm.

When the patient is receiving intravenous therapy for the sole purpose of maintaining adequate fluid intake, the nurse should observe for indications that he might be able to start taking fluids orally. She should consult with the physician concerning daily testing of the patient's ability to handle oral feedings. When oral feedings cannot be taken safely, consideration must be given to insertion of a nasogastric feeding tube or a feeding gastrostomy.

Tube feedings

Tube feeding formulas contain protein, fat, carbohydrates, minerals, and vitamins, all of which are essential to maintain an adequate nutritional state. There are several commercial tube feeding preparations that are available in most hospitals. The formula may also be prepared by the dietary department in accordance with the content of protein, fat, and carbohydrate prescribed for the patient [7].

Since patients who require tube feedings over prolonged periods of time are likely to develop electrolyte imbalances, it is important for the nurse to be aware of the proportion of protein, fat, and carbohydrate in the feedings as well as of the total fluid intake. When the protein content exceeds 1 gm per kilogram of body weight, the patient must be observed closely for excessive fluid losses, since the high solute feeding will cause diuresis, and dehydration may occur. More water must be provided to the patient receiving a high solute formula in order to replace the fluid losses. Thirst normally serves to regulate fluid intake. The patient with stroke may not perceive this, or he may be unable to communicate that he feels thirsty [7].

Diarrhea is a common complication in patients receiving tube feedings. It may be related to the content of fat, lactose, and carbohydrate in the formula, to the administration of an ice-cold mixture, or to the too rapid ingestion of the feeding. The technique of administration as well as content of the formula should be assessed if this complication arises. The most common treatment is prescription of such anti-diarrhea agents as kaolin with pectin (Kaopectate) or diphenoxylate with atropine (Lomotil). The addition of banana flakes or apple powder to the feedings is also effective [7].

Other causes of fluid loss are fever, copious respiratory tract secretions, and high atmospheric temperatures that increase the insensible fluid losses through perspiration.

INSERTION OF THE NASOGASTRIC FEEDING TUBE

Since insertion of the tube is an uncomfortable and frightening experience for the patient, every attempt must be made to allay his fears and enlist his cooperation. The nurse should explain why the tube is needed, how it will be inserted, and how it will be used. The patient's sense of well-being and confidence will be fostered by a calm and confident demeanor in the nurse who inserts the feeding tube. This procedure is most skillfully performed when the nurse has gained the patient's confidence, has all of the necessary materials for the procedure at hand, and is able to introduce the tube deftly, gently, and with a sense of knowing precisely what she is doing. The patient's resistance to insertion of the tube can be overcome best when the nurse is able to communicate to him that she not only understands and cares about his problem but also knows how to help him deal with it. Her gentleness in inserting the tube and the tone of her voice while explaining what is being done can serve to reassure the patient further. The nurse should remember that, in spite of an inability to communicate, the aphasic and/or comatose patient may be able to hear and comprehend what is going on around him. Such patients also deserve considerate care and gentle explanation.

In most hospitals, feeding tubes are routinely inserted by nurses. In some, however, it is the policy for the physician to do this. In others the physician performs the initial procedure, and thereafter the nurse is responsible for changing or replacing the tube. Regardless of who places the tube, the nurse is responsible for the preparation and teaching of the patient.

The feeding tube is prepared by lubricating the first six inches with a nonoily preparation. Oily substances such as glycerine and mineral oil should never be used for this purpose, since the patient may aspirate droplets of the oil. With the patient's head elevated so that he is at a 45—90-degree angle, the tube is inserted via the nostril, through the esophagus, and into the stomach. In an adult the tube will be introduced approximately 20—30 inches. If the patient is alert enough and able to swallow without danger of aspiration, he should be given sips of water or ice chips to aid in the passage of the tube. Each time the patient swallows, the tube is advanced. Between swallows he should be allowed to catch his breath and rest. The position of the tube in the pharynx should be checked frequently to make sure the tube is progressing into the esophagus and is not coiled in the mouth or entering the trachea. To test the position of the tube, the proximal end is placed in a glass of water. If the tube is in the trachea or lung, air bubbles will be produced. If this happens the tube should be withdrawn gently and reinserted. Once the tube is placed, it should be aspirated with a 20-cc syringe; if it is properly positioned, stomach contents will be withdrawn.

CARE OF THE NASOGASTRIC FEEDING TUBE
The tube must be anchored securely to prevent accidental removal or displacement. This can be accomplished with a minimal amount of tape strategically placed at the nares and another piece fastened at the side of the forehead or over the ear so as not to obstruct the patient's vision. The area around the nares should be cleansed frequently and kept lubricated in order to prevent irritation and the formation of crusts. While the tube is in place, oral hygiene procedures should be carried out every two hours to prevent stagnation of secretions in the mouth and pharynx. If the patient is able, he should be encouraged to brush his teeth. The lips should be kept lubricated to prevent dryness and cracking. The nasogastric tube should be changed at least every five days, since food particles remaining within the tube can undergo bacterial changes and cause gastrointestinal infection. All old tape should be removed at each change and the patient's face washed and dried carefully. The fresh tube is placed in the opposite nostril so as to prevent irritation and erosion of the delicate mucous membranes.

ADMINISTRATION OF NASOGASTRIC TUBE FEEDINGS
Being fed by this unnatural means can be extremely unpleasant and upsetting to the patient, particularly if it is required for a prolonged period. The nurse can help the patient to accept the tube feedings and tolerate the presence of the tube by keeping

it neatly and comfortably secured and providing frequent mouth care and bathing of the face [12].

During the first 24 hours following passage of the tube, approximately 100 cc of water is instilled through the tube every 2 hours. Feedings are then changed to 50 cc of water and 50 cc of formula every 2 hours. If the patient can tolerate this, the feedings can be increased to 200 cc of formula every 2 hours up to 400 cc every 4 hours to achieve a total daily intake of 2,000 to 3,000 cc per day. The amount of tube feeding given depends upon the needs and tolerance of the individual patient. The most nutritious formula is prepared by mixing the ingredients of three balanced meals of a regular diet in the blender. If the mixture is blended with liquid, it is less likely to cause diarrhea. Supplementary vitamins and oral medications can be administered via the tube as well [1, 12].

Before the formula is given, the tube should be tested to make certain it is still in the stomach. Three methods are commonly used: (1) aspirate for stomach contents; (2) place the proximal end of the tubing in a glass of water — if air bubbles escape, the tube is most likely in the trachea; and (3) inject 5 cc of air through the tube while listening with the stethoscope over the epigastric area. The air will be heard entering the stomach if the tube is still properly in place. All feedings should be preceded and followed by instillation of approximately 50 cc of water to clear the tube and prevent blockage, and this should always be recorded as intake. To prevent overdistention of the stomach, always aspirate stomach contents to ascertain the amount before giving the feeding. Then return the contents to the stomach and subtract that amount from the feeding to be administered.

The formula should be kept in the refrigerator, never left at the bedside, since it is an excellent culture medium for bacteria. A sufficient amount for a feeding should be removed from the refrigerator just before it is administered to the patient. Warming it to room temperature will help to prevent nausea, abdominal cramps, and diarrhea. This may be done by setting it in a pan of warm water. The feeding should never be warmed over direct heat because of the danger of overheating it and burning the patient.

The patient should be positioned on his back with his head elevated at a 45–90-degree angle for the feeding. Disposable tube feeding sets are provided in some hospitals. If such a setup is not available, the feeding should be introduced into the tube by means of a syringe barrel or funnel and allowed to flow into the stomach by gravity. Positive pressure should never be used. Pressure can be regulated slightly by raising or lowering the syringe. In order to prevent introduction of air via the tube, the nurse should clamp the tubing before refilling the funnel with water or formula. A patient should always be attended while being tube-fed because of the dangers of vomiting and aspiration. It is especially important to prevent patients with elevated blood pressure or cerebral aneurysm from vomiting.

The patient should remain in a sitting position for 15–30 minutes after feedings to prevent the possibility of regurgitation. Overfilling of the stomach can also produce regurgitation or even vomiting, with the possibility of airway obstruction and resultant aspiration pneumonia. Other factors that may lead to vomiting are the content or consistency of the formula, increased gastric motility, and decreased gastrointestinal absorption of the feedings. In addition to maintaining a patent airway the nurse should observe the patient with vomiting for signs of dehydration, acidosis, or alkalosis [7].

GASTROSTOMY TUBE FEEDING

If a patient has cranial nerve impairment with prolonged inability to swallow, a surgical procedure may be performed to insert a feeding tube directly into the stomach. This is usually done in the operating room under local anesthesia. The patient should be observed for signs of bleeding or infection during the immediate postoperative period. After the first 24 hours initial feedings of water are started. If these are tolerated, a tube feeding formula is prescribed by the physician. The procedure for administering the tube feeding, positioning of the patient, and temperature of the formula are the same as for patients with nasogastric tubes, with one exception. Before instilling the feeding the nurse should aspirate the contents of the stomach to find out the amount of absorption that is taking place. If the aspirate is greater than 100 cc, withhold the formula feedings and recheck the aspirate in 1 hour. If it is still greater than 100 cc, withhold the feeding and notify the physician. If the aspirate is between 50 and 100 cc, refeed it and give the formula in an amount that, when added to the amount of aspirate, will total the prescribed amount of feeding. Since the aspirate contains gastric secretions — including the intrinsic factor necessary for absorption of vitamin B_{12} — and undigested food, it should always be replaced into the stomach before the formula is given.

The skin surrounding the gastrostomy should be washed with soap and water daily and the skin protected to prevent gastric enzymes from causing local irritation. The tubing should be secured to the skin so as to prevent tension on it and accidental removal. Any tenderness, redness, drainage, or skin breakdown should be reported to the responsible physician.

The neurological deficits resulting from stroke frequently leave the patient with overwhelming losses, some temporary, many permanent, all damaging to the self-image and self-esteem. The patient with stroke is generally, and quite justifiably, frustrated and depressed with his dependent state. During the more acute stages of stroke the nurse's primary goals are short-term, related to maintaining the patient's basic respiratory and circulatory functions. When tube feedings are instituted at this stage, the main concern is restoring and maintaining hydration. Critical measures draw most heavily on the nurse's knowledge of the physical sciences and ability to keep precise records. Planning care for the management of the patient who requires long-term or permanent tube feedings presents a challenge to the nurse's knowledge of the behavioral sciences. In addition to whatever loss of independence or capacity for interaction with others he may have suffered from the stroke, this patient is also deprived of one of life's most basic pleasures: eating.

If the nurse is to help the patient to adjust to life with his disability she (or he) must realize the full extent of this loss. She cannot possibly help the patient to accept a tube feeding as a meal he wants and needs as opposed to a treatment that he must endure unless she understands the social ramifications of the situation as well. The patient requiring tube feedings will still feel hunger, experience cravings for certain foods, and respond to the sight and aromas of favorite dishes with a long-ing to taste them. However, the sight of even his favorite foods reduced to a lique-fied state in the blender may fill him with disgust and loathing at the thought of "eating" in such an unnatural manner. The risk of offending the sensibilities of his friends and loved ones will isolate him from the pleasures of social interaction that are usually associated with mealtimes. The nurse must appreciate the patient's fear of being offensive to others and respect his need for privacy and protection from curious onlookers during feedings. However, since the sharing of food is such an archetypal symbol for love and acceptance, thought must be given to establishing some form of socialization in association with feedings. This will require sensitivity and creativity on the part of the nurse and will have to be geared to each patient's temperament and life-style. Its success will depend greatly on the emotional stability and maturity of the patient and on that of the family members and friends involved [12].

Although they cannot taste their meals, some convalescent patients may enjoy selecting their own menus and seeing the food before it is placed in the blender. If this appeals to the patient's esthetic sense and contributes to his enjoyment, the nurse should arrange with the dietary department to have these foods served attrac-tively on a tray at mealtime, then taken away, put through the blender and adminis-tered. This may appear an inordinate waste of time and effort in a busy nursing unit, but the patient's sense of well-being and self-esteem will be well worth the effort. It should be noted that the blenderized food should always be brought to the bedside in an opaque container, since it will not be attractive and may be a distressing sight to the patient [12].

When patients are to be discharged with a permanent feeding gastrostomy, and sent home or to a nursing facility, instructions must be provided for preparing, storing, and administering the feedings as well as caring for the tube and mouth. If the patient is to receive a regular diet rather than a prepared formula, the following suggestions may be helpful to the person responsible for preparing the feedings. Meats should be boiled after all fat is removed, then put through a meat grinder before they are placed in the blender. Fruits and vegetables should also be cooked before being put in the blender. Broth or milk should be used to dilute the feeding to the proper consistency. Custards, puddings, and gelatins in a semisolid form should be thinned with milk. Soft ice cream may be given. Soups and fruit juices should be strained. Only cooked cereals should be used, and these should always be strained. The nurse should stress the importance of providing the daily requirement of basic nutrients. She should be certain that the caloric content of the various foods as well as any dietary restrictions are thoroughly understood, and should explain the dangers of overdistention of the stomach and serving foods that are too hot or cold [12].

Feeding difficulties

Good nutrition implies that the supply of food is adequate in quantity and quality to the needs of the cells and that the cells are able to utilize the nutrients provided in a physiological manner. A continuous supply of water, oxygen, and nutrients is essential for maintenance and replacement of cell structures and regulation of cell function. Although some nutrients can be stored, continued deprivation will result in an imbalance between essential nutrients available and cell requirements. This will pose a serious threat to health and survival [1].

Difficulties with digestion, absorption, and assimilation of nutrients due to gastro-intestinal disturbances will certainly have a deleterious effect on the patient's nutritional state. For patients with stroke, however, the major barriers to adequate nutrition are feeding difficulties that result from cranial nerve dysfunction, perceptual or motor and sensory impairment, and aphasia. It is not uncommon to find that patients become dehydrated and/or malnourished because of these difficulties. Careful planning, recording, and evaluation of nutritional intake can help in preventing such complications.

CHEWING AND SWALLOWING DIFFICULTIES
Paralysis of one or both sides of the mouth and an absent or diminished gag reflex may interfere with chewing and swallowing. It is recommended that the nurse test the gag reflex, the patient's ability to swallow, and the strength of his facial muscles prior to giving any oral feeding.

Gag reflex.   The nurse depresses the patient's tongue with a tongue blade and touches the posterior pharynx with a cotton-tipped applicator. If the gag reflex is intact, this will evoke a contraction of the palatal muscles.

Swallowing.   The patient is given a small amount of water to drink, preferably through a straw. If he has difficulty swallowing it, he is fed thicker fluids such as frappes or semisolids. Frequently patients can swallow semisolids successfully but have difficulty with clear liquids. Applesauce, hot cereal, and ice cream seem to have the best consistency for patients first attempting to swallow after a stroke. Suction apparatus should be available at the bedside in case the patient aspirates.

Facial paralysis.   When facial muscles on one side of the face are paralyzed or weak, a sagging will be noted on that side. The patient may also complain of facial weakness and numbness. Feedings should be given through the unaffected side of the mouth to reduce drooling and the chances of aspiration. If the patient is lying on his side, the paralyzed side, should be uppermost to facilitate easier swallowing and to avoid aspiration. Mouth care should be provided after each feeding to prevent food from lodging in the mouth on the paralyzed side. If a patient has brainstem stroke, which may mean bilateral involvement of the gag reflex and facial muscles and limitation of palate, tongue, and lip movements, oral feedings should not be attempted until there is adequate evidence of recovery.

PERCEPTUAL DIFFICULTIES
A patient with a visual defect such as hemianopsia may leave half the food on his tray because he has not seen it. The nurse should make certain that the patient's meal tray is arranged so that all the food is within his field of vision.

MOTOR AND SENSORY DIFFICULTIES
Due to paralysis and impaired sensation, the patient may not be able to reach for a glass of water or may spill it. He may not be able to butter bread or open containers of milk or condiments. Heavy china, lids, or utensils may be too cumbersome for him to manipulate. If his dominant hand is paralyzed or has a sensory deficit, he may be clumsy in hand-to-mouth movements and may voluntarily eliminate some foods because of embarrassing consequences. Apraxia of hand or mouth movements may severely interfere with independent feeding. Food that requires two hands for preparation, such as opening milk containers, buttering bread, cutting meat, and opening salt and pepper packs, should be prepared by the person who serves the tray. If the patient requires special eating utensils, such as builtup spoons or forks, plate guards, or devices to stabilize dishes, they should be readily available, and he should be encouraged to use them.

COMMUNICATION DIFFICULTIES
An aphasic patient may not be able to communicate his likes and dislikes, consequently, his daily caloric intake may be inadequate. The nurse should make every effort to obtain information about his food preferences from the patient's family and friends and to incorporate it into his care plan.

NURSING MEASURES FOR PATIENTS WITH FEEDING DIFFICULTIES
The following steps are recommended for the prevention of malnutrition and dehydration in stroke patients with feeding difficulties.

Fluid intake.   The patient should receive 2,000—3,000 cc per 24 hours; unless there is a medical contraindication. An accurate record of fluid intake is necessary.

Caloric count.   Caloric intake should also be computed and recorded to assure that the total calories consumed are sufficient. Carefully kept records will show a decrease in dietary intake, so that supplements may be added when necessary.

Dentures.   If a patient has dentures he should wear them at each meal to ensure adequate chewing.

Positioning.   The head should be elevated at a 45—90-degree angle to prevent aspiration of the food and allow gravity to assist in swallowing. Patients with hemiparesis or hemiplegia may have difficulty sitting. Their balance will be poor and they will tend to fall to the weak or paralyzed side. Therefore such patients should be positioned comfortably in a chair or in bed with the affected side supported. Patients with quadriplegia will require bilateral support.

Feedings.   Initial disability resulting from stroke varies from patient to patient and depends upon the extent and location of the lesion. Rate and degree of recovery also vary. Consequently, in planning care the nurse must evaluate each patient individually to determine how much assistance is required to provide adequate nutrition and how to motivate the patient to become more independent in feeding. The patient may require only supervision or limited assistance or, as in the case of quadriplegics, may always need to be fed. In addition to such physical limitations the patient may have to be fed to assure adequate nutrition because of lethargy or depression. The nurse must consider assignment of staff for feeding stroke patients in terms of their individual limitations and potential capabilities. She should supervise feeding in order to assess the adequacy of the patient's intake as well as his ability to progress to more solid foods and independence. This will also afford the nurse the opportunity to evaluate the expertise of her staff in this area and reinforce teaching concerning nutrition and assisting patients to achieve independence.

Eating should be a pleasurable experience. The nurse should make every effort to create a relaxed, comfortable atmosphere while feeding a patient. She should not appear rushed or anxious about the time required to assist the patient. If at all possible, she should sit rather than stand over the patient. Care should be taken to avoid anything that would make the patient feel like a child. Bibs should never be used.

Independent feeding. Patients should be encouraged to feed themselves as early as possible in their convalescence. With this independence they will take meals at their own pace and feel less helpless than if someone must feed them. Meal trays should be placed within a patient's reach and within his field of vision. Some patients may progress to independence more rapidly with the help of adaptive equipment prescribed by the occupational therapist.

Arrangement of food on meal tray. The primary goal in serving meals is to provide adequate nutrition. To encourage the patient to eat, the nurse should work with the dietary department to assure that meal trays are arranged so that the stroke patient, whose state of awareness, perceptual, and manual abilities may be severely impaired, is served reasonable portions of foods that he likes, can manipulate, can chew, and can swallow safely. It is most important that the tray not be cluttered with an endless array of separate dishes, heavy covers, and hermetically sealed containers that will only serve to confuse, frustrate, and depress him in his attempts to eat independently.

Occupational therapy. The therapist will evaluate a patient with self-feeding problems and may prescribe special utensils, such as a rocker knife and plate guard, or set up a specialized program to assist the patient in developing independence in this activity.

Nursing assessment of hydration, electrolyte balance, and nutrition

Laboratory tests are the most accurate means of assessing the patient's hydration status. These include determinations of serum and urine osmolality, determinations of serum sodium and blood urea nitrogen levels, and hematocrit [5] (Table 9-2). The following bedside procedures are also useful as indicators of disturbances in fluid and electrolyte balance and should be carried out by the nurse.

Table 9-2
Laboratory tests used in assessment of hydration

Test	Normal Value	Purpose	Significance of Findings
Serum osmolality	270–300 mOsm/kg water	Measures the osmotic pressure of body fluids. Reflects total body hydration.	*Elevated* value indicates dehydration. *Low* value indicates water excess.
Urine osmolality	38–1400 mOsm/kg water	Measures the osmotic pressure of urine. Reflects constituents of urine.	Values vary greatly with dietary changes. *Elevated* value may indicate dehydration. *Low* value may reflect excretion of large amounts of water or inability of the kidney to concentrate urine.
Ratio of serum osmolality to urine osmolality	4:1	Indicates the ability of the kidney to concentrate urine.	A ratio of less than 1 indicates excessive water. A ratio of 1 indicates inability to concentrate urine.
Serum sodium (Na)	135–147 mEq/L	Measures cellular hydration.	*Elevated* value indicates deficit of water, excessive fluid loss, solute diuresis. *Low* value indicates excessive water intake, excessive losses via G.I. tract or diuretic therapy, decreased renal perfusion, or inappropriate ADH.
Blood urea nitrogen (BUN)	6–22 mg/100 ml serum	Measures amount of urea from protein catabolism retained in the blood. Reflects rate at which urea is formed and rate at which it is excreted.	*Elevated* value may indicate decreased renal blood flow, dehydration, increase in protein intake, or compromised renal function with decreased production of urine.
Hematocrit (Hct)	37–47 ml/100 ml (F) 40–54 ml/100 ml (M)	Measures proportion of red blood cells to plasma. Reflects degree of hemoconcentration and amount of blood loss.	*Elevated* value may indicate dehydration, increased production of red cells. *Low* value may indicate water overload, blood loss, decrease in red cells.

Adapted from Grant and Kubo [5]. Copyright © 1975, the American Journal of Nursing Company. Reproduced with permission from *American Journal of Nursing*, Vol. 75 No. 8.

BODY WEIGHT

A rapid change in body weight can reflect a gain or loss in body fluids. A gain or loss of 1 kg is equivalent to the gain or loss of 1 liter of water. The patient should be weighed each time on the same scale under the same conditions, that is, at the same time, with the same clothing, and with an empty bladder.

MEASUREMENT AND RECORDING OF INTAKE AND OUTPUT

A record of the patient's intake and output reflects both increases and decreases in body fluids. Accurate recording will help to assure that the patient receives an adequate amount of fluid to prevent dehydration and that he is not retaining excess fluids.

RECORD OF STOOLS

A record of the number and consistency of stools is important in assessing the hydration of the patient. As the number and softness of the stools increase, so does the loss of body fluids. The dehydrated patient, however, will have hard stools, because water is absorbed in the large intestine to compensate for decreases in total body fluids [5].

MONITORING OF VITAL SIGNS

Temperature. An elevated temperature can reflect a decrease of total body fluids in a dehydrated patient. Fever can contribute to further loss of body fluids through perspiration.

Pulse. Both the character and rate of the pulse are important. A rapid pulse may indicate sodium excess, while a bounding pulse may reflect fluid volume excess. An easily obliterated pulse may indicate impending circulatory collapse.

Respirations. Rapid, deep respirations may reflect a potential fluid loss, while shortness of breath may denote a volume excess.

Level of consciousness. Symptoms of cerebral dysfunction, such as confusion, agitation, stupor, and coma, are seen with fluid and electrolyte imbalances. The most notable is hypernatremia due to inadequate intake of water.

MONITORING OF NEUROLOGICAL SIGNS

Changes in hydration can cause increased muscle weakness, muscle cramps, headaches, and even seizures.

INSPECTION OF MUCOUS MEMBRANES

To assess the condition of the mucous membranes, pull the patient's lower lip out gently and note the moistness of the membranes and the thickness of the secretions. Normal mucous membranes appear moist and glistening. Dry mucous membranes are associated with a fluid volume deficit.

OBSERVATION OF SKIN TURGOR

The elasticity and shape of the skin is related to the amount of body fluid. Turgor is checked by pinching the skin over the clavicle gently, releasing it and noting how long it takes to return to its original state. Decreased skin turgor reflects decreased body fluids [5]. With normal skin turgor there is an immediate return to the original state.

OBSERVATION OF VEIN FILLING

Select a small vessel in the hand or foot and see that the extremity is not in a dependent position. Occlude the vein distally, and empty it by stroking the vessel proximally. Then release the occlusion quickly and observe the degree and rate of blood return to the vessel. Under normal conditions the vein will fill immediately. If there is dehydration, the rate of filling will be slower, or the vein may remain empty. Flat neck veins are generally associated with a sodium depletion, while engorgement of the peripheral veins is associated with an excess of extracellular fluids [5].

REFERENCES

1. Beland, I., and Passos, J. *Clinical Nursing: Pathophysiological and Psychosocial Approaches* (3rd ed.). New York: Macmillan, 1975. Pp. 319–510.
2. Betson, C. Blood gases. *Am. J. Nurs.* 68:1010, 1968.
3. Betson, C. The nurse's role in blood gas monitoring. *Cardiovasc. Nurs.* 7:83, 1971.
4. Beyers, M., and Dudas, S. *The Clinical Practice of Medical-Surgical Nursing.* Boston: Little, Brown, 1977. Pp. 151–192.
5. Grant, M. M., and Kubo, W. M. Assessing a patient's hydration status. *Am. J. Nurs.* 75:1306, 1975.
6. Guyton, A. C. *Textbook of Medical Physiology* (5th ed.). Philadelphia: Saunders, 1976. Pp. 2–11; 424–437; 485–500.
7. Kubo, W., et al. Fluid and electrolyte problems of tube-fed patients. *Am. J. Nurs.* 76:912, 1976.
8. Kurdi, W. J. Refining your I. V. therapy techniques. *Nurs. 75* 5:41, 1975.
9. Lee, C. A., Stroot, V. R., and Schaper, C. A. Extracellular volume in balance. *Am. J. Nurs.* 74:888, 1974.
10. Lee, C. A., Stroot, V. R., and Schaper, C. A. What to do when acid-base problems hang in the balance. *Nurs. 75* 5:32, 1975.
11. Reed, G. M., and Sheppard, V. F. *Regulation of Fluid and Electrolyte Balance: A Programmed Instruction in Physiology for Nurses.* Philadelphia: Saunders, 1971. Pp. 3–207.
12. Smith, A. V. Nasogastric tube feedings. *Am. J. Nurs.* 57:1451, 1957.
13. Streeter, D. H. P., Moses, A. M., and Miller, M. Disorders of the Neurohypophysis. In G. W. Thorn, et al. (Eds.), *Harrison's Principles of Internal Medicine* (8th ed.). New York: McGraw-Hill, 1977. Pp. 490–501.
13a. Wade, J. F. *Respiratory Nursing Care* (2nd ed.). St. Louis: Mosby, 1977. Pp. 54, 76.
14. Welt, L. G. Disorders of Fluids and Electrolytes. In M. M. Wintrobe, et al. (Eds.), *Harrison's Principles of Internal Medicine* (7th ed.). New York: McGraw-Hill, 1977. Pp. 1343–1356.
15. Welt, L. G. Acidosis and Alkalosis. In M. M. Wintrobe, et al. (Eds.), *Harrison's Principles of Internal Medicine* (7th ed.). New York: McGraw-Hill, 1977. Pp. 1356–1367.

10. Assessment and reestablishment of bladder and bowel function following stroke

Following stroke the patient may be troubled with urinary and fecal incontinence or with constipation and fecal impaction. These problems are embarrassing to the patient and complicate nursing care and rehabilitation efforts. Unfortunately, nursing measures routinely initiated to deal with these problems often lead to more severe and even life-threatening complications. In this chapter we will discuss first bladder function, then bowel function, and the principles of restoring them in the stroke patient.

PHYSIOLOGY OF THE BLADDER

A basic understanding of the bladder physiology and rationale for bladder training is necessary for evaluation of bladder dysfunction following stroke and establishment of a bladder training program. The bladder is a smooth muscle vesicle composed of the *detrusor muscle,* or body of the bladder, and the *trigone,* or internal sphincter, which is a small, triangular area near the mouth of the body. The bladder has three openings or orifices, two for insertion of the ureters and one for the urethra. The ureters enter the bladder at an oblique angle, so that with contraction of the bladder the ureteral openings are blocked and reflux of urine back into the ureters is prevented. The muscle that forms the external bladder sphincter is called the *urogenital diaphragm.* The urethra, which carries urine out of the bladder and away from the body, passes through this muscle.

As urine collects within the bladder, the body of the bladder stretches until tension rises to a threshold level, at which a nervous reflex is elicited. This is referred to as the *micturition reflex* and it is mediated through the second, third, and fourth sacral segments of the spinal cord. Contraction of the detrusor muscle is perceived consciously as a desire to urinate, and with its contraction the external sphincter of the bladder relaxes to allow the bladder to empty [8].

The process of micturition is regulated by a highly coordinated set of reflexes. These are controlled by the parasympathetic and sympathetic divisions of the autonomic nervous system, the somatic nervous system, and certain cerebral pathways (Fig. 10-1). The *parasympathetic nerve fibers* cause contraction of the detrusor muscle and some opening of the internal sphincter. The sensory signals from the bladder are conducted by the afferent pathway to the sacral segments of the spinal cord through the pelvic nerve. Motor signals are conducted by the efferent pathway from the spinal cord to the bladder via motor fibers of the same nerves to cause contraction of the detrusor. *Sympathetic nerve fibers* pass from the thoracic and upper lumbar regions of the spinal cord through the hypogastric plexus to the bladder. Stimulation of these nerves causes the bladder to relax, which is opposite

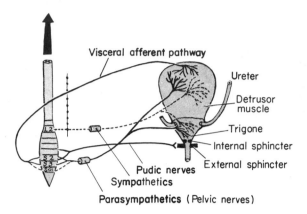

Figure 10-1
Schematic representation of the micturition reflex. (From A. G. Guyton, Textbook
of Medical Physiology *[5th ed.]. Philadelphia: Saunders, 1976.)*

to the effect of parasympathetic stimulation. However, sympathetic nerves do not
normally enter the process of micturition. The primary innervation of the sympathetic nerves is from the bladder trigone.

The *somatic nervous system* sends motor impulses to the striated muscle of the
external urethra through the pudendal nerve. This nerve, which has its origin in the
first and second sacral segments of the spinal cord, controls the external urinary
sphincter. In contrast to the smooth muscle of the detrusor, the external urinary
sphincter is a voluntary skeletal muscle. The external sphincter surrounds the urethra
and remains contracted to prevent constant dribbling of urine, but it can be relaxed
either reflexly or voluntarily at the time of micturition.

Although the micturition reflex is the basic cause of micturition, this reflex can
be inhibited or facilitated through *cerebral pathways* that carry signals to and from
the brain to permit voluntary control of bladder function. The cerebral centers
involved in this function are (1) a facilitory center in the upper pons, (2) a facilitory
center in the hypothalamus, (3) an inhibitory center in the midbrain, and (4) several
centers located in the cerebral cortex that are mainly inhibitory but can at times
function as excitatory centers. These higher centers exert final control of micturition: (1) they keep the micturition reflex inhibited at all times, unless there is a
conscious desire to void; (2) they maintain continued tonic contraction of the
external urinary sphincter until there is a convenient time and place to void; and
(3) they facilitate the activity of the sacral micturition center to initiate the reflex and
inhibit the action of the external urinary sphincter so it will relax and urination
can occur when there is a desire to urinate [8]. The *nerve fiber pathways* in the
spinal cord that carry signals to and from the brain for micturition have not been
positively identified. According to research in this area, it seems that the afferent
fibers travel in association with the lateral spinothalamic tracts and that the efferent
fibers lie below the lateral corticospinal tract [8]. Guttman reports that bilateral

section of the spinothalamic tract will result in immediate disorganization of the micturition reflex [7].

Micturition becomes involuntary when only the spinal reflex mechanism operates and the sensation of the need to void is not carried to the brain. This is the case in a young child who has not been toilet trained. Voluntary control of voiding involves inhibition of the spinal reflex by constriction of the external bladder sphincter. This is accomplished when the brain sends impulses to motor neurons in the sacral area of the spinal cord, causing parasympathetic efferent fibers of the pelvic nerve to stimulate contraction of the bladder muscle, and relaxation of the external sphincter takes place through inhibition of the pudendal nerve by the impulses from the micturition center [20].

When *nervous control of micturition* is intact, the act of micturition is a powerful reflex response at the spinal segmental level. The three phases of micturition are (1) contraction of the trigone, which depresses the posterior portion of the internal bladder orifice and allows it to open; (2) contraction of the detrusor, which originates in the area of the internal vesicle orifice, continues toward the dome of the bladder, and exerts a lateral pull on the internal orifice to open it even further; and (3) contractions of the abdominal muscles, which increase intraabdominal pressure and also the power of the detrusor contraction [7].

NEUROLOGICAL BLADDER DYSFUNCTION DUE TO STROKE

Neurogenic bladder dysfunction can result from lesions of the cortex, hypothalamus, midbrain, pons, and medulla or damage of the spinal cord at, above, or below the level of the spinal micturition center in the sacral cord [7]. Representation of bladder function in the cerebral cortex is bilateral. Therefore cortical and subcortical lesions that occur on one side only will have a transient effect on bladder sphincter control, making it relatively easy, in terms of bladder physiology, to establish bladder training for a patient with a unilateral stroke. However, if the patient has a language disorder, the establishment of a bladder training program will be complicated by his communication difficulties.

Upper motor neuron bladder

Bladder dysfunction resulting from central nervous system lesions is usually classified as either an upper motor neuron bladder or a lower motor neuron bladder depending upon the level of damage to the central nervous system. With an upper motor neuron lesion the sacral reflex center remains intact. However, the nerve damage that occurs above the spinal cord, as in stroke, frees the bladder from voluntary control. This is referred to as a *reflex bladder,* because it will empty abruptly, independent of the patient's wish, as soon as the stretch receptors in the bladder muscle reach their threshold. Voiding in this case will be completely involuntary and the patient will have no sensation of the bladder filling [20].

An upper motor neuron bladder may also be referred to as an *automatic* or *spastic bladder.* If the damage is above the micturition center, the micturition reflex still occurs. The reflex patterns via the pelvic nerves (autonomic) and internal pudendal (somatic) nerves remain intact, since those sections of the cord through which the micturition center is mediated have not been damaged. However, the brain will no longer control micturition, because the pathways leading to the brain will have been completely or partially interrupted. The bladder then functions in reflex fashion, with little or no cerebral inhibiting or controlling influences to regulate its activity. The reflex arc for micturition is intact, but its action is deranged secondary to interruption of cerebral control. Thus the bladder may empty abruptly when stretch receptors reach threshold level and trigger the reflex arc. For some patients the micturition reflex will be elicited by approximately normal amounts of urine, while for others the threshold may be either high or low. Factors causing this difference are related to early bladder management. If the bladder is kept completely emptied by continuous drainage, contracture of the bladder muscle can result, causing a low threshold for the micturition reflex. On the other hand, if the bladder is kept overly stretched, large volumes of urine will be required to initiate the micturition reflex. The patient may have little or no sensation of the bladder filling but may experience other sensations mediated by the autonomic nervous system that are usually associated with a full bladder. Examples are sweating, restlessness, and abdominal discomfort.

The major symptoms of an upper motor neuron bladder are frequency, urgency, and incontinence. The bladder capacity is usually small (100–300 cc), and voiding contractions may not be sustained long enough to allow complete emptying. The external sphincter may be spastic, and prevent adequate emptying. Consequently residual urine may be present in varying amounts at all times. Expulsion of urine will be determined mainly by the amount of fluid the patient drinks. He may void spontaneously whenever there is increased abdominal pressure, as when he laughs, coughs, attempts to exercise, or changes position. The spread of skeletal spasms to striated muscles of the pelvic floor may cause interruption of the urinary stream during voiding. Although voluntary control is lost, voiding may be initiated by stimulating the reflex arc through stimulation of areas innervated by the sacral centers. The patient will usually discover "trigger areas" for induction of micturition that work for him. Methods that seem to be effective are suprapubic percussion, scratching the inner thigh or genitalia, tapping the abdomen, and anal stimulation.

Lower motor neuron bladder

A lower motor neuron bladder occurs with damage to the sacral reflex center, resulting in denervation of the bladder muscle and external sphincter. The bladder muscle loses its normal tone, and reflex emptying will not occur. Since the bladder is constantly distended, the walls become flabby. Urine in amounts of up to 1,000 cc can be retained without sensation. Overflow incontinence may occur, with the patient voiding in small amounts. This will usually be noticed when the patient moves, for example, from bed to chair.

This type of bladder dysfunction is often called a *flaccid* or *autonomic bladder.*

The symptoms of a lower motor neuron bladder are urinary retention, distention of the bladder, and overflow incontinence (dribbling), which are the result of a lesion of the sacral centers involving the reflex micturition center in the cord or its peripheral nerves. Even though the neurogenic connections with the brain remain intact, the patient loses control of his bladder. Because the damage is to the innervation of the bladder muscle and external sphincter, the reflex pattern via the autonomic and somatic nerves is absent; the reflex arc is broken, and no spontaneous activity can take place. Since the bladder is isolated from the spinal cord, there is no way to effect cerebral control. The bladder empties, in small amounts, only when the mechanical pressure in the bladder overcomes the forces of external urethral resistance. The constant residue of urine in the bladder predisposes to infection. Stroke is not a common cause of a lower motor neuron bladder; however, neurogenic bladder dysfunction does not always occur as purely either an upper or a lower motor neuron bladder. When there is cortical infarction following stroke, a mixed type of dysfunction usually occurs, with partial sensation and partial voluntary control [20].

Types of dysfunction after stroke

The patient with hemispheric stroke will have what is called an *incomplete* upper motor neuron lesion. Since the lesion is unilateral, the patient has partial sensation and partial control of the bladder. The patient with a brainstem stroke will have bilateral damage to the pathways and resultant upper motor neuron bladder. Stroke causes urinary disturbances according to the location of the lesion. The internal capsule, which is supplied by the middle cerebral artery, is commonly involved. The result of a unilateral lesion is long-lasting frequency, urgency, and incontinence. The symptoms are those of an incomplete upper motor neuron lesion with a hyperactive detrusor of reduced capacity. Bilateral lesions lead to loss of all facilitation and inhibition of the micturition reflex [4].

The prognosis for return of normal bladder function is excellent for the patient with hemiplegia due to stroke because (1) the reflex arc remains intact, (2) partial sensation of bladder filling remains, and (3) he maintains partial voluntary control over voiding [20]. Such a patient can be bladder-trained quite easily, and this training should start immediately. This requires close nursing observation and accuracy of recording to reflect the amount of intake and output, frequency of urination, force of urinary stream, and any subjective sensations the patient is aware of.

Patients should not be catheterized for incontinence in the early phase of stroke, as initial incontinence does not mean there will be a permanent problem. They must be allowed a supervised trial period without a catheter, to determine voiding ability. Peszczynski states that "unnecessarily hurried application of an indwelling catheter in a patient with recent stroke is common practice, unnecessarily prolonged use of an indwelling catheter is poor practice" [15]. When a patient with stroke is admitted, an indwelling catheter is often inserted with the best of intentions to keep the skin dry and protected from irritation. Unfortunately this is a misguided nursing measure. About the time deep tendon reflexes become hyperactive, the urinary bladder becomes spastic. Thus a continuously open urinary drainage system invites the development of a small, spastic, contracted bladder that cannot retain much urine after the catheter is removed. Frequency and precipitous voiding result [15].

Urinary incontinence that persists after the patient has regained consciousness is rarely the result of neurological impairment, unless the patient has suffered widespread bilateral infarction or brainstem involvement. It is not uncommon for the medical and nursing staff to relate all forms of dysfunction to the stroke, even though there may be other perfectly obvious causes that are amenable to treatment. Incontinence at this stage may be due to a urinary tract infection resulting from catheterization. It may also be a manifestation of prostatic hypertrophy, cystocele, or other pelvic disorders [6]. Before inserting an indwelling urinary catheter for incontinence, the nurse must evaluate the patient's ability to express his need to void, his ability to get to a urinal, bedpan, commode, or toilet in time, and his ability to summon assistance readily if he cannot function independently.

Complications resulting from bladder dysfunction

The most frequent complications of bladder dysfunction are urinary tract infections, urinary stones, and vesicoureteral reflux. In addition, use of an indwelling catheter to drain a paralyzed bladder can predispose to hydronephrosis, bladder diverticula, and urethral fistulas.

Prevention of urinary tract infections is the most important aspect of treatment of the neurogenic bladder. Infections potentiate bladder dysfunction, because an inflamed bladder increases activity of the detrusor. Infections may be caused by bacteria of the urethra and external urinary meatus, urinary retention, indwelling catheters, and improper care of an indwelling catheter. Long-standing urinary tract infections may result in chronic pyelonephritis and consequently in renal insufficiency.

Formation of urinary tract stones may be due to bone dimineralization from decreased weight bearing, alkaline urine with resulting phosphatic deposition, stasis of urine, and dehydration with oliguria. The presence of stones may cause bladder and skeletal spasticity, which will further complicate the neurogenic bladder.

Vesicoureteral reflux may be caused by damage due to overdistention of the bladder muscle. Regurgitation of urine in the bladder up into the ureter can result in pyelonephritis and hydronephrosis and thus bring about progressive renal failure. The following regimen is suggested for care of patients with bladder dysfunction to prevent the development of these complications.

URINARY TRACT INFECTION

1. Avoid indwelling catheters, since a catheter is a foreign object and its introduction into a sterile cavity may lead to infection. It provides for introduction of bacteria as the catheter is inserted, a route for the bacteria to travel through the lumen, and a route for bacteria to travel between the catheter and the urethra [1]. If a catheter must be used because the patient's medical condition requires strict measurement of urinary output, it should be changed every 2 to 3 days or when crystals are forming in the tubing.

2. Use strict aseptic technique. Inspect for proper placement of the tubing.
3. Prevent undue tension on the tubing by securing the catheter to the inner aspect of the thigh for women and taping the tubing to the abdomen for men. This reduces the possibility of pressure necrosis at the penoscrotal angle, which can result in abscess and fistula formation. Avoid placing the tubing under the buttocks or thighs and allowing it to dangle over the bedside.
4. Place the drainage bag to prevent reflux of urine back into the bladder. It should never be raised above the level of the bladder. This is particularly important to remember when positioning a paralyzed patient. The drainage bag should be changed every 8 hours and should never be allowed to fill to capacity, since this can cause reflux of urine into the bladder. Aseptic technique should be used when disconnecting the tubing.
5. Maintain acid urine, since microorganisms cannot survive in acid urine. Acidifying agents such as ascorbic acid may be prescribed by the physician. The pH of the urine should be kept at an acid level of 5.5.
6. Antimicrobial agents may be prescribed, and when a urinary tract infection has been documented by culture, antibiotic agents will be prescribed according to the appropriate sensitivity studies.
7. Urinalysis and culture and sensitivity studies should be provided if there are signs and symptoms of an infection [4].

The two most important defenses against infection are blood supply and integrity of the cells. Blood supply to the bladder is markedly decreased when the bladder becomes distended with urine. If the patient is unable to void, a program of intermittent catheterization should be instituted to reduce the development of cystitis.

STONE FORMATION
1. Avoid residual urine in the bladder.
2. Encourage weight-bearing activity to help prevent loss of calcium from the bones due to immobilization.
3. Provide a high fluid intake to dilute urine.

VESICOURETERAL REFLUX
Avoid large residuals of urine and overdistention of the bladder. This may require intermittent catheterization. Avoid placement of urinary drainage receptacles above the level of the symphysis pubis.

Establishing a bladder retraining program

Under normal circumstances the forces that regulate retention and expulsion of urine are in balance so that no residual urine remains in the bladder. When this balance is disrupted by infection, obstruction, neurological impairment, pharmacological action, or any combination of these factors, residual urine is left in the bladder. Any one of these factors also has an effect on the neurological function of the bladder muscle, resulting in inactivity, hyperactivity, or hypoactivity. For example, inflammation of the mucosa secondary to infection will stimulate hyperactivity of the detrusor, producing stronger and more frequent contractions. When the primary problem is of neurological etiology, the smooth muscle of the detrusor will respond to various lesions along the neuroaxis with areflexia, hyporeflexia, or hyperreflexia. Interruption of bladder function may be due to trauma, infection, neoplasm, or a degenerative or vascular problem. It may be due to either a central or peripheral lesion, which may be limited to involvement of only efferent or only afferent pathways. For these reasons one must not automatically assume that any bladder dysfunction is the result of stroke. It may be due to a preexisting condition such as prostatic hypertrophy or to some aspect of the existing therapeutic regimen [4].

The most common form of bladder dysfunction with stroke is *incontinence* due to loss of inhibition from the higher centers and consequent impaired voluntary control. It is important to remember that in the acute stage of stroke this can occur whether the patient is conscious or not. The first step in bladder training should take place during this early stage of stroke by analyzing the patient's voiding pattern. During this initial trial period the nurse must also be alert to any signs of overdistention: restlessness, perspiration, chills, flushing or pallor, marked elevation of blood pressure, coldness of the extremities, or severe headache. If there is overdistention, palpation of the lower abdomen will reveal a firm distention of the bladder wall directly above the symphysis pubis [21].

Rationale and purpose of bladder training

The purpose of a bladder program is to establish a regular voiding pattern, to eliminate the need for a catheter, and to prevent urinary complications such as infections, retention, and incontinence. If the bladder is kept completely empty by a catheter, drainage contracture can occur, resulting in a low threshold for the micturition reflex. If the bladder is allowed to remain overly filled for long periods of time, it will stretch, and eventually large volumes of urine will be necessary to initiate the micturition reflex. Continued overdistention of the bladder will decrease the blood supply and predispose to infection. The existence of either of these conditions will make subsequent bladder training difficult.

ASSESSMENT
The first step in bladder training is *assessment of bladder function.* This involves determining the current voiding pattern and cause of incontinence and is best accomplished by preparing a 24-hour record of fluid intake, urine output, and the specific methods used in establishing bladder control. This information can serve as baseline data to analyze existing patterns and assess progress in bladder training. A sample chart is shown in Figure 10-2. The *record of fluid intake* should include the type of fluid, the amount, and the exact time it was taken. *Urine output* should be recorded by specifying both the amount at each voiding and the times of voiding. It is important to determine whether a relationship exists between fluid intake and output and between fluid intake and incidence of incontinence. Voidings should be related to the amount of fluid intake during the intervals between them. For example,

Date	Fluids	Voidings					Facility	Comments
	Type and Amount	Time	Description	Continent	Incontinent		(1) bedpan (2) commode (3) urinal (4) toilet (5) standing	

Figure 10-2
Bladder training chart. A day-to-day record of voiding pattern provides a cumulative summary. This record will alert the nurse to the patient's progress and to any need for changes in the program.

it may be noted that a patient voids less than an hour after drinking tea, coffee, or cola, or it may be noted that after approximately 400 ml of any fluid voiding will take place in about two hours. To establish the patient's *voiding pattern,* the nurse must record whether the patient is incontinent or not, whether he has any sensation of a full bladder, or whether he is aware of spontaneous voiding. It is also important to note what position the patient assumes for urination and whether he is able to use the toilet or commode or must depend upon urinals and bedpans. It is difficult to relax the perineal muscles and external sphincter when using a bedpan or urinal in the supine position. Consequently, micturition may fail to occur, resulting in bladder distention with overflow incontinence. Some people cannot void in the supine position because of the psychological conditioning involved in establishing habits of toileting. Lack of privacy can be a strong deterrent to initiating voiding also [1].

The following figures can be used to estimate the amount of urine when there has been an *incontinent voiding* [17]:

```
 9-inch stain =   50- 75 cc
12-inch stain = 100-125 cc
18-inch stain = 150-175 cc
24-inch stain = 200-300 cc
```

Note must be made of whether incontinence is continual, occasional, only at night, or at another specific time. To determine the cause of incontinence the nurse must know (1) if the patient has any medical cause for incontinence apart from his stroke; (2) what the patient's voiding pattern was prior to the stroke; (3) if he is lethargic from cerebral insult or medication; (4) if there is dribbling or difficulty in initiating urination, urgency, frequency that could be due to retention, a urinary tract infection, or cerebral inhibition; (5) if he is aware of the need to void; (6) if he is able to ask for help; (7) if he is able to reach for the urinal, bedpan, or call bell; and (8) whether the patient is assuming a correct position for urination.

SCHEDULE
Once the current voiding pattern and apparent cause of incontinence have been considered, a program can be instituted that will meet the specific needs of the patient. It may be necessary to follow closely and modify such a program for days or even weeks. On the other hand a solution is sometimes found on the first day. The following steps are designed to help in establishing a schedule:

1. Encourage awareness of environment and body functioning, so that the patient will become more alert to bladder stimulation.
2. Provide the optimal position for urination to allow for relaxation of the perineal muscles and the external urinary sphincter. A sitting position is best for females and a standing position for males. The best way to obtain this is by using a commode or toilet.
3. Offer the bedpan or urinal every two hours initially, then increase or decrease the time intervals accordingly. Establish a voiding schedule by offering the bedpan or

urinal or an opportunity to use the toilet or commode at specific times – for example, upon awakening in the morning, before and after meals, before any scheduled activity such as physical therapy, or at bedtime.

4. Once the voiding schedule has been established, place the patient on the bedpan or provide the urinal or opportunity to use the commode or toilet before the anticipated time.

5. Establish a fluid intake schedule, and give the patient 200 cc of fluid every hour from 7:00 A.M. until 6:00 P.M., unless there is a fluid restriction because of medical reasons. Record the fluid intake carefully.

6. Suggest measures to stimulate voiding.

TECHNIQUE

Some trigger areas for induction of micturition have already been discussed in relation to the upper motor neuron bladder. Pouring water over the perineum, using a warm bedpan, and running water from the tap are also useful in helping the patient to relax and void. When there is a spastic bladder, the micturition reflex can also be stimulated by stroking the thighs, pulling on the pubic hair, and stimulating the anal sphincter.

When the patient first begins to void spontaneously, residual catheterization may be used to determine the ability of the bladder to empty completely. A residual of more than 75 cc indicates that the bladder is emptying poorly and bears close observation.

When none of the methods just described produces a normal voiding pattern, other methods must be considered. First, of course, possible medical problems must be ruled out. Unfortunately, the common solution to such a problem is usually placement of an indwelling catheter. In addition to the complications of catheter use already discussed, it should be noted that long-term use of an indwelling catheter can cause dilation of the urethra, requiring an ever-increasing size of catheter. Spinal cord specialists recommend intermittent catheterization for patients with neurogenic bladders [7, 16]. This approach can be used for the stroke patient as well.

INTERMITTENT CATHETERIZATION

Catheterizing intermittently helps to regulate bladder activity regularly and prevents bladder distention from occurring. Because the approach involves complete emptying of the bladder, it also helps to reduce the chance of an infection. This procedure also reduces the constant pressure and ischemia that may occur with an indwelling urethral catheter and is particularly helpful in preventing development of pressure sores at the penoscrotal angle of the urethra in men [7].

Over the past 7 years, research by Lapides and his associates at the University of Michigan has suggested that decreased blood flow to the bladder caused by overdistention and high intravesical pressure is the most common physiopathological mechanism in the development of cystitis and pyelonephritis. To test this idea, the effectiveness of nonsterile, intermittent self-catheterization as therapy for vesical dysfunction in 100 patients with neurogenic disease has been studied. In all cases improvement has been observed and sterile urine maintained without antibacterial medication for up to 3 years [12]. Lapides states that "infection results from inter-action between bacteria and host resistance and that invasion of body tissues occurs only when defense mechanisms are weakened" [10]. With respect to the urinary tract, factors that affect the integrity of the urothelium lead to infection. These include stones, tumors, indwelling catheters, rough instrumentation, and decreased blood flow. The most common cause of decreased blood flow to the bladder is overdistention related to infrequent voiding in women and increased intravesical pressure due to obstruction in men. Lapides advocates emptying the bladder every 2—3 hours during the day and once or twice a night while the patient is consuming a normal amount of food and fluids. If the patient is unable to void, intermittent, clean catheterization should be carried out. It is most important, however, that the bladder not be allowed to overdistend between catheterizations, since catheterization of the overdistended bladder can lead to cystitis [13].

Guttman states that with proper aseptic precautions, the bladder can be kept sterile with intermittent catheterization [7]. The interval between catheterizations is usually 4 to 6 hours. Because overdistention can affect bladder tone, it may be necessary to limit fluids for those patients who have retention. The patient's intake can be adjusted according to the amount of urine obtained. The bladder should not hold more than 400 cc, and the time interval between catheterizations should be decreased if this amount is exceeded. Sudden, rapid decompression of the bladder can produce hemodynamic changes that may result in hemorrhage or shock [1]. Therefore, only 500 cc should be removed at a time. If there is more urine in the bladder, the catheter should be clamped for about a half hour before the remainder is removed.

INDWELLING CATHETER

Intermittent catheterization may be used as a temporary measure to control reten-tion and overdistention in the stroke patient. This method seems to afford the best protection against the complications usually associated with long-standing use of indwelling catheters. At times indwelling catheters may be required for hourly measurement of urinary output or analysis of constituents — for example, when there is renal impairment or another medical condition that warrants close super-vision of kidney function. The frequency with which the catheter is changed is very important. Guttman has found, in his work with patients who have neurogenic bladder dysfunction, that leaving an indwelling catheter in place for 1—2 weeks leads inevitably to such complications as stone formation and damage to the mucosa of the bladder and urethra, even with the newer plastic catheters, which are much less irritating to the urethra than the rubber ones. He recommends changing the catheter every other day initially, then two to three times per week. While it may be neces-sary to use a larger catheter in female patients, in males he recommends that no size larger than a 14—16 French gauge catheter be inserted and that no balloon larger than 5 cc be used [7].

Insertion of a urinary catheter. A urethral catheter should always be smaller than the external urinary meatus to minimize trauma to the delicate tissues. If an indwelling catheter is to be inserted, a triple lumen tube should be used to provide for a sterile closed drainage and irrigation system. One channel serves to inflate the retention balloon, one serves to irrigate the catheter and bladder, and the third drains urine from the bladder. Surgical asepsis is mandatory for insertion of the catheter, which should be well lubricated with an antimicrobial preparation then passed gently in order to minimize trauma and prevent infection. It should be attached to a closed sterile drainage system. Disposable units with drip chambers and drainage bags with a valve opening are available commercially. The drip chamber serves as an airlock to prevent bacteria from ascending from the collection container. The valve opening at the end of the bag allows measurement of output without disruption of the drainage system.

An antibacterial preparation is generally used to rinse the bladder thus limiting multiplication of organisms. The bladder should be irrigated every 2–4 hours with approximately 20–30 ml of a solution that is allowed to flow into the bladder at about 30–60 drops per minute. The irrigating fluid should be accounted for when the output is recorded. For alkaline urine 0.5% acetic acid, 4% boric acid, and Zephiran 1:1,000 are among the irrigating solutions that may be prescribed; for acidic urine, normal saline or potassium permanganate 1:2,000 may be given [7]. The area around the urethral meatus should be cleansed regularly with soap and water, and a gauze square soaked with hydrogen peroxide should be used around the catheter at the meatus to prevent encrustations from forming. In male patients, the foreskin should be cleansed and repositioned gently to prevent paraphimosis.

To maintain safe and adequate drainage of urine, kinking or twisting of tubing must be prevented, as well as dangling loops of tubing in which the urinary drainage can pool and flow back into the bladder. It is most important that the catheter drain freely. If it becomes obstructed, the bladder can become overdistended, and bacteria in the urine can be disseminated readily into the systemic circulation. Sepsis can ensue in minutes [13]. Unless cardiac or renal impairment necessitates fluid restriction, the patient should have an intake of about 3000 cc of fluid daily to assure adequate dilution of urine and decrease the chance of stone formation.

Because of the many disadvantages of keeping an indwelling catheter in place for prolonged periods, disposable condom urine collecting appliances may be used for male patients when bladder training has been unsuccessful. They can be used when there is no infection, obstruction or danger of ureteral reflux. Before applying the condom, the shaft of the penis should be washed and dried thoroughly and the skin checked for signs of edema, irritation, discoloration or breaks. The condom is rolled onto the penis with some slack left at the connection to the tubing to prevent irritation. It is secured with an expandable adhesive strip which is placed around the penis about an inch beyond the head of the penis. The appliance should be checked periodically for twisting which may cause irritation or interference with drainage.

BOWEL FUNCTION

Bowel function can be impaired by stroke because of immobility, lethargy, or coma. It is not uncommon for the patient to become *constipated,* with a severe fecal impaction from prolonged retention of stool in the bowel. The major causes of constipation are immobility, decreased oral intake, inability to communicate the need to defecate, and lack of response to the defecation reflex. *Diarrhea* may be precipitated by tube feedings, drugs, or fecal impaction. *Incontinence* may be due to decreased cerebral inhibition, but this is rare. To evaluate bowel function and develop a program for bowel training the nurse must understand the physiology of the bowel.

Physiology of the bowel

The two primary functions of the gastrointestinal system are digestion and absorption of nutrients. The upper gastrointestinal tract conveys food to the lower tract, breaks it up into smaller particles and mixes them with the digestive juices, and begins the process of chemical digestion. The midportion of the gastrointestinal tract extends from the duodenal papilla to the midtransverse colon. It is here that digestion is completed and absorption takes place. The lower tract extends from the midportion of the transverse colon to the anus. Its primary function is storage of the end products of digestion until they can be expelled [1].

The pattern of intestinal activity is complex and depends on pendular, circular, and segmental movements of the various sections of the intestinal tract *(peristalsis)*. The speed of intestinal activity varies widely: it is greatest in the duodenum and jejunum and slowest in the ileum. The gastroileal reflex stimulates the ileum to move semifluid contents into the cecum and gradually fill the ascending and transverse colon. The propulsive movements of peristalsis are stimulated by distention. As food progresses through the tract, collections causing distention in any area will cause peristalsis. Absorption of salts and water takes place in the transverse colon. This slows down the process for long intervals, until a powerful mass movement of the transverse colon propels the contents into the lower colon. All these processes take place without conscious awareness. The act of defecation, however, is initiated voluntarily after the urge to defecate is felt through afferent impulses, to the sacral spinal center and cerebral stations, that occur after filling and distention of the sigmoid and upper rectum. Efferent impulses from the sacral center then start the opening mechanism by evoking contractions of the sigmoid and rectum and relaxing the two rectal sphincters. Passage of stool is assisted by straining. Once the anal canal has been emptied, closure of the sphincters is caused by contraction of the levator ani. Intestinal activity relies on the coordinated action of various parts of the nervous system, including the intramural plexus in the bowel wall, the autonomic nervous system, and the voluntary nervous system [7] (Fig. 10-3).

The *intramural plexus* of the alimentary tract provides the nervous supply. It is composed principally of two layers of neurons with connecting fibers. The outer, more extensive, layer is the myenteric or Auerbach's plexus; and the inner, which lies within the submucosa, is the submucosal or Meissner's plexus. Stimulation of the plexus increases activity of the intestines, causing increased muscle tone, increased intensity and rate of rhythmic contractions, and increases the speed with which excitatory waves are conducted along the intestinal wall. A few of the fibers in the plexus

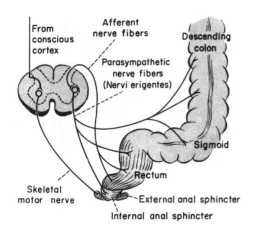

Figure 10-3
Schematic representation of the defecation reflex. (From A. G. Guyton, Textbook
of Medical Physiology *[5th ed.]. Philadelphia: Saunders, 1976.)*

are adrenergic and have an inhibitory effect. Therefore administration of atropine
can paralyze the intramural plexus. Parasympathetic nerves constitute the major
source of neurological control of peristaltic function, and any parasympathetic
stimulation can influence the intensity of peristalsis and its speed. Effective peristalsis
cannot occur without active involvement of the intramural plexus [8].

The *autonomic nervous system* influences gastrointestinal activity through both
sympathetic and parasympathetic innervation. The cranial division of the parasympathetic system provides stimulation, by the vagus nerve, of the esophagus, stomach,
pancreas, small intestine, gallbladder, and first half of the large intestine. The sacral
division of the parasympathetic system controls the lower portion of the large bowel.
These fibers are especially important in the defecation reflex. Gastrointestinal
activity is inhibited by sympathetic innervation, which originates in the thoracic
section of the spinal cord and primarily causes effects that are opposite to those of
the parasympathetic system. The sympathetic system also elicits excitatory effects
on the ileocecal sphincter and the internal anal sphincter, however, so that strong
stimulation of this system can block the movement of food through the gastrointestinal tract. These effects are usually transient. However, when the parasympathetic system has been denervated, the resultant decreased activity of the alimentary
canal can persist for months or years. When this occurs, the intramural plexus compensates by gradually increasing its excitability, so that bowel function returns
almost to normal [8].

Cerebral influence can inhibit the sacral spinal center to decrease peristaltic
activity by voluntarily increasing anal sphincter tone and relaxing the colon. This
will cause the urge to defecate to disappear [7].

The functions of the *colon* are (1) absorption of water and electrolytes, which
occurs mainly in the upper section, and (2) storage of fecal material, which takes
place in the lower colon. *Mass movements* propel the fecal material forward. These

are caused principally by the duodenocolic reflex, which is initiated when the duodenum is filled. Mass movements are most active for about 10 minutes each day within one hour of the first meal. When they have been sufficient to force a mass of stool into the rectum, the desire to defecate is felt. These reflexes are transmitted through the intramural nerve plexus and intensified by the parasympathetic system or overdistention of the colon [8]. When feces enter the rectum, the distention of the rectal wall initiates afferent signals that spread through the myenteric plexus to initiate peristaltic waves in the descending colon, sigmoid, and rectum that force feces into the anus. With relaxation of the external anal sphincter, defecation will occur.

However, the defecation reflex is weak, and to be effective it must be fortified by another reflex that involves sacral segments of the spinal cord. Voluntary inhibition and initiation of defecation is made possible by cerebral control through transmission of impulses to and from the brain. Stroke can affect the cerebral areas responsible for control and cause fecal incontinence. Bowel dysfunction that occurs following stroke, however, is usually due to constipation caused by the patient's restricted physical activity, limited fluid intake, and failure to respond to the defecation reflex. When fecal incontinence does occur, it is rarely due to the stroke itself, although a decrease in cerebral inhibition may add to the problem.

Establishing a bowel training program

The nurse should anticipate problems in reestablishing a normal pattern of bowel movements following stroke. A bowel training program should be started early to prevent complications. There are many patterns of bowel habits among healthy individuals. Most patients' life-style is altered significantly by the stroke, and it may not be easy to reestablish the former pattern in all cases, but the nurse must attempt to determine former bowel habits to plan for the bowel program. The timing of peristaltic activity in the small bowel and mass movements in the large bowel must be considered. Most programs are more successful when they are planned around the first meal of the day.

The purpose of the bowel program is to establish regular bowel habits that will be safe and meet the particular needs of the patient. This can be accomplished by establishing voluntary control through regularity and diet or by setting up a program for a controlled pattern with the use of suppositories, stool softeners, and laxatives. If successful, the program will eliminate irregularity, constipation, fecal impaction, and involuntary evacuations. The three most important factors influencing the efficiency of bowel function are diet, intake of fluids, and physical activity. Once the patient is able to take solids by mouth safely he should have a well-balanced diet with three regular meals a day. Roughage such as salads, whole grain breads and cereals, fruits, and vegetables should be included as soon as they can be chewed and swallowed adequately, to help stimulate peristalsis and to prevent constipation. Prolonged recumbency has an adverse effect and tends to cause fecal retention. The patient who can be out of bed and involved in physical activities will have return of bowel function more quickly. Patients should drink 2–3 quarts of liquid daily, unless fluid intake has been restricted for medical reasons. Some patients find that hot water, prune juice, or hot coffee every morning for breakfast is helpful in initiating a bowel movement.

Defecation can be stimulated by a suppository or by digital rectal stimulation, with no need for enemas [17]. Suppositories are given to potentiate the activity of the defecation reflex. Success is dependent upon giving the suppository at the time when motility of the bowel is greatest. The suppository should be inserted daily or every other day, 15–20 minutes after a meal, preferably breakfast. The patient should be on his left side with the right knee flexed. The suppository is inserted as high as possible above the internal sphincter and then gently pushed against the rectal wall to either side. It is important that the suppository be in contact with the rectum. The suppository will not be effective if placed in stool. Sometimes it will be necessary to give an enema before starting the program, to provide a clean bowel. Fifteen to twenty minutes after the suppository is inserted, the abdomen may be massaged from right to left and down, following the course of the large intestine, several times. If he is physically able, the patient should be in a squatting position for evacuation, to allow for proper use of the abdominal muscles. If he is able, he may lean forward and strain. Use of the bedpan should be avoided, as much as possible.

The following measures should be taken in establishing a program for bowel function.

1. Follow the bowel pattern that existed prior to illness. Some patients normally have a movement every two or three days; others have one daily.
2. Provide a good diet adequate in roughage.
3. Give fluids adequate to stimulate reflex activity and to assure enough liquid in the stool.
4. Obtain a physician's order to give stool softeners such as Colace daily.
5. Establish a time for a bowel movement. It should be the same time each day.
6. Begin the program with an enema to assure that the rectum is not filled with stool.
7. Give a glycerine suppository to initiate the defecation reflex. If the suppository is not effective the first day, let the patient rest, then insert another suppository the next day. If this is effective, continue the program. If after two days the suppository has not been effective, obtain an order for a Dulcolax suppository and continue the regimen with that. If this is unsuccessful, give an enema and begin the regimen over again, using Dulcolax suppositories. Obtain an order for a laxative which can be used as needed. For long-term use glycerine suppositories are preferred, since they are milder. The goal is to eliminate the need for long-term use of suppositories.

A written record of bowel function is necessary to determine progress and to initiate the appropriate changes. In some cases it may take a week or longer to establish a satisfactory bowel pattern. For regularity, stools should be of a fairly firm consistency. If stools are too soft or loose, eliminate laxatives and decrease roughage. If stools are too hard and constipated, increase fluid intake and roughage. These difficulties may be caused by certain foods, laxatives, or fecal impactions or

Date	Fluids	Diet	Enemas	Medications						Time	Evacuation		Comments
				Laxatives, Stool Softener		Suppositories					Facility (bedpan, commode, toilet)	Stools	
				Time	No. and Name	Time	No. and Name					Description: consistency, amount	

Figure 10-4
Bowel training chart. This chart, like the one on bladder training (Fig. 10-2), keeps track of the patient's progress on a day-to-day basis and alerts the nurse to any need for changes in the program.

by medical problems not directly related to the stroke. If these suggestions are not effective in establishing bowel function, this should be reported to the responsible physician. Figure 10-4 is an example of a bowel training chart and cumulative record of progress.

REFERENCES

1. Beland, I. L., and Passos, J. Y. *Clinical Nursing: Pathophysiological and Psychosocial Approaches* (3rd ed.). New York: Macmillan, 1975. Pp. 962–966.
2. Bergstrom, D. *Care of Patients with Bowel and Bladder Problems: A Nursing Guide.* Minneapolis: American Rehabilitation Foundation, 1968.
3. Beyers, M., and Dudas, S. *The Clinical Practice of Medical-Surgical Nursing.* Boston: Little, Brown, 1977. Pp. 469–521.
4. Bors, E., and Comarr, E. *Neurological Urology.* Baltimore: University Park Press, 1971. Pp. 223–237.
5. Cleland, V., et al. Prevention of bacteriuria in female patients with indwelling catheters. *Nurs. Res.* 20:310, 1971.
6. Friedland, F. Physical Therapy. In S. Licht (Ed.), *Stroke and Its Rehabilitation.* Baltimore: Williams & Wilkins, 1975. Pp. 221–225.
7. Guttman, L. *Spinal Cord Injuries, Comprehensive Management and Research.* Oxford, Engl.: Blackwell, 1976. Pp. 458–473.
8. Guyton, A. G. *Textbook of Medical Physiology* (5th ed.). Philadelphia: Saunders, 1976. Pp. 501–504; 850–866.
9. Herr, H. W. Intermittent catheterization in neurogenic bladder dysfunction. *J. Urol.* 113:477–479, 1975.
10. Lapides, J. Urinary tract infections in women. *J. Practical Nurs.* 25, 19–20, 1976.
11. Lapides J., Diokno, A. C., Gould, F. R., and Lowe, B. S. Further observations on self-catheterization. *Trans. Am. Assoc. Genitourin. Surg.* 67:15–17, 1975.
12. Lapides, J., Diokno, A. C., Lowe, B. S., and Kalish, M. D. Follow-up on unsterile, intermittent self-catheterization. *Trans. Am. Assoc. Genitourin. Surg.* 65:44–47, 1973.
13. Lapides, J., Diokno, A. C., Silber, S. J., and Lowe, B. S. Clean intermittent self-catheterization in the treatment of urinary tract disease. *Trans. Am. Assoc. Genitourin. Surg.* 63:92–95, 1971.
14. Perkosh, I. Intermittent catheterization: The urologist's point of view. *J. Urol.* 111:357–360, 1974.
15. Peszczynski, M. Rehabilitation in Hemiplegia. In S. Licht (Ed.), *Rehabilitation and Medicine.* Baltimore: Williams & Wilkins, 1975. Pp. 390–410.
16. Rossier, A. B. Neurogenic bladder in spinal injury. *Urol. Clin. North Am.* 1: Pp. 125–137, 1974.
17. Rossier, A. B. Rehabilitation of the Spinal Cord Injury Patient. *Acta Clinica.* No. 3, J. R. Geigy, S. A. Basel, Switzerland, 1964. Pp. 21–45, 46–49.
18. Sauerland, E. Infection control urological care. The Nervous Control of the Bladder. *Curr. Prac. Perspect.* 1: Pp. 3–5, 1976.
19. Shafer, K., Sawyer, J., McCluskey, A., Beck, E., and Phipps, W. *Medical Surgical Nursing* (6th ed.). St. Louis: Mosby, 1975. Pp. 173–184.
20. Stravino, V., and Delehanty, L. Achieving bladder control. *Am. J. Nurs.* 2:312–316, 1970.
21. Stryker, R. *Rehabilitation Aspects of Acute and Chronic Care.* Philadelphia: Saunders, 1972. Pp. 66–80.

11. Maintaining the integrity of the skin and personal hygiene

During the acute stage of stroke the patient is completely dependent upon the nursing staff for maintaining his personal hygiene and protecting his skin from injury. Because of the various neurological deficits resulting from stroke, the nurse must remain constantly vigilant as the patient's condition stabilizes, to assure that bathing, mouth care, and grooming are carried out adequately and that every effort is made to ensure integrity of the skin. The patient should be taught to carry out his own personal care as soon as possible, but he needs continued supervision of these important functions.

Each year hundreds of thousands of dollars are spent on lengthy hospitalizations, repeated debridements, skin grafting, and antibiotic therapy to treat tissue necrosis resulting from pressure sores. Substantial amounts are also spent on restorative dentistry required because of poor oral hygiene during hospitalization. Although the cost to society, the patient, and his family is staggering, the cost to the patient in terms of agony, disfigurement, and threat to life is incalculable. To be sure, every case is not one of willful or wanton neglect on the part of the nursing staff. Sometimes overwhelming complications lead to problems in spite of the finest care. In other cases lack of knowledge concerning the principles of skin care and oral hygiene can foster practices that aggravate rather than prevent pressure sores and disease of the teeth and gums.

Care of the patient's comfort is also a uniquely nursing function. There are many times when a good massage will contribute to the patient's sense of well-being, improve circulation to the tissues, relieve pressure, and still allow the nurse an opportunity to assess the patient's neurological and physical functioning. As significant as it may be for the nurse to detect a life-threatening cardiac dysrhythmia, change in neurological status, or disturbance of acid-base balance, she will not have discharged fully her professional responsibility if the patient's skin and mouth are inadequately cared for and he is suffering from sustained pressure because he is paralyzed or too weak to shift his own body weight.

In this chapter we will discuss the anatomy and care of the skin in some detail, outline the principles of good dental hygiene, and discuss eye care briefly.

THE SKIN

Anatomy

The skin of an adult covers about 20,000 cm^2 of body surface, has an average thickness of 2.5 mm, and thus is the largest organ of the body. It is nourished by the capillary system, through which blood circulates, carrying oxygen and nutrients to the tissue and carrying away the products of cell metabolism [4]. Healthy skin is one of the body's first lines of defense against infection. Every effort must be made therefore to keep the patient's skin scrupulously clean and intact. Numerous bacteria and fungi are present normally on the surface of the skin and are harmless there but may have deleterious effects within the body. A break in the skin can give entry to these organisms and set up an infectious process. Since the body is particularly susceptible to systemic infection when afflicted with a chronic debilitating illness, prevention of skin breakdown as a potential focus of infection is very important [6]. It is also important to keep the bacterial population of the body surface at a safe level. The significance of good hygiene and skin care for the patient's morale, comfort, and self-esteem also must not be overlooked.

Figure 11-1 shows a cross section of the skin, divided into two distinct parts: the epidermis, or superficial layer, and the dermis, or deeper section. The *epidermis* is composed of stratified epithelial cells that have become flattened as they have matured and risen to the surface. This outer layer protects against invasion of microorganisms and aids in heat regulation [12]. It is particularly thick over the palms of the hands and soles of the feet. The *dermis* is composed of dense connective tissue containing many blood vessels, lymphatic vessels, and nerves. This layer of the skin is connected to the underlying deep fascia or to the bones by means of the *superficial fascia,* which is usually referred to as *subcutaneous tissue.* It is a mixture of loose areolar and adipose tissue. The *deep fascia* is a membranous layer of connective tissue that covers the muscles and other deep structures. The two fascial layers

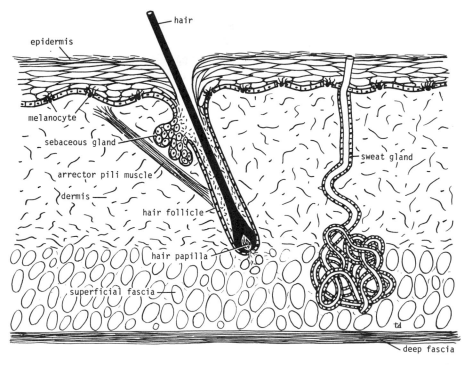

Figure 11-1
Cross section of the skin. (From R. S. Snell [12].)

lie between the skin and the underlying muscles and bones [12]. Nails, hair follicles, sebaceous glands, and sweat glands are all appendages to the skin. They are common sites through which pathological organisms such as *Staphylococcus aureus* gain entrance into the underlying tissues [12].

Factors predisposing to pressure sores

Much has been written about the seriousness of pressure sores and the prevention and treatment of this common problem; but relatively little has been published concerning a systematic assessment of the patient's potential for developing pressure sores and tissue necrosis [8]. At the time of admission, when the nurse checks the condition of the patient's skin, she should note the presence of any of the following factors that may predispose to breakdown of the skin.

1. Dry skin, which may crack and peel, allowing harmful bacteria to enter
2. Improperly cared for nails, which can in themselves become a focus of infection or can lead to abrasions of the skin due to scratching
3. Paralysis, which limits the patient's ability to move independently and thereby concentrates pressure over a limited body area for prolonged periods
4. Impaired sensation, which decreases the patient's appreciation of extremes of temperature or the need to redistribute weight to relieve prolonged pressure on one spot. Heating pads, hot water bottles, cigarettes, and hot beverages can cause severe burns without the patient's awareness when sensation is impaired.
5. Incontinence of urine, which can lead to breakdown because skin that remains wet for long periods soon becomes macerated
6. Spasticity, which can lead to breakdown of the skin because of the friction of the affected extremity against the bedclothes
7. Decrease of muscle bulk over the bony prominences with little subcutaneous tissue to protect the skin from the pressure over these areas
8. Edema, which interferes with cell nutrition
9. Traction, casts, crutches, or braces, which are a potential source of friction and sustained pressure over bony prominences
10. Existing redness, sores, or skin infection
11. Absent or diminished peripheral pulses, which may indicate inadequate circulation to the extremities
12. Dryness or lesions of the gums, tongue, and mucous membranes of the mouth and lips
13. Impaired sensation and/or paralysis of the mouth, which may lead to poor oral hygiene and pooling of food particles and secretions in the paralyzed side
14. Diabetes mellitus, which makes the patient more prone to skin infection and prolonged tissue healing
15. Drugs that interfere with tissue healing, such as cortisone, or emergency parenteral drugs like norepinephrine, which can lead to tissue necrosis if the intravenous solution extravasates into the surrounding tissues

16. Poor nutrition. An adequate supply of protein and vitamins is essential to the integrity of the skin. A negative nitrogen balance will lead to tissue wasting and weight loss. If a pressure sore is established, good nutrition is essential to promote tissue healing and replacement of protein loss from wound drainage.

Maintenance of intact skin requires vigilance and careful planning. Because the stroke patient is immobile, pressure sores will develop unless preventive measures are taken. The nurse must familiarize herself with the causes of skin breakdown, its stages, the susceptible areas, proper nursing measures for preventing it, and measures of treatment should it occur in spite of preventive efforts.

Causes of skin breakdown

A pressure sore is an area of cellular necrosis caused by lack of blood flow. Although many factors predispose to the development of such a sore, the actual cause is *sustained pressure*. The amount of pressure and how long it is sustained are both important. Intense pressure can be tolerated for very brief intervals without skin breakdown. Breakdown is more often the result of a slight to moderate degree of pressure, sustained for an extended period of time, and eventually causing ischemia of the skin and underlying tissues, when skin and subcutaneous tissue are compressed between an underlying bone and the firm surface of a mattress or chair [8, 9]. This continued pressure on the delicate tissue expresses blood from the area, preventing it from reaching the cells. The result is anoxia and tissue necrosis [4].

Impaired sensation, spasticity, and paralysis, which frequently accompany stroke, can contribute to prolonged pressure and ischemia. Normally, afferent impulses arising from an area exposed to pressure that impedes blood flow will elicit a protective sensation of "pins and needles," numbness, and eventually pain. These are the earliest symptoms of impending ischemia, and the person with intact motor and sensory function will respond by changing position, thus restoring blood flow to the area [9]. The patient with stroke may be unconscious or unable to appreciate or express a sensation of discomfort. If he is paralyzed, he will be unable to change his position without help. Body build is an important contributing factor to skin breakdown. A heavy patient puts greater weight on pressure points. The less padding there is between the weight-bearing bony prominences and the skin, the greater is the resulting compression of the skin and subcutaneous tissue. It is important to remember that motor paralysis will eventually lead to muscle atrophy, thereby reducing muscle mass in the involved extremities. When the patient remains lying or sitting in one position, pressure is concentrated on several small areas of skin.

While pressure sores over the bony prominences resulting from sustained pressure are the most significant cause of skin breakdown, it can also be caused by trauma, friction, shearing forces, tape burns, cracking of dry skin, maceration due to moisture, medications, constriction, and dependent edema.

Trauma to the skin can result from improperly trimmed toenails and fingernails scratching the skin. The patient with hemiplegia, perceptual deficits, or impaired sensation may injure the skin while attempting to change position, cut food, pour a hot beverage, or perform numerous other activities of daily living.

Friction can result from involuntary movement such as spastic motion of a paralyzed limb. Sores resulting from the stress of continual rubbing due to spasticity may be seen on the inner surface of the knees and ankles. This type of tissue damage can also be inflicted if a nurse or attendant attempts to position a patient in a bed or chair without adequate assistance. Dragging the patient's limbs, torso, and buttocks over the bed linens or chair seat, rather than lifting him off the surface to move or position him, can abrade his skin. The breasts, male genitalia, heels, sacrum, knees, and elbows are most vulnerable.

Moving the patient in this manner can also inflict *shearing pressure.* When the patient is pulled up in bed or slides down while sitting up in bed or in a chair, friction between the surface and the skin causes the skin to move more slowly than the underlying structures [10]. The layers of skin and subcutaneous tissue are pulled over each other as the bony prominences move over them. The force applied to the tissues is referred to as shearing pressure. It is directed diagonally rather than vertically, and the pressure exerted can damage blood vessels and impair blood supply over much larger areas than the pressure resulting from immobilization. Improper technique in massaging the skin can also exert shearing force on the skin and subcutaneous tissues.

Adhesive tape burns are another source of skin breakdown. Unless a protective coating is placed on the skin before the tape is applied, the outer layer of skin cells will be pulled away when the tape is removed. Patients with sensitive skin can develop severe local reaction to the adhesive, which will result in redness, weeping, and excoriation. If tape is applied too tightly, the skin can be pinched, causing impairment of circulation.

Dry skin can crack and peel, allowing pathogenic bacteria to infect the deeper layers. Lack of regular lubrication and adequate hydration and nutrition, as well as prolonged contact with bed linens that have been laundered with harsh chemicals, can contribute to dryness of the skin.

Excessive moisture can also have deleterious effects. When the skin remains wet, the tissues become soft and swollen and much more vulnerable to injury. Wound drainage, excessive perspiration, exudation from pressure sores, and urinary and fecal incontinence are all sources of moisture that can soften and irritate surrounding tissues and lead to skin breakdown.

Harsh chemicals in topical antiseptic preparations or irrigating solutions such as Dakin's solution or hydrogen peroxide, which may be beneficial in cleansing open wounds, can be caustic or irritating to the surrounding skin and should be used with caution. The healthy skin can be protected from these solutions temporarily during wound irrigations by a layer of petrolatum or petrolatum gauze.

Constriction of blood vessels is often the result of measures instituted in good faith to prevent pressure sores or enhance venous flow. "Donuts," rubber rings, and similar cut-out devices designed to eliminate pressure over the bony tuberosities divert more pressure onto the surrounding tissues, thereby decreasing further the blood supply to the affected area. Elastic hose and bandages, when improperly applied, are another source of constriction that may decrease circulation and lead to formation of pressure sores. Arm boards and tape used to prevent an intravenous needle or catheter from displacement are a source of constriction as well as pressure, friction, and tape burns. Hand splints that have not been properly fitted or have been secured too tightly are another potential cause of skin breakdown resulting from constriction of circulation. Restraints of any kind can impose trauma, friction, shearing forces, tape burns, and constriction. They should be used only when absolutely necessary for the patient's protection, and then with utmost caution and constant vigilance for signs of pressure and skin breakdown.

Dependent edema can result whenever an extremity is allowed to dangle. The presence of increased amounts of interstitial fluid interferes with the supply of essential nutrients to the cells, thus contributing to tissue necrosis.

Areas most susceptible to breakdown

Figure 11-2 illustrates the areas most susceptible to skin breakdown. When the patient is in the *prone position,* the anterior superior iliac spines, patellae, tibial surfaces, and facial bones will exert sustained pressure. In the *supine position* the posterior surface of the head and the skin over the scapulae, vertebrae, sacrum, elbows, and heels are most vulnerable to breakdown. When the patient is *lying on one side,* the ears, shoulders, hips, and areas over the head of the fibula, ribs, and lateral and medial malleoli are most susceptible to breakdown. It is important to remember that tissue necrosis — erosion of the nares and trachea and breakdown

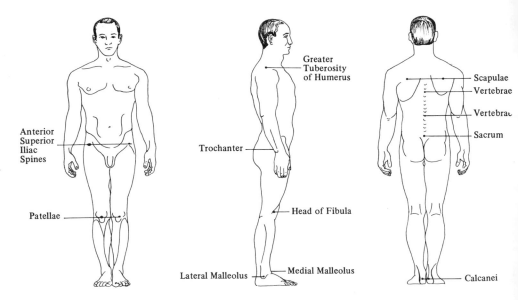

Figure 11-2
Areas most susceptible to skin breakdown. (Adapted from Sister Kenny Institute. Nursing Care of the Skin *[Rehabilitation Publication #711]. Minneapolis: Sister Kenny Institute, 1975. Published by permission of the Institute.)*

of the penoscrotal angle — can also result from the pressure exerted by drainage tubes, feeding tubes, and airways, as discussed in Chapters 7, 9, and 10. Adhesive tape used to secure drainage and feeding tubes can also cause irritation of the skin and predispose to breakdown.

Stages of breakdown

Guttman has described six stages of pathological change in cutaneous and subcutaneous tissue that occur in skin breakdown [9].

In the *first stage* there is a transient disturbance of circulation due to pressure. The result is erythema of the area with some edema. There is no destruction of tissue, and the situation can be reversed promptly by relief of pressure and gentle massage of the involved area.

The *second stage* involves permanent damage to cutaneous tissue. Guttman has classified three types of damage at this stage: (1) that characterized by erythema and congestion of the skin, which does not disappear with relief of pressure but progresses to induration and discoloration; (2) that which resembles an abrasion and is due to destruction of superficial skin layers from excoriation; and (3) damage of the deeper layers of skin, resulting in necrosis and ulcer formation beneath the area of sloughed tissue. The border of the resulting ulcer may be pigmented.

Deep penetrating necrosis occurs in the *third stage,* with destruction of subcutaneous tissue and involvement of fascia, muscle, and bone. The necrotic area is highly infected and is usually surrounded by an inflammatory zone, which will not disappear unless the slough is excised and the deep area of underlying fascia and muscle is exposed. This type of pressure sore is most common over the sacrum and trochanters.

In the *fourth stage,* sinuses develop that communicate with the joint bursae. This stage is most commonly seen with pressure sores over the trochanters and ischial tuberosities. In the latter case, the appearance of the skin breakdown may not reveal the actual extent of destruction to the underlying tissues, since the resulting sinuses may be quite deep.

The *fifth stage* is specific to paralyzed patients who are confined to wheelchairs. Closed ischial bursa formation occurs secondary to continual pressure or trauma when the patient transfers in and out of the chair. A cavity forms which, if not treated, will cause impairment of circulation to the skin, necrosis, and sinus formation.

The *sixth stage,* which is extremely rare, involves cancerous degeneration of long-standing pressure sores and sinuses.

Once necrosis of the tissues occurs, a distinct margin between it and the healthy tissues becomes apparent. The necrotic area becomes dehydrated and blackened, and the surrounding skin is inflamed. If the pressure is relieved, the patient's general condition is conducive to wound healing, and infection is not present, granulation can begin once the eschar has sloughed away; and spontaneous healing may take place. With a large pressure sore, healing may take many months. If there is a low-grade inflammation, and bacterial invasion takes place, damage to the underlying muscle, tendon, and bone can follow and prevent wound closure. In such cases surgical intervention will be required to close the wound, and skin grafting or flap closure may be necessary. Scar formation, bleeding, hematoma formation, or edema can also interfere with wound healing. Insufficient vitamin C and protein, the presence of diabetes mellitus, and the use of corticosteroids will also delay wound healing [4].

The most significant *complications* resulting from pressure sores are related to infection and interference with rehabilitation. Pressure sores always become infected and are a common source of sepsis. If vigorous treatment is not instituted immediately, the infection can extend from the skin and subcutaneous tissue into the bone causing periosteitis, osteitis, and osteomyelitis [9]. The development of pressure necrosis over the trochanteric and ischial regions is particularly dangerous because of the potential of joint involvement. The entire joint may be destroyed [9]. Pressure sores over the heels and sacrum can make ambulation impossible and retard rehabilitation significantly. Pain resulting from sores may increase spasticity and impede ambulation still further.

Care of the skin to prevent and treat pressure sores

PROTECTION FROM PRESSURE

The most important principle in skin care is prevention of pressure necrosis by *protecting the vulnerable bony prominences from undue pressure*. Miller and Sachs observe that pressure sores seldom occur over the occipital bone. They attribute this to the use of pillows and the fact that the head is the most likely member of the body to move freely [10]. The stroke patient who is not able to change his position independently should have a *program of scheduled position changes* to prevent sustained pressure. Until he is able to move on his own, he should be repositioned at least every two hours. It is important to note, however, that improper positioning can lead to development of pressure sores just as readily as no position change. If the knee gatch on the bed is elevated, undue pressure may be applied under the knees. Allowing one extremity to rest directly on the other in the sidelying position can also create undue pressure.

The patient who uses a chair or wheelchair must also be positioned and repositioned properly, since sustained pressure can be just as hazardous in the sitting position. Consideration must also be given to the effects of pressure exerted by drainage and feeding tubes, restraints, respiratory equipment, and intravenous or arterial lines. Equipment used to support the body in proper alignment, such as trochanter rolls, footboards, and sandbags, can also put prolonged pressure on the skin. Rubber rings, "donuts," and other devices designed to decrease pressure over bony prominences have already been indicted for actually fostering ischemia to the area by concentrating more pressure on the surrounding tissue.

The program of position changing must be tailored to each patient's needs. Scheduling should take into account the patient's other pre-set activities, such as bowel and bladder training, meal times, physical therapy and speech therapy sessions, exercise programs, and visiting hours, so that the patient's position will allow him to interact with others and participate in therapeutic activities to his fullest capacity [13].

It may become necessary to eliminate certain positions to protect an area where a skin problem has already started. Pillows, foam rubber (4 inches thick), and padding can be used liberally to *cushion all surfaces that potentially might cause pressure.* Gel or water cushions provide a good padding for wheelchairs but are very heavy to lift.

Elastic hose that are too tight, wrinkled, or left in place too long only serve as tourniquets and hide the color, temperature, and condition of the skin of the feet and legs from the nurse's view. When elastic bandages are required, they should be applied in a spiral fashion, starting at the toes and including the heel. They should be wrapped firmly but not tightly. The ends must be fastened very carefully so as not to abrade the skin. If they are fastened in place with adhesive, rather than metal clips, the strip of adhesive must never completely encircle the leg. As with the elastic hose, the bandages must be removed frequently to observe the condition of the feet and legs. This should include a *check of the pulses, color, temperature, presence of edema, and integrity of the skin.* It is recommended that this be done at least four times a day and that the hose or bandages be left off for about a half hour each time.

Water beds, water mattresses, and air mattresses are often recommended to prevent pressure sores. The water bed or mattress is based upon the principle of flotation and displacement of weight. It does have the disadvantage of limiting muscular activity, thereby interfering with the rehabilitation process. Because neither the water mattress nor the water bed offers much resistance, it is difficult to carry out activities of daily living or range of motion exercises on them. The water mattress and bed are too unstable for a paralyzed patient to sit up on or transfer from. The air mattress has the disadvantage that the noise of the air flow is extremely disturbing to most patients. As a result of his studies of measures of prevention and treatment of pressure sores in paralyzed patients, Guttman has concluded that neither device is successful in preventing pressure over the bony parts [9]. It is our opinion that in the majority of cases neither the water bed nor the air mattress is necessary when there is a systematic program for turning, positioning, and skin care. A water mattress may be necessary in the extreme case, such as long-standing paralysis, when the patient cannot be positioned in such a manner as to keep pressure off existing areas of tissue necrosis. A 4-inch foam rubber mattress pad placed over a firm mattress seems to afford the best cushioning for relief of pressure.

PROTECTION FROM EDEMA AND TRAUMA

Dependency of the limbs and infiltration of intravenous infusions both may contribute to an increase of interstitial fluid. This can progress to edema and tissue breakdown. Intravenous infusions should be supervised and the extremities properly supported to *prevent dependent edema.* With loss of sensation and motor function due to stroke, the mechanisms that usually protect against mechanical injury are absent. The patient may be unaware that any trauma has occurred to his affected extremities during transfer from one place to another. He should be instructed to guide and *protect these paralyzed limbs.* Mobilization of the patient is an important factor in prevention of pressure sore formation, because it promotes circulation to all areas and involves shifting of body weight.

PREVENTION OF BREAKS AND INFECTION

The significance of *maintaining cleanliness and adequate lubrication of the skin* over the bony prominences has already been discussed as an important nursing responsibility for prevention of breaks in the skin and development of local infection in all areas of the body. It is also important for prevention of skin breakdown of the paralyzed arm and hand. Tightness of the joints and spasticity will lead to skin irritation within flexed areas and between skin folds. Dead skin and debris will continue to collect within a tightly flexed hand unless measures are taken to improve its position and hygiene. Warm soaks can be used to reduce tension to clean the hand. The hand should be dried thoroughly. Powders and ointments should not be applied, because they tend to macerate the skin, but a lubricating hand lotion should be used as necessary to prevent cracking due to dryness. When a splint is used to bring the hand and wrist into a functional position it should be removed regularly to cleanse the hand.

Daily observation of the skin, to check for evidence of breaks in the skin and reddened or ischemic areas, is essential. Special attention should be given to the skin over bony prominences and under splints, braces, restraints, and other equipment that can exert pressure and/or irritate the skin. Any areas of redness or impaired circulation should be considered the beginning of a pressure sore. *Massage and range of motion exercises* to promote circulation should be an integral part of the program for prevention of pressure necrosis. A program of range of motion exercises is outlined in Chapter 12.

TREATMENT

Once a pressure sore has become established, a vigorous treatment program must be undertaken to promote healing and reduce the likelihood of infection and other complications. The severity of the pressure sore may vary from a loss of a small area of the superficial skin to a deep ulcer formation with necrosis of underlying structures [7]. Treatment will depend upon the depth of the lesion and the structures involved. Attention should be directed to alleviating the cause and promoting healing. Local treatment of the wound often avails little if the patient is not in good general condition [9]. *Adequate nutrition* with a high protein and high vitamin content is essential.

A simple ulcer will usually heal by granulation if it is kept clean and protected from injury [3]. Wet or greasy dressings should be avoided, since they macerate the skin and provide a good medium for bacterial growth. Powders should also be avoided, since they macerate the skin. A protective film of *tincture of benzoin* may be spread over small abrasions. It should be applied lightly with gauze and allowed to dry thoroughly before the patient is positioned, so that it does not adhere to the bedclothes and cause skin loss.

Although *ultraviolet treatment* has been advocated by some, Guttman warns that there is a great possibility of burns, because it is difficult to regulate the dosage of ultraviolet light directed to the devitalized tissue of the pressure sore [9]. *Wet to dry saline dressings* are effective for superficial debridement of infected tissue, if applied carefully. Warm soaks to ischemic extremities are contraindicated, because the increased metabolic rate induced by heating cannot be met by increased blood flow, and an increase in the area of ischemia and further cell damage will occur.

SURGICAL DEBRIDEMENT

If there is no response to conservative therapy, surgical debridement may be necessary. Whenever pressure sores occur over bone, such as on the heels, sacrum, or ankle, there is the risk of bone infection. The patient must be observed carefully for signs and symptoms of osteomyelitis. Because pressure sores generally become infected, slough should be excised as soon as the area becomes demarcated. If the underlying fascia is also necrotic and appears infected, the tissue should be excised and the area incised to allow drainage of the infected material. Often there are localized abscesses that must be drained [9]. When a closed septic wound covered with slough is thus transformed into an open draining wound, the immediate improvement of the patient's general condition is usually quite dramatic. Guttman advises against leaving the slough untouched until it falls off or becomes liquefied. He considers this form of conservative therapy both time-consuming and hazardous to the patient. He states that most of the deeper tissues are necrotic and infected by deep penetrating pressure sores, but that even if the necrotic material remained uninfected, absorption of the dead tissue would have a toxic effect on the patient manifested by loss of appetite, listlessness, and a bad taste in the mouth.

Daily wound care after surgical debridement should include (1) cleansing with an oxidizing agent such as hydrogen peroxide to encourage separation of slough, (2) dressing the sore with antibiotics in saline solution, and (3) covering and sealing the wound. In dressing the sore, preparations containing heavy metals should not be applied, since they inhibit growth of granulation tissue and thereby delay filling in of the defect that resulted from the debridement. These preparations can also cause further damage to the tissues. Once infection has been controlled, saline or Dakin's solution can be used. To cover the wound, several layers of gauze are placed over the wet dressing and the entire dressing is then sealed off with a porous elastic tape. With sacral pressure sores, one must be careful to prevent fecal contamination of the dressings and wound [9]. Granulation tissue will grow inward from the boundaries of the cavity. Once it has reached the level of the skin, and epithelialization has begun, skin grafts may be placed if the area is large [5, 9]. Surgical excision is the most common procedure for treatment of tissue necrosis due to pressure. However, biological debridement may be employed when sharp debridement cannot be performed. This involves application of digestive enzyme preparations.

MOUTH CARE AND DENTAL HYGIENE

Healthy teeth and gums require thorough cleaning at regular intervals. Effective cleaning of the teeth can be accomplished only by using a toothbrush and dental floss. Unfortunately even nurses who are conscientious about proper brushing and flossing of their own teeth often fail to apply these principles of dental hygiene to the patients in their care. Since the end result of neglected or improper mouth care will not often become apparent to the nurse or the patient during the course of hospitalization, this component of personal care is frequently assigned a low priority.

Problems

When the mouth has been neglected, plaque, which is a film of mucus and bacteria, builds up on the teeth, and debris from food collects around the teeth and in the gingival crevice. If this material is not removed, local inflammation and swelling of the gums will occur, with recession and pocket formation. The inflammatory process can extend so that the entire gingiva and alveolar bone are involved. Patients who are unconscious or have difficulty swallowing are also susceptible to infection of the parotid gland due to blockage of the duct. This can be prevented by promoting cleanliness of the mouth, stimulation of the flow of saliva, and adequate hydration [11]. Weak and debilitated patients may develop a monilial infection of the mouth and throat, if this area is not kept scrupulously clean. Such an infection can be extremely painful and will interfere with nutrition, hydration, and speech.

Keeping the patient's mouth clean and moist requires planning, time, and continued effort. The patient may have a long history of poor oral hygiene, improper nutrition, and lack of regular dental care. The teeth may be in a state of disrepair. The edentulous patient may have ill-fitting or improperly cared for dentures. Deterioration of the gums, mucous membranes, and teeth can progress quite rapidly without a good program of care regardless of the original state of the mouth and teeth. Before an oral hygiene routine is established, the patient's mouth should be inspected to ascertain the condition of the oral tissues. Care should be directed toward preventing complications, promoting comfort, teaching the patient about the importance of regular dental care, proper oral hygiene, and good nutrition, and assisting him with referral for continued supervision of his dental care needs and denture care.

Care

It cannot be emphasized enough that the patient's teeth *must be brushed.* Glycerine and lemon swabs, sponges, and applicators simply will not remove plaque and will not prevent gingivitis [11]. Unfortunately some health care facilities do not provide toothbrushes, thus thwarting the best care plan of the most well-intentioned nurse. Most hospitals, however, do have a patient care coordinator, procedure committees, and/or a supervisor who is responsible for provision of patient care equipment. The nurse should make an effort to establish policy and procedure and provide proper equipment to foster good mouth care. A soft nylon brush with tufts of equal length should be used. An electric toothbrush is highly recommended. If the patient has an electric toothbrush or a waterpick, the family should be encouraged to bring the appliance, since this will facilitate mouth care.

During the acute stage of stroke, the patient may be unable to brush his own teeth or even to assist the nurse because of coma, confusion, or paralysis. He should be positioned on his side to prevent aspiration, and suction should be readily available at the bedside. A bulb syringe can be used to rinse the mouth, and suction applied to clear the mouth of fluid when the patient is unable to expectorate. The toothbrush should be placed at the margin of the gingiva at a 45-degree angle and vibrated horizontally about ten times; then the front and back surfaces of the teeth brushed by drawing the toothbrush up from the gums over the crowns in a series of upward strokes. An electric toothbrush is most effective in providing mouth care for the unconscious patient. Dental floss can be used to clean the areas between the teeth. A lubricant should be applied to the lips to prevent dryness and cracking.

Mouth care, including brushing, should be provided at least four times a day and more frequently for the patient who is intubated or receiving tube feedings. (Special mouth care needs for these patients are discussed in Chapters 7 and 9). For the patient with facial paralysis, it is important that mouth care be provided after meals and at bedtime, as a pocket of food usually remains in the paralyzed side of the mouth. As the patient learns to brush his own teeth, he should be instructed to check for this after all meals.

If the unconscious or severely debilitated patient's oral hygiene is neglected for a period of time, debris will collect in the mouth and crusts form over the tissues. The most effective way of removing this material is to put on gloves, apply a 3% solution of hydrogen peroxide to the entire area with moistened gauze sponges, and then rinse the foam and debris away. The tongue must not be neglected. As the crusts become softened, they can be removed. The nurse must be very gentle in doing this so as not to injure the delicate mucosa, which has already been irritated by lack of attention. This procedure can be followed by application of a solution of milk of magnesia to the tongue and oral mucosa.

The brushing action is more important than the type of dentifrice used, although the flavor of most commercial preparations is refreshing. If the patient wears dentures, they should be removed, brushed, and replaced regularly, after the mouth is cleansed. When dentures are not worn for a period of time, the facial contour will change, and dentures will require adjustment to fit properly. Proper fit is essential for mastication of food and prevention of irritation and tissue breakdown. A clean, moist mouth is beneficial to the patient's comfort and self-esteem. It also contributes to his enjoyment of food and fluids and helps to prevent inflammation, infection, and loss of teeth. Suggestions for helping the hemiplegic patient learn self-care techniques are discussed in Chapter 13.

EYE CARE

Eye care is particularly important for the comatose patient or the patient with facial paralysis that prevents complete closure of the lid. If corneal reflexes are absent or the eye is partly open, the cornea may become scratched on a pillow, injured by dust particles, or excessively dry due to diminished secretions. To prevent corneal ulceration, keratitis, and even blindness, drops should be used to lubricate the eye and protect the cornea from lint, dirt, and drying. Methylcellulose ophthalmic solution is most frequently prescribed.

Eyes should be inspected daily for irritations and inflammation. If the eyelids do not close completely, eye pads may be used for protection, but cautiously. The pad should be elevated away from the eye so that it does not touch the cornea, for the eyelid cannot be guaranteed to stay closed under the patch. If the eyelid opens, the cornea may be damaged. In some cases the lids are sutured closed temporarily to afford adequate corneal protection.

REFERENCES

1. Beland, I. L., and Passos, J. Y. *Clinical Nursing: Pathophysiological and Psychosocial Approaches* (3rd ed.). New York: Macmillan, 1975. Pp. 108–112; 889–890.
2. Bergersen, B. *Pharmacology in Nursing* (13th ed.). St. Louis: Mosby, 1976. Pp. 511–523; 637–641.
3. Beyers, M., and Dudas, S. *The Clinical Practice of Medical-Surgical Nursing.* Boston: Little, Brown, 1977. Pp. 5–148.
4. Cosman, B. Physiology of the Skin. In J. A. Downey and R. C. Darling (Eds.), *Physiological Basis of Rehabilitation Medicine.* Philadelphia: Saunders, 1971. Pp. 317–349.
5. Elson, R. *Practical Management of Spinal Injuries for Nurses.* Baltimore: Williams & Wilkins, 1965. Pp. 69–91.
6. Falconer, M. *The Drug, the Nurse, the Patient* (5th ed.). Philadelphia: Saunders, 1974. Pp. 376–397.
7. Fowkes, W., and Hunn, V. *Clinical Assessment for the Nurse Practitioner.* St. Louis: Mosby, 1973. Pp. 35–36.
8. Gruis, M., and Innes, B. Assessment: Essential to prevent pressure sores. *Am. J. Nurs.* 76: pp. 1762–1764, 1976.
9. Guttman, L. *Spinal Cord Injuries. Comprehensive Management and Research* (2nd ed.). Oxford, Engl.: Blackwell, 1976. Pp. 512–542.
10. Miller, M., and Sachs, M. L. *About Bedsores: What You Need to Know to Help Prevent and Treat Them.* Philadelphia: Lippincott, 1974.
11. Reitz, M., and Pope, W. Mouth care. *Am. J. Nurs.* 73:10, 1973.
12. Snell, R. S. *Clinical Anatomy for Medical Students.* Boston: Little, Brown, 1973. Pp. 5–8; 34–35.
13. Stryker, R. *Rehabilitation Aspects of Acute and Chronic Nursing Care.* Philadelphia: Saunders, 1972. Pp. 127–145.
14. Talbot, H. S. Adjunctive care of spinal cord injury. *Surg. Clin. North Am.* 48: pp. 1–21, 1968.

12. Care of the patient with impaired neuromuscular function

The stroke patient may be devastated when he becomes aware that his neuromuscular functioning is impaired. The nurse must help the patient to understand why the impairment occurred and what modalities of treatment will be used to help it. The nurse should not give the patient false hope about his recovery, since it is impossible to predict whether or not function can ever be fully restored. However, it is important to maintain a positive attitude and encourage the patient to participate as actively as possible in the exercise program that has been scheduled for him. If the patient has aphasia as well as paralysis, the nurse should be sensitive to his inability to express his questions, fears, and lack of knowledge about his condition. Even though the patient cannot give any outward sign that he understands what is said, the nurse should explain simply and clearly what she (or he) is doing and why she is doing it when positioning the patient and performing range of motion exercises.

ASSESSMENT OF NEUROMUSCULAR FUNCTION

The neuromuscular status of the patient with stroke must be assessed early, so that an appropriate program of exercise and positioning can be established promptly. The functioning of all four extremities should be evaluated for restrictions in either passive or active range of motion, abnormalities of muscle tone, and incoordination.

RANGE OF MOTION

Any restriction in passive or active range of motion indicates a need for institution of an exercise program and careful positioning of the affected limbs. The muscular, skeletal, and nervous systems are all involved in movement and exercise. The cardiovascular and respiratory systems are affected by exercise and have a direct influence on its performance. Bed rest, required during the initial stage of stroke because of the patient's neurological condition, will have a deleterious effect on his neuromuscular state, which may already be impaired by his upper motor neuron lesion. Skeletal muscles are usually the first body system affected by bed rest, with muscle atrophy beginning almost immediately. Muller found that muscle strength could decrease by about five percent each day that a muscle was immobilized. If muscle contractions are not maintained by a regular exercise program, disuse atrophy of the muscles will eventually result. Two changes will occur with immobilization of a joint — (1) shortening and eventual fibrosis of the muscles that are maintained in a flexed position, and (2) loss of lubrication between the moving parts. When these changes occur, therapy to restore mobility will be painful and difficult.

MUSCLE TONE

Muscle tone is assessed to detect spasticity or flaccidity. *Spasticity* is characterized by a sudden, sustained, involuntary muscle contraction. A spastic limb has a greater possibility of contracture that could become permanent. The patient with spasticity, therefore, should be given frequent range of motion exercises. *Flaccidity* is characterized by a toneless and flail muscle with decreased or absent resting muscle tone. Flaccid extremities require particular support. To prevent subluxation of the humeral head out of the glenoid cavity, a flaccid arm should be supported on pillows when the patient is in bed and supported with an arm sling when the patient is transferring or ambulating. In many cases a spastic arm will not need an arm sling, because the muscle tone will support the shoulder joint in place. The spastic arm, like the flaccid arm, should be supported on pillows and abducted when the patient is in bed or sitting in a chair.

COORDINATION

Coordination of the extremities should be assessed, so that the nurse will be aware of any lack of control that might lead to injuries during transfers or self-care activities. Incoordination frequently prevents or limits independent bathing, feeding, and dressing.

TERMINOLOGY

The terms *rotation, flexion, extension, abduction,* and *adduction* are used to describe the position of an extremity or the range of joint movement. The nurse must clearly understand the meaning of each of these terms before attempting to assess the patient's neuromuscular status or initiate exercises. For illustrative purposes, consider the joint as the center of a circle and the extremity as the radius of that circle. *Rotation* refers to a turning about a center or axis. Theoretically, full rotation of the joint would involve turning the limb through a complete 360-degree revolution. *Flexion* refers to a bending of the joint to form an acute angle. This involves contraction of the muscles, bringing the portions of the extremity on either side of the joint into closer proximity. To visualize this, consider the elbow as the center of the circle and the arm as its diameter. With flexion of the elbow the two radii of the circle converge to form an increasingly more acute angle. *Extension* refers to the stretching, lengthening, or straightening of a flexed or bent joint. With extension, one radius of the circle will be brought from an acute angle back to the 180-degree position, or a straight line along the diameter of the circle. When the elbow is in full extension, the arm is in a straight line from shoulder to wrist. In *neutral position* an extremity is in its normal resting position. With *abduction* the extremity is drawn away from its normal resting position. For example the hip is abducted when the extended leg is drawn away from the center of the body. With *adduction* the limb is returned to or brought closer to the neutral position or center of the body.

POSITIONING

In the initial stage of stroke the affected extremities may be flaccid and without tone, but it is unusual for them to remain in this state. The rate and degree of

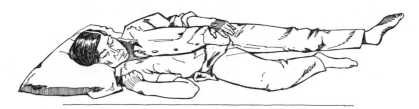

Figure 12-1
Characteristic position assumed by the hemiplegic patient.

recovery of muscle tone will vary for each patient. Following the initial flaccid phase, some degree of spasticity will be observed in the paralyzed extremities. Most patients will assume the characteristic hemiparetic posture: adduction and internal rotation of the affected shoulder, with flexion of the elbow, wrist, and fingers. The involved leg assumes a position of external rotation, with the knee slightly flexed and the foot in plantar flexion and inversion. It is important to note that for many patients in the early phase of stroke, initially the affected limbs will be flaccid (Fig. 12-1).

Careful attention to positioning is essential for stroke patients who are unable to move all their joints actively. Restricted range of motion and contracture deformities will limit progress in rehabilitation and can prevent the patient from gaining independence with activities of daily living in one or more areas. The body must be kept in proper alignment, since deformities will occur whenever normal joint range is restricted. The objectives of positioning are to (1) maintain full passive range of motion, (2) prevent contractures, (3) prevent pressure necrosis, and (4) improve circulation.

Problems of positioning

The following problems frequently affect patients with stroke. The deformities they cause are preventable with elimination of the contributing factors, proper attention to positioning, and an exercise program.

1. *Flexion of the neck* can be caused by keeping too many pillows under the patient's head while he is in bed, failing to support his head while he is in a sitting position, and neglecting the head and neck in the range of motion exercise program. Forgetfulness of this area, which often happens, leads to a flexion contracture which can be exquisitely painful and difficult to treat. This position restricts the patient's interaction with others and his awareness of his surroundings. It poses a significant problem in the case of the depressed patient.
2. *Hyperextension of the neck* can result from improper positioning and failure to provide necessary support for the head. When the patient is unconscious for a long time and requires intubation or a tracheostomy, the neck may be maintained in hyperextension to guarantee patency of the airway.

3. *Flexion of the trunk* may be due to poor mattress support and use of a pillow behind the patient's back when he is sitting in a chair.
4. *Restricted shoulder range* or *frozen shoulder* will be seen when the arm is left close to the patient's body at all times or under his body when he is placed on his side.
5. *Subluxed shoulder* can occur if the shoulder joint of a flaccid arm is not supported with pillows when immobile or with an arm sling during transferring or ambulation.
6. *Flexion contracture of the elbow* can occur when an arm is left in adduction and placed across the chest.
7. *Wrist flexion* or *wrist drop* will result if proper support is not provided to maintain the wrist and hand in normal alignment.
8. *Flexion contractures of the fingers* will occur if the fingers are not supported in slight extension by handrolls or splints.
9. *Flexion contractures of the hip* may be caused by allowing the patient to remain in a sitting position for prolonged periods or maintaining flexion of the hip to keep the patient on his side while in bed. A sagging mattress can also contribute to this condition.
10. *Abduction and external rotation of the hip* are seen when the hips are not supported by trochanter rolls while the patient is lying supine in bed.
11. *Adduction of the hips* is due to failure to align the legs properly and support the position with pillows placed between the legs. This occurs most often when there is spasticity of the leg muscles.
12. *Flexion contracture of the knee* will occur with inappropriate use of pillows under the knee or elevation of the knees by means of the foot gatch of the bed.
13. *Plantar flexion of the ankle* or footdrop may result when neutral alignment of the foot is not maintained with footboards or sandbags. With hemiplegia the affected ankle will assume the footdrop position. Every effort must be made to position and support the ankle, since this deformity precludes normal ambulation.

Figures 12-2 through 12-6 illustrate the positioning that should be used to prevent contracture deformities in the patient with hemiplegia.

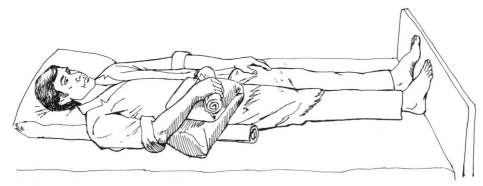

Figure 12-2
Proper supine position.

SUPINE

Figure 12-2 shows the proper positioning for the patient while lying *supine.* The head is in a neutral position or placed so that the neck is slightly extended. A small pillow supports the head and shoulders. The weight of the head will encourage flexion of the neck. Therefore, attention must be given to preventing the head and neck from remaining in flexion, since contractures will form quite readily. Often the head is forced into flexion by the use of too many pillows. The trunk should be supported by a firm mattress, using a bed board if necessary, to maintain the normal curvature of the spine. The supine position is not recommended for comatose patients because it does not allow for drainage of saliva and secretions.

ARM

Figures 12-2 and 12-3 show the proper positions of the paralyzed arm while the patient is supine. The paralyzed limb should be placed alternately in the three positions illustrated, being repositioned each time the patient is turned. In the first position (Fig. 12-2) the affected arm is abducted, in partial external rotation, with the elbow in slight flexion and the wrist extended. The fingers are slightly flexed, with the thumb placed in opposition to the fingers. A firm roll or splint should be used to position the hand, and the arm should be supported by pillows. The second position is shown in Figure 12-3A. Here the arm is abducted and placed in external rotation, with the upper arm at shoulder level. The elbow is flexed, and the palm of the hand is facing upward. The hand is supported on a pillow placed above the shoulder. The wrist is extended, and a hand roll or splint is used to support the

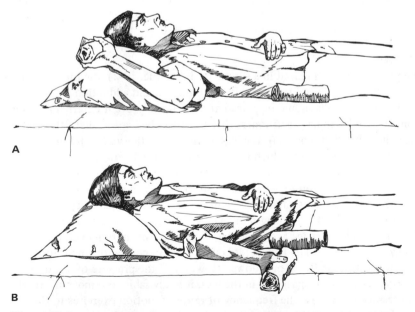

A

B

Figure 12-3
Proper placement of the paralyzed arm. A. Affected arm abducted and in external rotation. B. Affected arm abducted and in internal rotation.

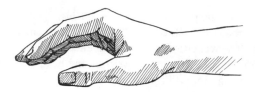

Figure 12-4
Functional position of the hand.

fingers and thumb. The third position for the paralyzed arm is shown in Figure 12-3B. The affected arm is abducted partially and extended at the patient's side. The elbow is extended, the forearm supinated, and the wrist extended. A hand roll or splint is in place to maintain the functional position of the hand.

HAND
The functional position of the hand and fingers is illustrated in Figure 12-4. The wrist should be hyperextended slightly, with the fingers in extension about 15 degrees and the thumb in opposition to the fingers. This position can be achieved by placing a hand roll in the patient's hand with the fingers curved around the roll and the thumb placed opposite to the index finger, and it can be maintained by applying a hand splint constructed to fit the patient. Care must be taken to trim the fingernails regularly to prevent abrasion of the skin and to remove the splint or hand roll for skin care at frequent intervals. Usually the splint is kept in place for two hours, then removed for two hours, alternating throughout the day.

HIPS AND KNEES
When the patient has been placed in a supine position (Fig. 12-2), the hips and knees should be extended in neutral rotation. Both abduction and adduction are to be avoided. Trochanter rolls should be placed at each hip to prevent external rotation. It is recommended by some practitioners that the knees be kept in slight flexion, since it is believed that extension of the legs increases spasticity. Stretching of or pressure on the peroneal nerve, which is exposed under the lateral aspect of the knee, can predispose to footdrop, and pressure on the popliteal area is known to predispose to thrombophlebitis. Therefore, we suggest caution in placing pillows or rolls under the knees. However, it seems advisable as a measure to reduce spasticity to place a pillow lengthwise under the full length of the leg, taking great care to prevent undue pressure on the popliteal space and providing extra range of motion exercises to the limb to prevent footdrop. The feet can be maintained in neutral or slight dorsiflexion by using a footboard, sandbags, or pillows. However, if the pressure of a footboard or sandbag causes extensor spasticity in the legs, it is advisable to remove it. It will then be necessary to increase the frequency of range of motion exercises to the ankle in order to prevent tightening of the heel cords that may lead to a permanent deformity and prevent normal ambulation. The bedclothes should be draped over the footboard rather than tucked tightly over the patient's feet, since even the weight

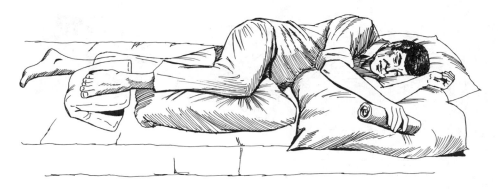

Figure 12-5
Side-lying position.

of a single sheet can encourage the development of plantar flexion of the ankles. If a footboard is not used, pillows can be placed to support the bedclothes. A posterior splint may also be used to maintain proper position of the ankle. For some patients, a high-laced sneaker may be used for this purpose. In either case, the foot should be inspected regularly and skin care provided to prevent pressure and skin breakdown.

SIDE-LYING

Figure 12-5 shows the proper side-lying position for the patient with hemiplegia. Unless the condition of the patient's lungs or skin necessitates rotating him from side to side, it is suggested that the patient with hemiplegia not be placed on his affected side because of the tendency of the venous blood to pool due to a lack of muscle action. If, for medical reasons, it is necessary to place the patient on the affected side, he should not remain on that side for more than an hour at a time. The patient's head should be maintained in a neutral position, supported by a small pillow. To maintain normal curvature of the spine, after turning the patient on his side the nurse should pull the patient's hips and shoulders far enough back toward her to allow the weight of the patient's body to maintain his side-lying position. The uppermost arm is placed in forward flexion with the elbows lightly flexed. This arm should be supported with pillows, and the wrist should be extended with a hand roll in place. The opposite arm should be flexed and supinated, with the wrist supported on the mattress or pillow. The patient's weight should not rest on this arm. The upper leg should be flexed and placed on pillows in front of the bottom leg. It should not be allowed to rest on the bottom leg. The bottom leg should be extended so it will rest on the mattress behind the top leg. The feet should both be placed in neutral or slight dorsiflexion of the ankle. Sandbags or other supports may be placed to prevent footdrop of both feet.

PRONE

Figure 12-6 shows the proper prone position. Because of potential respiratory embarrassment the patient should not be placed in this position until the responsible

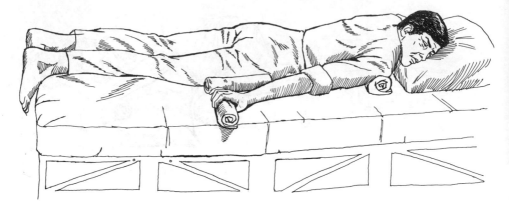

Figure 12-6
Prone position.

physician has been consulted, and never when an artificial airway is in place. The neck should be slightly extended and the head placed in lateral rotation. The nurse should make certain that the patient's face is not buried in the pillow or mattress and that there is no respiratory embarrassment. The trunk should be extended. A small pillow may be placed under the patient's abdomen. Small pillows can be placed under each shoulder for support. The lower body should be positioned to allow the feet to hang over the edge of the mattress in neutral position at right angles to the legs to prevent footdrop. The hips and the knees should be extended in neutral rotation to prevent abduction and external rotation. Trochanter rolls should be placed at each hip. Pillows may be positioned between the legs to prevent adduction. The unaffected arm can be placed in any comfortable position. However, the affected arm should be placed alternately — with each turning — in the two following positions. First, the affected arm is internally rotated and abducted, with the elbow extended, the wrist extended, and a hand roll or splint in place. Second, the shoulder of the affected arm is externally rotated, with the arm extended away from the body, the elbow placed in flexion with the wrist extended, and a hand roll or splint in place.

SITTING
To maintain a proper sitting position, the patient's head should be kept in a neutral position. If the patient has poor control of his head, a headrest is required. A small pillow can be used, but with extreme care to prevent the shoulders from falling forward. Pillows should not be placed behind the shoulders or lower back, since this will encourage flexion contractures. The lower back should be positioned against the back of the chair. The involved shoulder should be abducted and in slight external rotation, the elbow flexed, and the arm supported. Armrests are usually not wide enough to keep the affected arm in the proper position: the flaccid arm frequently slides off the rest and remains dangling at the side of the chair. The patient may be unaware of the position of his arm, and, if sensation is impaired, he

may be injured without realizing it. A table or lapboard is preferable, therefore, since it provides a broader base of support than the armrests of the chair and will allow for greater abduction and elevation, but it must be the proper height. A sling can also be used to support the arm. The wrist should be extended and supported, and a hand roll should be placed in the palm of the hand, or a splint worn. The fingers should be in slight flexion. The hips and knees should be at approximately right angles with the feet, which are placed flat on the floor. If the feet do not touch the floor, a footstool may be used to maintain the position of the legs. Pillows placed between the patient's legs will help to prevent tight adduction of the hips.

RANGE OF MOTION EXERCISES

Range of motion (ROM) exercises should be instituted in the acute phase, when the patient is unable to move his extremities actively. Normal range varies from joint to joint, depending on anatomical structure, and ordinarily is maintained by the motion of daily activities. With a weak or paralyzed limb the patient may lose normal joint range due to immobility. This may result in deformities caused by fibrotic changes in muscles, joint capsules, and connective tissues. Prevention of contractures requires constant vigilance on the part of the nursing staff, but it is much easier than treatment of contractures, which involves prolonged mechanical stretching and may necessitate surgical intervention, and is certainly much less painful for the patient.

Before starting the exercise program, the patient should be placed in a comfortable and relaxed position. If he is conscious, the purpose of the exercises should be explained to him, the program outlined, and the goals explained. He must understand that if he experiences pain due to tightness or spasticity, the nurse will terminate the exercises. During the exercises the nurse should talk to the patient and let him know of any progress that is made. He should be reassured, if progress is not seen, that restoration of function is a slow process and that even a slight return of function is a positive outcome. It is important to recognize that the patient will not usually be aware of slight improvements of function that the nurse and other members of the health team will recognize. The patient needs continued encouragement. Often this can be conveyed nonverbally by the nurse's supportive attitude.

Range of motion is the extent of movement of a given joint. It can be achieved in any of the following ways.

1. *Passive.* Passive ROM exercises are performed by the nurse with the patient not actively involved and even unconscious. The joint is firmly supported and brought through the normal range of motion passively by an outside force such as a nurse or therapist.
2. *Active.* Active ROM exercises are performed by the patient under the direction of the nurse or therapist. The patient independently brings his joint through the normal range of motion by the action of muscles or groups of muscles.

3. *Active-Assistive.* The joint is brought through the normal range of motion assisted either by the nurse, the therapist, or by the patient himself, who uses his normal extremities to assist the movement of the weaker ones or helps himself with a device such as an overhead pulley.

The purposes of range of motion exercises are as follows.

1. To prevent the tightening of ligaments and muscles that may cause contractures. Contractures are painful and unattractive and limit performance in activities of daily living, such as dressing, bathing, and feeding.
2. To improve circulation. Range of motion prevents or reduces edema by enhancing venous flow.
3. To assist in rehabilitation. If joints are kept "free" or "loose" during the acute stage of illness, motion can be performed as soon as recovery begins.

The following principles should be observed in carrying out a range of motion exercise program.

1. Never go beyond the point of pain. However, if there is tightness in the musculature, there will be discomfort associated with joint movement. Hot packs to the involved joint prior to initiation of the exercise will help to promote some degree of muscle relaxation, thus decreasing the discomfort and allowing an increased range of movement. If this measure does not permit the extremity to pass through its normal range without significant discomfort, the physician should be contacted. If medication has been prescribed for pain, the nurse should see that he receives adequate analgesia to allow maximum range of motion.
2. Carry out all motions slowly and smoothly.
3. Be sure there is a complete stop at the beginning and end of each motion.
4. Encourage the patient to perform any motion that he can do for himself.
5. Exercise both paralyzed and normal sides.
6. It is necessary to move a joint approximately four times a day to prevent contractures.
7. If spasticity or rigidity is present, range of motion exercises should be carried out more often than four times a day.

Passive range of motion exercises

Figures 12-7 through 12-15 show how the nurse should conduct range of motion exercises. As illustrated, the patient is placed in the supine position and the exercises usually start with the head, progressing to the upper extremities and on to the lower extremities. The sequence can be varied if necessary, so long as every joint is taken through its full range of motion at least four times a day.

NECK

Figures 12-7A–C show the nurse exercising the patient's neck muscles. This area is forgotten quite frequently. It is not uncommon to find a stroke patient who has had

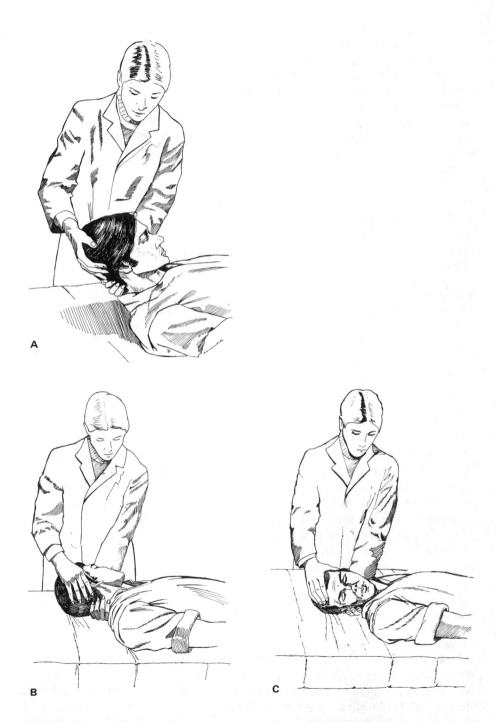

Figure 12-7
Neck exercises. A. Neck flexion and extension. B & C. Lateral neck rotation.

careful attention to his paralyzed limbs but has a severe contracture of the neck.
Many factors, including hemianopsia and perceptual disorders, can contribute to this.
The patient who lacks awareness of one side of his body may not turn his head to
that side. The patient with visual field defects may also favor one side in order to
accommodate his limited field of vision. A patient who has had an airway or an
endotracheal, or tracheostomy tube in place for some time may have had head and
neck movement restricted to safeguard the airway and will find it painful to move
his neck. The depressed and withdrawn patient will often sit with his head hanging
down.

As shown in Figure 12-7A, the nurse should remove the pillow from under the
patient's head, place her two hands on either side of the patient's head, lift his head
off the bed, touch his chin to his chest, gently return his head to the neutral position, then extend the neck and return the head to the neutral position again. The
nurse then gently rotates the head in neutral position, first to one side, then to the
other (Fig. 12-7B and C).

SHOULDER

To flex and *extend* the shoulder, the patient's arm is positioned so that it lies close
to his side. The nurse then supports the elbow and wrist to keep these two joints
extended and gently raises the patient's arm over his head as shown in Figure 12-8A.
When there is no limitation in the shoulder joint, the arm can be brought to rest on
the mattress in straight flexion of the shoulder. This can be facilitated by holding
the arm so that the patient's palm is facing the center of his body. The arm is then
gently lowered to its original position at the side of the body.

Abduction and *adduction* of the shoulder are performed in the following manner.
With the patient's arm lying at his side, the nurse cradles his elbow and forearm,
places her other hand on his shoulder to prevent it from hiking up, and then gently
abducts the shoulder by drawing the arm out to form a right angle with the body,
as shown in Figure 12-8B. She adducts the shoulder by guiding the arm back to its
original position at the patient's side. To *rotate* the shoulder, the nurse first abducts
it so that the arm is at shoulder level. She then supports the patient's wrist and
elbow, flexes his elbow, and rotates the shoulder externally by bringing the forearm
back toward his head. When there is no joint resistance, the forearm can be rested
on the mattress at a right angle to the upper arm (Fig. 12-8C). To perform internal
rotation of the shoulder, the nurse then brings the forearm back toward the patient's
feet, as shown in Figure 12-8D, so that it again is placed at a right angle to the upper
arm in the opposite direction.

ELBOW

Before exercising the *elbow*, the patient's arm is placed along the side of his body
with the palm facing up. The nurse supports the patient's elbow and wrist and
gently flexes the elbow as shown in Figure 12-9A, by drawing the forearm up toward
the patient's head while the upper arm remains flat on the surface of the bed. She
extends the elbow by returning the forearm to its original position (Fig. 12-9B). To
supinate the patient's forearm, the nurse grasps the patient's hand as in a handshake

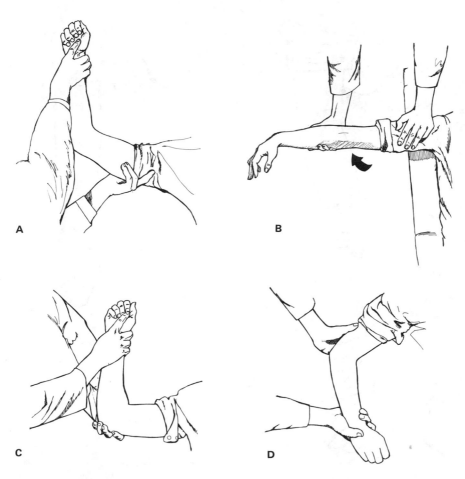

Figure 12-8
Shoulder exercises. A. Flexion and extension of the shoulder. B. Abduction and adduction of the shoulder. C. External rotation of the shoulder. D. Internal rotation of the shoulder.

and supports his elbow with her other hand. She then rolls the forearm so that the patient's palm is facing upward (Fig. 12-9C). To pronate the forearm, she rolls it back so that the palm is facing down (Fig. 12-9D).

WRIST
Range of motion exercises for the *wrist* are illustrated in Figures 12-10A–C. The nurse supports the patient's wrist with her hands and gently draws the hand downward from the wrist to flex it (Fig. 12-10A), then upward and back toward the wrist to extend it (Fig. 12-10B). The wrist is then placed in a neutral position, so that the hand is in a straight line with the forearm. The nurse supports the patient's hand on hers (Fig. 12-10C) and draws it toward its outer aspect. This is referred to as *ulnar*

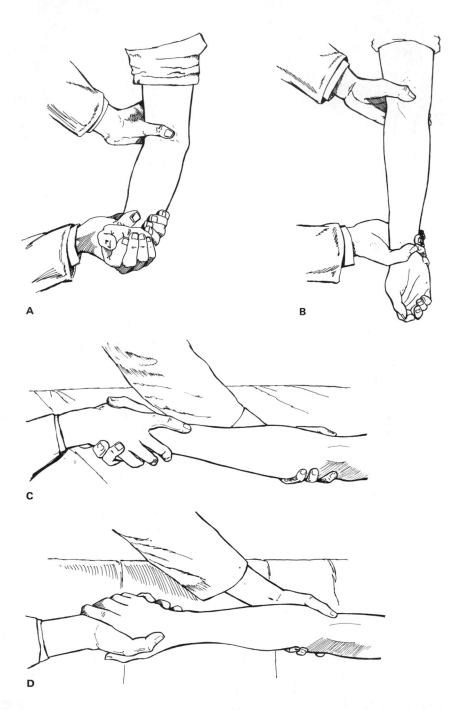

Figure 12-9
Elbow exercises. A. Elbow flexion. B. Elbow extension. C. Forearm supination.
D. Forearm pronation.

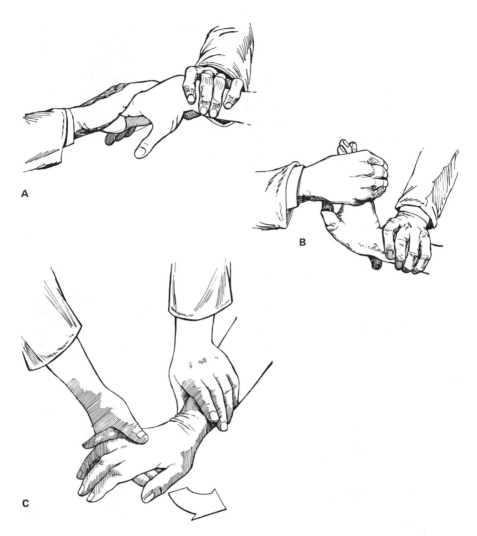

Figure 12-10
Wrist exercises. A. Wrist flexion. B. Wrist extension. C. Ulnar and radial deviation.

deviation. She then draws the hand in toward its inner aspect or thumb side in *radial deviation.*

THUMB AND FINGERS

Exercising the thumb and fingers is time-consuming but extremely important. The ability to grasp objects varying in size from a large carton to a needle, and to carry out many fine, coordinated activities upon which self-sufficiency and means of livelihood depend, is determined by the ability to flex and extend the fingers and bring them into opposition with the thumb. When this is lost, the function of the hand is lost, and with it independence for many activities of daily living. Although the extent of brain damage resulting from stroke may preclude the possibility of complete restoration of function of the hand, every effort must be made to prevent the formation of flexion contractures and to maintain the hand in a functional position. If this is done, even if the patient does not fully regain voluntary control of the hand, he can be taught to use the paralyzed hand to assist the unaffected hand in some self-care activities; whereas contractures can render the paralyzed hand totally useless.

Figures 12-11A—C illustrate range of motion of the fingers and 12-12A and B illustrate range of motion of the thumb. The nurse supports the patient's wrist and hand with her hand. With her opposite hand she flexes all the fingers by closing the

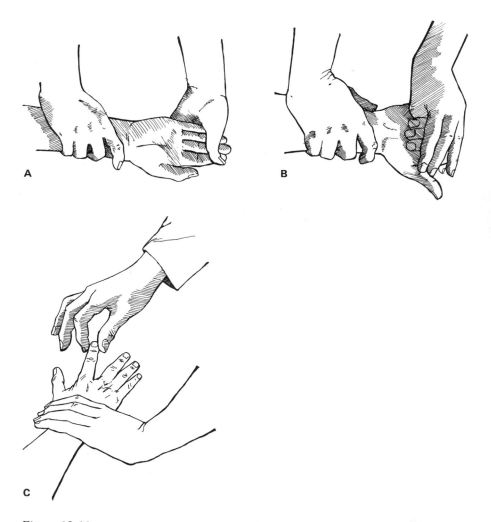

Figure 12-11
Finger exercises. A. Finger extension. B. Finger flexion. C. Abduction and adduction of the fingers.

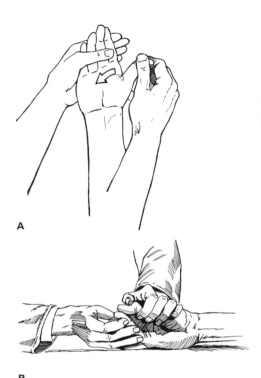

A

B

Figure 12-12
Thumb exercises. A. Extension of the thumb. B. Thumb opposition.

hand (Fig. 12-11A), then extends the finger joints by straightening all the fingers (Fig. 12-11B). To abduct and adduct the fingers, the nurse positions the patient's hand on a flat surface with the palm down so that all the fingers are straight, then spreads the fingers apart. Each finger is moved sideways away from the adjacent finger and then back toward it, as shown in Figure 12-11C. To exercise the thumb, the nurse supports the patient's hand in hers, grasps the patient's thumb between her thumb and index finger with her opposite hand, and extends it away from the patient's hand (Fig. 12-12A). She then flexes the patient's thumb by drawing it in toward the center of the palm. She then touches the tip of the patient's thumb to the tip of each of his fingers (*opposition*, Fig. 12-12B).

HIP AND KNEE
Figure 12-13A–D illustrates range of motion exercises for the hip and knee. To flex the hip, the nurse places one hand under the patient's knee, the other under his heel, gently raises the lower leg while flexing the patient's knee, and moves the knee toward the patient's head. This brings the thigh closer to the abdomen. Flexion of the hip and knee are shown in Figure 12-13A. To *extend* the hip and knee joints the leg is brought back down to its original position resting flat on the bed.

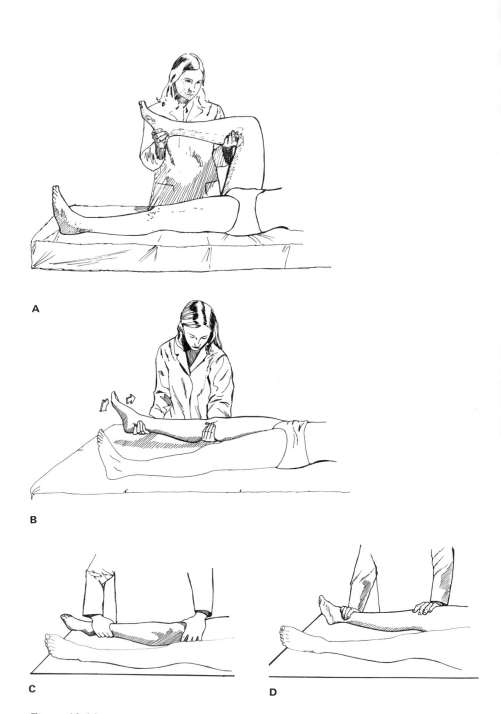

Figure 12-13
Hip and knee exercises. A. Flexion and extension of the hip and knee. B. Abduction and adduction of the hip. C. Internal rotation of the hip. D. External rotation of the hip.

As shown in Figure 12-13B, to *abduct* the hip the nurse slides one hand under the patient's knee and the other under his ankle and draws the leg away from the midline of the body, taking care to keep the leg at the level of the mattress. To *adduct* the hip, she brings the leg back in toward the midline of the body. To *rotate* the hip, the nurse places one hand over the patient's knee and the other hand over his ankle. For internal rotation (Fig. 12-13C) the patient's thigh is rolled inward, toward the center of the body. For external rotation (Fig. 12-13D) the thigh is rolled outward, away from the midline of the body.

FOOT

With hemiplegia the paralyzed foot will assume the position of plantar flexion and inversion. Unless there is a constant effort to maintain the feet at right angles to the legs and to stretch the muscles and tendons of the ankle regularly, footdrop with shortening of the Achilles tendon will occur very rapidly. This deformity makes it difficult to walk, since the patient is unable to place his foot flat on the floor or to accomplish the flexion action of the ankle involved in walking.

To exercise the foot, the nurse places one hand over the patient's ankle, supports his foot with her other hand, and brings the foot up toward the knee in dorsiflexion. She then draws the foot back downward to plantar flexion and returns the ankle to the neutral position as shown in Figure 12-14. *Inversion* of the ankle is accomplished by turning the foot inward. The foot is then returned to the midline and drawn outward in eversion of the ankle. The *toes* should not be neglected, since flexion contractures will prevent the patient from wearing shoes and walking normally. As shown in Figure 12-15A the nurse grasps the patient's toes and extends them, then curls them downward to flex them as shown in Figure 12-15B, then returns them to a neutral position.

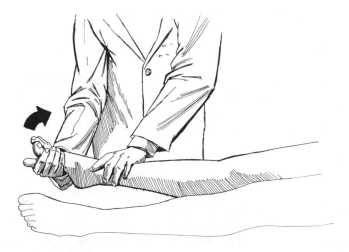

Figure 12-14
Ankle exercises. Plantar flexion and dorsiflexion.

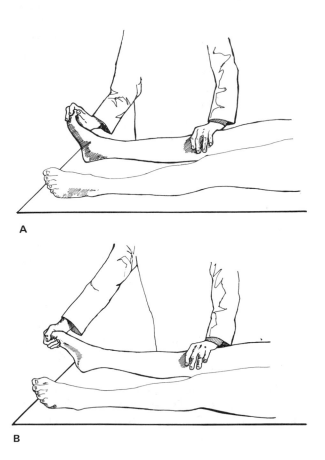

Figure 12-15
Toe exercises. A. Extension of the toes. B. Flexion of the toes.

Active range of motion exercises

Passive range of motion exercises are started by the nurse early in the course of illness to maintain suppleness of the joints and prevent contracture deformities from developing. As the patient's condition stabilizes, an active therapy program will be instituted. The physical therapist or occupational therapist will establish goals for the patient and, as his strength and control of movement increase, he may progress from passive to active range of motion exercises. It is important that the patient learn to carry out these exercises correctly, under the supervision of the therapist, since he may have to continue the exercise program at home for a long time.

In the acute stage of illness it is not always apparent how much return of function can be expected. If the prognosis for return is good, the patient's joints should be kept as supple as possible and his muscles in tone, so that he will be able to use them as soon as function returns. When the prognosis is poor, intensive efforts are necessary to prevent contractures that will be painful, unsightly, and a barrier to independent self-care activities. Patients with little or no chance of eventual return of voluntary muscle control must keep up range of motion exercises indefinitely to reduce pain and prevent disuse atrophy. Such patients often become discouraged at seeing no functional return and discontinue the exercises. It is important to encourage them to continue, in order to keep the affected extremities looking as normal as possible and in as flexible a state as possible to facilitate dressing and other self-care activities. Exercise will also improve circulation, reduce edema, decrease pain in the affected limbs, and benefit the patient's overall physical condition.

The self-ranging exercises illustrated in Figures 12-16, 12-17, and 12-18 should be carried out at least once daily. It is recommended that each exercise be repeated ten times.

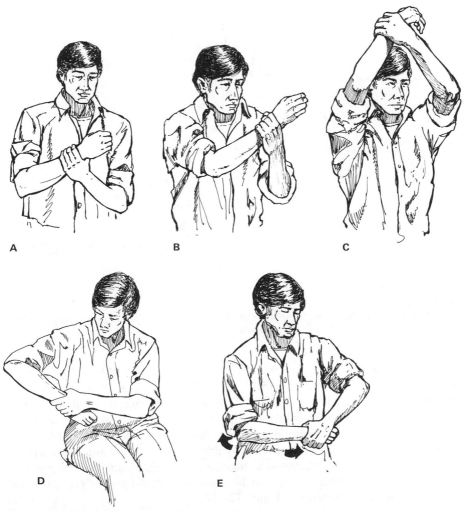

Figure 12-16
Shoulder exercises. ABC — flexion, D abduction, and E adduction.

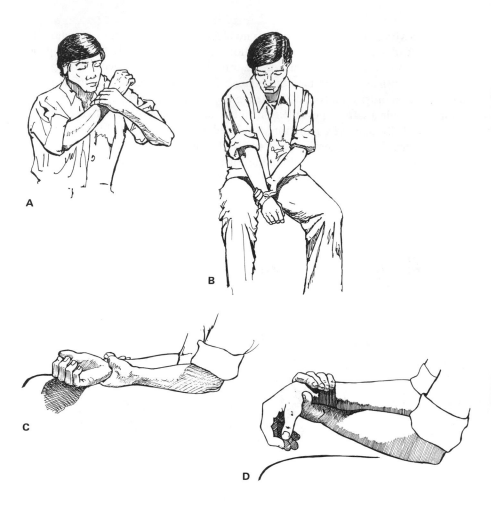

Figure 12-17
A—D. Elbow and forearm exercises — A flexion, B extension; C supination of the
forearm, and D pronation of the forearm.

To *flex the shoulder* the patient is taught to grasp the wrist of his affected arm
(Fig. 12-16A), lift the arm to shoulder height (Fig. 12-16B), and then raise the arm
straight up over his head (Fig. 12-16C). To *abduct and adduct the shoulder,* he is
instructed to place the affected arm on his lap, grasp it at the wrist, flex the affected
elbow, and move the arm from side to side as shown in Figure 12-16D and E.

Flexion of the elbow is accomplished by grasping the affected arm at the wrist
and raising it so that the affected hand touches the opposite shoulder as shown in
Figure 12-17A. The hand is then brought down between the patient's legs, thereby
extending the elbow as shown in Figure 12-17B.

Supination and *pronation* of the forearm (Figs. 12-17C and D) are best accomplished
with the patient seated. He is instructed to place his affected arm on his lap, then to

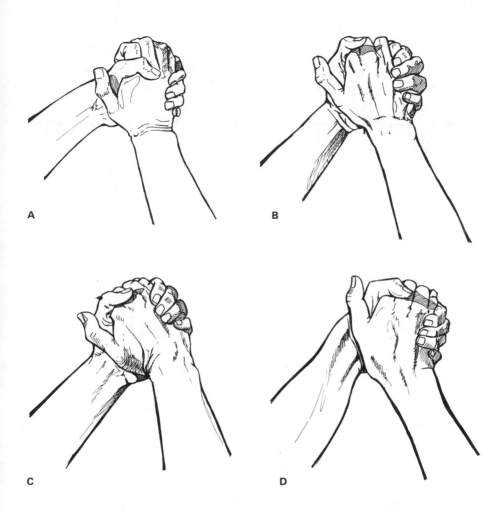

Figure 12-18
A–D. Wrist exercises – extension and flexion, radial and ulnar deviation.

grasp the forearm above the wrist and turn it so that his palm is facing up in supination, then to turn it so that the palm is facing down in pronation.

For *extension of the wrist* (Fig. 12-18A) the patient grasps his involved hand at the palm and pushes it back against the forearm. He then bends the wrist downward (Fig. 12-18B) to *flex* it, then returns it to the neutral position.

Figure 12-18C shows the patient grasping his affected hand to bring it toward the thumb side in radial deviation. Then it is drawn away from the thumb side in ulnar deviation (Fig. 12-18C).

To flex and extend the fingers, the patient should rest the affected arm on a table in front of him with the palm up. First he *flexes the fingers* by bending them into a fist with his unaffected hand (Fig. 12-19A). He then *extends the finger joints* by straightening them (Fig. 12-19B). The patient is taught to *abduct his thumb by*

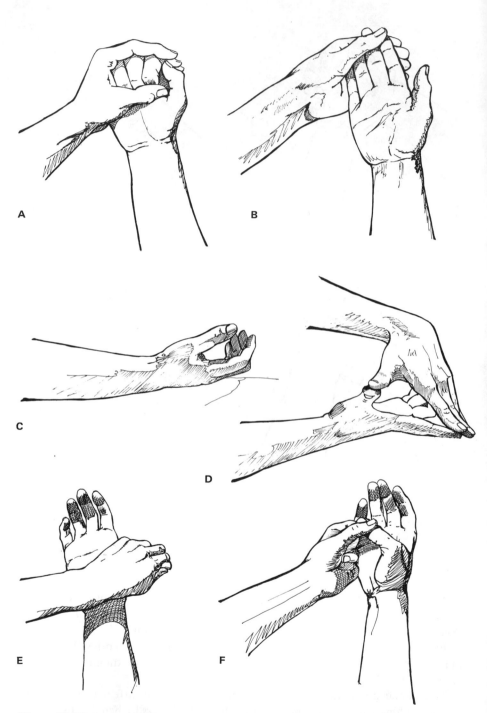

Figure 12-19
A—F. Finger exercises. A. Finger flexion. B. Finger extension. C and D. Abduction of the thumb. E and F. Opposition of the thumb.

placing his affected hand on his lap or a table (Fig. 12-19C) and placing the thumb and index finger of his unaffected hand against the thumb and index finger of the affected hand to spread the web space (Fig. 12-19D). *Thumb opposition* is exercised by grasping the thumb of the affected hand between the opposite thumb and index finger and bringing it over to touch the fifth finger of the affected hand (Figs. 12-19E and F).

Self-assisted range of motion exercises for the lower extremities are difficult to perform. Adequate range of motion of the lower extremities can usually be provided through transfers and ambulation for those patients who would be candidates for self-ranging of the legs.

REFERENCES

1. Darling, R. C. Exercise. In J. A. Downey and R. C. Darling (Eds.), *Physiological Basis of Rehabilitative Medicine.* Philadelphia: Saunders, 1971. Pp. 167–181.
2. Levenson, C. Rehabilitation of the Stroke Hemiplegia Patient. In F. Krussen et al. (Eds.), *Handbook of Physical Medicine and Rehabilitation* (2nd ed.). Philadelphia: Saunders, 1971.
3. Muller, E. A. Influence of training and inactivity on muscle strength. *Arch. Phys. Med. Rehabil.* 51:449–462, 1970.
4. Rusk, H. *Rehabilitation Medicine.* St. Louis: Mosby, 1977. Pp. 93–122; 601–620.
5. Stryker, R. *Rehabilitative Aspects of Acute and Chronic Nursing Care.* Philadelphia: Saunders, 1972. P. 163.

13. Rehabilitation and long-term care

In the preceding chapters the various deficits resulting from stroke were discussed with an emphasis on assessment, prevention of complications, treatment, and preliminary restorative efforts during the acute stage of stroke. This chapter will address the establishment of a rehabilitation program in detail. Disorders of language and perception were both dealt with completely in their respective chapters and will be referred to in this section only to emphasize their effect on the process of physical rehabilitation and long-term care.

Rusk has defined *rehabilitation* as "a program designed to enable the individual who is physically disabled, chronically ill, or convalescing to live and to work to the utmost of his capacity" (cited by Stryker, p. 13) [26]. Stryker describes rehabilitation as "a creative process that begins with immediate preventive care in the first stage of an accident or illness . . . [and is] continued through the restorative phase of care [that] involves adaptation of the whole being to a new life" [26]. Rehabilitation is not something that follows after everything else has been done for the stroke patient. Nor should it be isolated from acute and convalescent care. It must be integrated into the total care of the patient. To be most effective, a rehabilitation program must be started early in the course of illness.

Cerebrovascular disease is the third leading cause of death and disability in the United States and affects half a million Americans yearly. Approximately two million people are currently suffering with long-term disabilities resulting from stroke [9]. Some of these disabilities can be reduced or prevented by conscientious application of rehabilitation principles. In other cases a rehabilitation program can assist the patient to live a more comfortable and productive life in spite of deficits that cannot be cured or altered. The first step in developing a rehabilitation plan for the patient with stroke is a complete evaluation of his strengths and limitations. Rehabilitation planning should begin with institution of both short- and long-term goals as soon as the stroke is diagnosed. Even though it may not be possible to predict the patient's rehabilitation potential at this early stage of illness, it is imperative that the nurses caring for the patient with stroke understand techniques of preventing complications that will retard rehabilitation if the patient does have the potential for it. Complications that have a direct effect on rehabilitation, such as contractures, pressure sores, incontinence, and urinary tract infections, have been reviewed in preceding chapters.

It is important to remember that rehabilitation does not necessarily mean achievement of complete independence in all areas of activity, but rather that each individual reaches his maximum potential within his physical and mental limitations. For some this means becoming fully independent in all areas, including employment. For others it means achieving only partial independence for self-care. There are patients who will always require a wheelchair and may only be able to feed themselves with help, but this is a definite improvement over being confined completely to bed and receiving nourishment through a feeding tube. With stroke it is likely that many deficits will occur in varying combinations. No two rehabilitation programs can be the same; each must be tailored to the individual patient's abilities and disabilities. Since a patient with receptive aphasia may not be able to follow many verbal instructions, it will be necessary to use a different approach in teaching him an exercise program. When a patient has weakness or paralysis accompanied by a perceptual disorder, he will need to use a very different technique for dressing from another patient with the same physical deficit who has no perceptual impairment. A patient may perform poorly in ambulation training even when he has good functional ability, if he is fearful of spontaneous incontinence. Patients with hemianopsia will experience much more difficulty in transferring from bed to chair than patients who have no visual problems.

Because of the variety and complexity of deficits resulting from stroke, multidisciplinary involvement in the management of these patients has been the accepted approach. The Joint Commission for Stroke Facilities in its report on stroke rehabilitation states that the stroke patient's complex problems require specialized attention by persons with detailed knowledge and specific learning. The Commission described ten disciplines as components of the rehabilitation team, the primary physician, medical specialists, nurse, physical therapist, occupational therapist, social worker, dietitian, speech therapist, psychologist, and rehabilitation counselor [24]. The multidisciplinary team concept was developed to assure care for the whole patient. Unfortunately, however, fragmentation of care is often the result of this approach. The more people who are involved with care, the greater the danger there is of lack of coordination. The nurse has the most prolonged direct contact with the patient and is in a unique position to identify problems and evaluate progress in overall functioning. The primary functions of the nurse in rehabilitation should include evaluation and coordination to ensure continuity of care. Without continuity much of the effort by team members can be lost.

The nurse must know the patient's deficits and be aware of any therapy program that he is involved in, so that appropriate measures can be instituted on the patient care division to reinforce the therapeutic regimen. The patient usually is expected to practice the techniques for self-care and ambulation that he has learned in the physical medicine and rehabilitation unit when he returns to the nursing division. It avails little for the therapist to teach the patient new techniques if he is not given the opportunity to practice between therapy sessions or if he is not supervised adequately to assure that he is carrying out the newly learned techniques properly. If, for example, a patient is being taught by the occupational therapist to feed himself using special devices or to bathe himself using special techniques, then the nurse should not only be familiar with these techniques and how to apply and use the devices but should also understand the principles involved, so that she can determine that the patient is following through with what has been taught. It is important for her to know that usually she should allow the patient to struggle through his initial efforts at a newly learned activity, but that there are also times to intervene when the patient needs guidance or is completely frustrated in his attempts to carry out an activity. This type of professional judgment relies heavily on her sensitivity and knowledge of the factors influencing the patient's performance.

REHABILITATION POTENTIAL

The prognosis for functional recovery following stroke is limited by the coexistence of such chronic illnesses as hypertension, cardiac decompensation, obesity, emphysema, and diabetes mellitus [12]. The time that elapses between onset of stroke and institution of rehabilitation efforts is also important, since in most cases of long-standing, untreated disability, the results of even the most intensive therapy are poor [12].

Although it is difficult to predict just how much functional improvement can be expected for any given patient, a number of predictor items have been identified to assist in establishing rehabilitation potential. The following factors are associated with a *good prognosis* for functional recovery: (1) positive acceptance of the disability on the part of the patient, (2) presence in the home of a spouse or other family member to assist the patient, (3) good bladder control, (4) good visual-motor coordination, (5) early return of muscle tone, (6) early return of tendon jerks, (7) early return of voluntary motion, (8) good strength in muscles of hands and trunk, (9) skill in feeding, (10) strength of scapular retractors and hip abductors on the affected side, (11) strength of trunk flexors, (12) strength of forearm supinators on the unaffected side, and (13) some degree of passive wrist extension on the involved side [12]. Factors associated with a *poor prognosis* for functional recovery include: (1) a long period of time between onset of illness and entry into an active rehabilitation program, (2) lack of a spouse, other family member, or friend in the home to provide assistance, (3) excessive flaccidity or spasticity, (4) muscle contracture, especially with regard to limitation of hip abduction or ankle dorsiflexion, (5) evidence of diffuse cortical involvement, nystagmus, or history of a previous stroke, (6) severe sensory deficit including visual field defects, (7) severe motor involvement, (8) severe disturbances of visual perception, (9) presence of constructional apraxia, and (10) accompanying illnesses [12].

Patients who have failed to show any return of motor function within one to two months after onset of stroke cannot be expected to recover muscle control to any appreciable degree. Unless rehabilitation has been neglected or medical problems have caused delay or interruption of the rehabilitation program, maximum achievement of functional performance generally occurs within four to six months of start of therapy [11]. The majority of patients with stroke can be rehabilitated adequately by focusing on ambulation and self-care activities in the standard hospital setting. About fifteen to twenty-five percent may require a more extensive organized physical medicine and rehabilitation program [8]. Gordon and Kahn have reported on the value of a trained rehabilitation team in the community hospital. It is their conclusion that nurses in general hospitals should assume an active role in initiating a restorative program for hemiplegic patients [13].

RECOVERY OF MOTOR FUNCTION

Evidence indicates that motor recovery for the hemiplegic patient is a spontaneous process that occurs chiefly within the first two to three months following nonhemorrhagic stroke. There will, of course, be exceptions to this [21]. What is considered a classic study of motor recovery in hemiplegia of cerebral origin was carried out by Twitchell in 1951 [27]. His study involved patients with lesions of the cerebral hemispheres, mostly of the internal capsule or subcortical white matter. He found that recovery of motor function followed a regular sequence of reflex changes and that the process of recovery might become arrested at any stage in this sequence. Partial restoration of motor function followed the same pattern as full restoration but ended at an earlier point.

On the basis of data from the group of patients he studied, he reported the following sequence. The development of hemiplegia was followed immediately by a loss of voluntary movement and diminution of tendon reflexes in the involved extremities. At this time, resistance to passive movement was decreased on the affected side. More active tendon reflexes could be elicited in the involved limbs within 48 hours. A short time after this, a minimal increase in resistance to passive movement of the extremities was detectable. This increased resistance was first noted in the palmar flexors of the wrist and fingers and the plantar flexors of the ankle, then spread to the adductors and flexors of the arms and the adductors and extensors of the legs. During this period tendon reflexes were brisker, and clonus of the involved muscles appeared within 1—38 days following the onset of hemiplegia.

Twitchell noted that immediately after hemiplegia occurred the limbs were flaccid and would remain in whatever position they were placed or posture they assumed due to the forces of gravity. As spasticity developed, however, distinctive postural abnormalities were seen. These initially affected the foot and hand, with increased flexion of the fingers and plantar flexion and slight inversion of the ankle. As tendon reflexes became more active in the affected extremity, there usually was increased resistance to passive movement. At first this increased resistance could be demonstrated only by taking the muscle through its full range of motion, but within 5—10 days resistance to passive movement was quite obvious and affected even the resting position of the limb [27].

It is well known that recovery from hemiplegia occurs first in the proximal muscles of the extremities and is usually more complete for the proximal than for the distal muscles. Voluntary movement of the hand and foot is usually last to return; and, when it does, the movements are usually weaker, resulting in a severe loss of dexterity. Twitchell found that initial evidence of voluntary movement of the arm was observable within 6—33 days from the onset of hemiplegia. This involved a flexion of the shoulder which was very slow and had limited range and power. Elbow flexion returned within 1—6 days following this and also was slow and weak. What is most significant is that elbow flexion occurred only in association with shoulder flexion and could not be performed as a separate action. At this stage of recovery all attempts to flex the shoulder, elbow, or fingers voluntarily only resulted in a complex flexion synergy of the whole arm, that is, a simultaneous flexion of the shoulder, elbow, and fingers. Approximately 2—5 seconds elapsed between the time the patient was asked to attempt flexion and the time the movement started. The movement began slowly and became more rapid as it progressed. At the end of the movement there was a 2—3 second delay in relaxation of the flexed muscles. Some of the patients studied never progressed beyond this stage of recovery. The next stage in the recovery process was extensor synergy involving the shoulder, elbow, wrist, and fingers [27].

Return of voluntary movement of the leg began with development of flexor and extensor synergies similar to those of the arm. Willed or voluntary flexion of the hip was noted within 1–31 days following the onset of paralysis. Voluntary flexion of the knee and dorsiflexion of the ankle followed. Any attempt to flex the knee as a separate movement was seen to result in a combined flexion of knee and hip. An extensor synergy of the leg appeared next, involving extension and adduction of the hip, extension of the knee, and plantar flexion of the ankle and toes. As in the upper extremities, complete extensor synergy of the leg began approximately 2–5 seconds after the patient was requested to extend a portion of his lower extremity [27].

The ability to flex one portion of the affected limb voluntarily without bringing the full synergy into play returned gradually in both the upper and the lower extremity as the power of movement increased. Spasticity of the involved muscle groups could be intense at this stage but lessened as the power of the movements increased. For those patients who progressed to a considerable degree of recovery, the increased power of movement was accompanied by an abrupt lessening of spasticity and the ability to perform isolated voluntary movements of the extremities without eliciting the movement synergy [27].

Twitchell used two techniques to evoke voluntary muscle contractions in the hemiplegic patients he studied, proprioceptive facilitation and proximal traction. In *proprioception,* stimulation of sensory nerve endings in the various body tissues conveys information to the brain about movement, posture, and the relationship of various body parts to one another. Twitchell demonstrated that before the hemiplegic patient was able to perform movements voluntarily, the patient's willed effort to carry out a movement such as flexing the fingers and the therapist's stimulation of certain proprioceptive reactions in the patient, such as tapping the patient's fingers to elicit finger jerks, facilitated each other. This combination resulted in flexion that occurred slowly but powerfully. Voluntary efforts on the part of the patient alone were unsuccessful; and when the therapist ceased tapping the patient's fingers, flexion promptly relaxed in spite of the patient's willed efforts to continue it. The *proximal traction* response was defined by Twitchell as the facilitation of the total flexor synergy by passive stretch of the corresponding muscles. Passive traction upon the flexor muscles of the affected arm, for example, could cause an active contraction of all the flexor muscles of that limb. He concluded in his study that the most reliable prognostic sign for recovery from hemiplegia was occurrence of proprioceptive facilitation within 9 days of onset of hemiplegia and proximal traction response within 13 days. Patients in Twitchell's study who made complete recoveries demonstrated proprioceptive facilitation. These same reactions could not be elicited until at least 15 days following onset of hemiplegia in patients who only achieved partial recovery of function [27].

Late return of tendon reflexes and delayed onset of spasticity are both considered poor prognostic signs for return of voluntary movement, although there are exceptions. Twitchell observed that spasticity was first noted 1–9 days after onset of hemiplegia in those patients who eventually recovered complete functional use of the arm. He found that the increasing intensity of spasticity paralleled the development of proprioceptive facilitation and that spasticity decreased as the power of voluntary movement increased. This increase of power with lessening of spasticity began in the shoulder and eventually worked down to the fingers [27].

THERAPEUTIC PROGRAMS AND TECHNIQUES USED IN REHABILITATION

Prior to initiation of a therapeutic program an evaluation of overall muscle function is usually carried out. In Chapter 4 the standard grades used to classify muscle strength were presented (Fig. 4-3). These grades are based upon whether or not the muscle can move against gravity and maintain a position against manual resistance. These classifications, however, are of limited value in muscle testing for purposes of stroke rehabilitation. Loss of muscle strength with hemiplegia resulting from stroke is only one feature of the total muscle dysfunction. Results of muscle testing for these patients are influenced greatly by the presence of spasticity and rigidity. Values of zero, trace, poor, fair, good, and normal strength fail to take into consideration spasms, ataxia, and mass motions. Frequently these values are not reproducible because of the inconstancy of spasm and the inability of the patient with stroke to cooperate fully. A more meaningful recording of motor function can be made by expressing performance of individual muscles and muscle groups in descriptive terms of "zero function," "mass motion," "isolated muscle function," "useful function," and "normal function" [11].

"While the lower extremity acts as a pillar of support, the upper extremity needs to have fine and intricate function with preservation of distal motor function and intact sensation in order to be serviceable. There is a vast difference between a hand with a closed fist which can act only as a paperweight and a hand with thumb and index finger dexterity sufficient to repair a watch mainspring" [21]. This statement by Mossman vividly illustrates the difference in degree of difficulty of restoring function to the upper as compared to the lower extremities. Ambulation, the principle function of the legs, is possible with only minimal hip extension, whereas the arm with a comparable degree of shoulder extension is virtually useless.

The therapeutic objective for the upper extremity is most often to develop the involved hand as an assistive member, since success in functional recovery of the distal extremities is usually not good [17]. The return of upper extremity function is influenced by numerous factors, including the extent of motor return, degree of spasticity, primitive reflex patterns, apraxia, development of contractures, degree of peripheral sensory deficits, presence of perceptual disorders, and impairment of intellectual functioning [21].

Carroll found that the hemiplegic patient was unlikely to recover full use of his affected arm if no return of function was in evidence within one week of the onset of hemiplegia [4]. Carroll's definition of use was serviceable function including sensation, coordination, and voluntary movement. He stated that loss of precise finger movement constituted the major functional impairment of hemiplegia and noted that the patient who is left with only a weak or ineffective pinch will usually give up altogether trying to use the affected hand in his daily activities [4, 21]. Assessment of upper extremity functioning should take into account sensation, position sense, two-point discrimination, stereognosis, degree of flaccidity or spasticity, and voluntary movement. The various functional units should be assessed also, that is, the shoulder and elbow for placing and the hand and wrist for grasping and stabilizing [21].

Initially the exercise program consists of passive exercises of both the upper and the lower extremities. Active exercises of the uninvolved side are then added, followed by assistive exercises in which the patient uses his uninvolved arm to move the paralyzed one. Later, assistive exercises that require overhead pulleys may be added. For passive exercises of the hemiplegic shoulder, a shoulder wheel may be used in conjunction with the overhead pulleys. Most exercises are introduced to improve mobility and balance in preparation for ambulation. Ambulation training is discussed later in this chapter [17].

A series of graduated exercises may be prescribed to bring the patient up to his maximum potential, which may of course be only minimal serviceability of the upper extremity. Deliberate practice of picking up progressively smaller objects may be instituted to increase coordination. For patients with fairly good upper extremity function, handwriting exercises may be used. If it is found that writing is still not possible within about 12–15 months following onset of hemiplegia, a serious attempt should be made to train the patient to write with the opposite extremity [21].

Since development of a fixed flexion contracture of the hand and fingers interferes with performance of activities of daily living, hand splints are prescribed to prevent such deformities, which are painful as well as troublesome. For some patients a splint that is fashioned to fit across the extensor surface of the forearm may help to reduce undesirable flexor spasticity [21]. The splint should be constructed so that the patient can apply and remove it himself, for example, with Velcro fasteners.

Traditional and neurophysiological approaches to treatment

Treatment programs for the patient with hemiplegia are commonly designated as either "traditional" or "neurophysiological" [21]. The *traditional approach* relies heavily on active-assistive exercise programs. In active-assistive exercises the patient is instructed to concentrate on the activity and attempt to perform the movements voluntarily while the therapist carries out the range of motion exercises [23]. The aims of the *neurophysiological approach* are to inhibit abnormal reflexes and facilitate more normal muscle tone, thereby gradually developing more normal muscle responses [1]. Several treatment programs based upon this approach are used by physical therapists. These include (1) the *Brunnstrom approach,* which follows the stages of recovery from hemiplegia described by Twitchell and takes advantage of the recovery synergies which are facilitated by sensory stimulation; (2) the *Bobath method,* which is a treatment program using proprioceptive and tactile stimuli as reflex inhibiting patterns to control spastic synergies and thus help to relearn normal movement; and (3) the *Rood technique,* in which cutaneous stimulation is applied by fast stroking, brushing, and application of ice to modify muscle response [10, 21]. Flanagan describes the common elements of the various neurophysiological programs as follows. Each uses some degree of sensory input to facilitate or inhibit movement. Each uses reflex mechanisms to inhibit or facilitate the patient's voluntary efforts. Concepts of motor learning, such as repetition of activity, frequency of stimulation, and use of sensory cues, are relied upon to facilitate learning in each of the programs [10, 21]. The reader is referred to texts describing these programs for a complete description of the specific modalities of treatment involved in the neurophysiological technique. Opinions regarding the value of this technique differ sharply, and treatment plans based upon it remain controversial. Mossman states "Since no superiority of one method over the other has yet been demonstrated, selection of a treatment program must employ other criteria of which simplicity should be a main consideration. One must be cautioned not to give credit to technique when spontaneous recovery has naturally occurred" [21]. Peszczynski believes that there is no proof that complex reflex neurophysiological reaction facilitates recovery any better or more quickly than active-assistive exercises [22].

Activities of daily living

The term *activities of daily living* (often abbreviated ADL) refers to those activities involved with personal care, ambulation, homemaking, transfer, and transportation that allow us to function as independent persons. The purpose for which an ADL program is established is to train the patient who has been disabled by stroke to achieve his maximum level of performance in these activities in his home and social life as well as at work [18]. Such a program is aimed at assisting him to resume his previous role in each of these three areas and is geared toward conserving his strength, facilitating mobility, and providing any assistive equipment necessary to allow for independence. Each patient's program should be designed to train him to function as effectively as possible within his own physical environment. Therefore it is important to explore the general layout of his environment, including placement of furniture, before setting up a program, so that the necessary adaptations can be made to foster independent activity.

The patient who has been disabled by stroke may need to relearn many activities that he has carried out independently for years. It is most important that principles of learning and teaching be followed in the treatment program. Lawton recommends that, in teaching the patient activities of daily living, the therapist work from providing maximum support and help toward minimum assistance. The therapist should analyze the component motions of each activity, then have the patient practice each of these component motions as exercises until he is able to practice the activity as a whole [18]. The major factors that limit the patient's ability to perform these activities are brain damage, resulting in cognitive deficits, and loss or impairment of motor function. Brain-damaged patients may be physically able to perform daily activities but lack the understanding to follow a procedure. Impaired memory, short attention span, and poor judgment can prevent the patient from carrying over skills previously mastered as components of another activity. Paralysis, impaired sensation, poor muscle control, easy fatigability, and visual deficits with all interfere with learning [21].

Mossman identifies these *principles of teaching* that should be followed in an ADL program.

1. Know the procedure thoroughly before starting to work with the patient on it.
2. Know the patient's ability and limitations so as not to expect him to achieve beyond his ability. Expect to provide extended supervision, since he may forget part of the procedure from one day to the next.
3. Provide encouragement, but do not pressure the patient to perform. When he has difficulty, help him or try another activity that he can perform, then return to the first procedure later.
4. Some patients may not be able to perform certain tasks without assistive devices. Provide the proper equipment for the activity, and allow sufficient time and space for its performance, so that he will not feel rushed or restricted.
5. Be flexible. Some procedures will have to be adapted for each patient.
6. Make certain everyone who works with the patient is aware of what he is being taught. Everyone should teach him the same way, following the same steps and using the same terms.
7. Give instructions as simply as possible, using short sentences and repeating them often. If the patient has difficulty understanding, the sentence should be reworded. Gestures should be used to make directions clearer, especially for patients with language problems.
8. Repeat the procedure each time the patient would normally perform the activity [21]. To promote better learning when comprehension is impaired, teach one step at a time, use short commands, repeat instructions often, use gestures for demonstration, allow plenty of time to respond, and always praise the patient for trying.

Most therapists will follow a sequence of demonstration, practice, and evaluation. Patients who cannot learn new material readily will require repeated demonstrations from one day to the next. A patient with severe cognitive limitations will need to have the therapist initiate the activity, tell him what to do next in the sequence of the activity, and remind him of the safety precautions that he must take. Some patients become confused or disoriented when they receive many stimuli at the same time. They must have a quiet, private place with no distractions in which to learn their activities of daily living [13].

Transfer activities

The term *transfer* refers to movement of the patient from one surface to another: for example, from one place to another in bed, from bed to chair, and from chair to bathtub or toilet. Two basic considerations are fundamental to all transfers. The levels of the two surfaces between which transfer will be made should be the *same height*. For example, when the toilet seat is lower than the patient's wheelchair, an elevated toilet seat can be installed to facilitate transfer. Ease of transfer will be enhanced by having the *smallest possible distance* between the two surfaces. Frequently a sliding board can be used to bridge two surfaces [26].

As soon as the patient's medical condition permits, he should be gotten out of bed. The hemiplegic patient will need specific instructions on how to perform this transfer independently. Factors that may influence a patient's ability to perform a transfer are paralysis or weakness, impaired sensation, impaired vision, and perceptual deficits. Patients generally perform a better transfer when they lead with their uninvolved side. Hemiplegic patients should wear an arm sling on the involved arm, when it is flaccid, for all transfers, when getting out of bed, being transported by wheelchair or stretcher, or ambulating. The purpose of the sling is to support an involved, sagging shoulder and flaccid arm and hand. When a flail shoulder is not supported, there is a pull on the soft tissues of the shoulder joint, which may result in subluxation of the humeral head out of the glenoid cavity. An arm sling should support the shoulder, elbow, and wrist. It is most important that the wrist be supported in order to prevent wristdrop. Figure 13-1 illustrates proper arm support provided by a sling that the patient can apply himself with only one hand. The therapist should evaluate the patient with the sling in place to be certain that the weight of the arm does not exert undue pressure on the cervical vertebrae and cause damage. If necessary the therapist can construct a sling for an individual patient, to assure that it provides the proper support.

Each patient's deficits should be evaluated in terms of how they will influence transfer, so that the mode of transfer selected will meet the needs of the particular patient. We shall discuss here the basic techniques used by most nurses and therapists. However, just as no two patients are alike, neither are their responses to illness, disability, or a given situation. Therefore, due to any number of variables, techniques found to be effective for most patients with similar disabilities may not

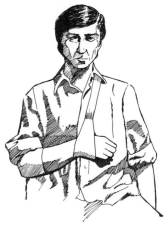

Figure 13-1
Hemiplegic arm sling.

prove effective for all patients. If the individual patient's condition is evaluated carefully and accurately, his need for modification of technique will become apparent.
First consideration should be given to the patient's physical condition. The presence
of a myocardial infarction would contraindicate any extra effort put into a specific
transfer. The patient who suffers from postural hypotension must not be allowed to
come up to a sitting position too abruptly. Aside from the very obvious difficulty
presented by hemiplegia, factors that influence transfers for the stroke patient include
(1) impaired sensation, which prevents the patient from identifying where his extremities are; (2) hemianopsia, which limits vision to one side, thereby preventing the
patient from seeing where he is going without assuming a distorted position and
possibly throwing himself off balance; (3) perceptual problems, which result in distortion of body parts and space, thus interfering with his judgment of distance; and
(4) language disorders, which may prevent him from understanding directions or
asking questions to clarify his understanding of them.

SHIFTING POSITION IN BED
In order to perform a transfer, the first requirement is that the patient be able to
get to a sitting position, either with assistance or independently. For a successful
transfer the mattress should be firm. If necessary, a bed board can be placed under
the mattress, since the firmness will give greater stability and maximize the effect
of the patient's effort. With a soft mattress the physical effort is dissipated into the
mattress and is not available for movement. The patient is taught first to move from
one place to another in bed. This sequence is begun in a supine position. The patient
bends his uninvolved knee, moves his uninvolved foot under the ankle of the involved
leg, lifts the involved leg with the uninvolved leg, and moves the involved leg to one
side of the bed (Fig. 13-2). Next the patient pushes his uninvolved elbow into the
mattress to raise his head and shoulders and slides the upper portion of his body to
the side of the bed. Using the unaffected arm the patient lifts and positions his
paralyzed arm. Short bedside rails can help the patient greatly in transfers, since he
can grasp the rail to turn, sit up, or steady himself.

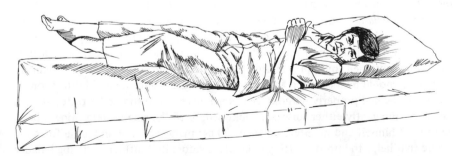

Figure 13-2
Moving from one place to another in bed.

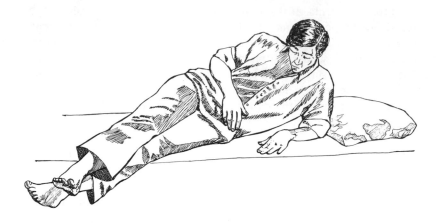

Figure 13-3
Supine to sitting transfer.

TRANSFERRING FROM SUPINE TO SITTING

To transfer from the supine to the sitting position, the patient places his involved
arm across his chest, slides his uninvolved foot under his involved ankle so that the
involved ankle rests on top of his uninvolved foot, pushes his uninvolved elbow into
the mattress and raises his head and shoulders. Resting on his uninvolved elbow,
the patient raises his torso, turns his hips, and swings his legs over the side of the bed
by lifting his involved leg with the uninvolved leg (Fig. 13-3). Once the patient is
seated on the edge of the bed, he can support and steady himself by placing his uninvolved hand behind him on the bed. Initially the patient usually needs assistance
in performing these motions. With supervised practice he can progress to independent
performance. Once he has come to a sitting position, the nurse should evaluate his
ability to maintain balance in a sitting position. The patient with hemiplegia must be
able to maintain fairly good sitting balance before he can transfer or stand safely.

BALANCING

Most patients with hemiplegia tend to slump toward their affected side when sitting
and will need *balancing exercises*. To begin, the patient should be seated at the edge
of the bed with his feet dangling over the side. To support himself, he places his
unaffected arm behind him or to his side with his hand flat on the bed. This sitting
position is maintained for approximately five to ten minutes. If the patient leans to
one side, he should be instructed to correct his posture. Once he is able to sit on
the edge of the bed properly without assistance, his balance should be tested further
by pushing him gently either forward, backward, or to the side to determine if he is
able to right himself and maintain balance. These maneuvers are, in fact, a form of
exercise that helps to improve sitting balance. Factors that influence sitting balance
include paralysis of one side, impaired sensation, and such perceptual defects as
spatial neglect, distorted body scheme, and disturbances in vertical sense.

Once the patient has become independent in sitting, he is ready to attempt *balancing in the standing position.* To begin, the patient sits on the edge of the bed. His affected arm should be in a sling, and he should have a belt around his waist. If there is any question about the patient's balance, or if he is in a debilitated condition, the nurse should not attempt to have him stand without being fully aided by two other people. The nurse should assist the patient in coming to a standing position by grasping the waist belt and giving him support as needed. To attain an upright position, he must have enough strength in one or both legs to sustain his weight. Once he is standing, he should remain upright for several minutes. If he slumps to one side, he should be instructed to correct his posture and remain standing. If he is unable to do so or shows any signs of weakness or alteration of pulse, he should be helped to sit down.

Once the patient is able to assume a standing position with adequate support, this procedure should be repeated several times daily. Since the physical therapist will also be working with the patient on an exercise program, the nurse and therapist should confer regularly to ensure a comprehensive program and reinforcement of the principles taught. Several activities are helpful in preparation for standing transfers. These include sitting on the edge of the bed, standing in parallel bars while practicing locking the knee, exercising to strengthen the muscles on the unaffected side, and exercising to improve the ability to roll, balance, and shift weight [17].

TRANSFERRING FROM SITTING TO STANDING

To teach the patient to transfer from a sitting to standing position or from the bed to a chair, the back of the chair should be placed parallel with the head board of the bed on the patient's unaffected side. The patient should wear a waist belt and arm sling. The patient sits at the edge of the bed, and the nurse stands in front of him, a little to the involved side, with her knee supporting the patient's involved knee. The patient is instructed to bend forward and to reach for the floor with his unaffected foot. Most of his weight should be on his unaffected leg as he rises from the bed. The nurse should support the patient by grasping the waist belt to assure protection without restricting his arm movement. She gives the patient a boost to help him come to a standing position. It is not recommended that the nurse support the patient under the arms, because this will prevent him from using his unaffected arm to help with the transfer. The nurse assists the patient to keep his involved knee extended by supporting it with her knee. When the patient needs less support, he is instructed to reach for the far side of the chair with his unaffected hand and pivot around. The patient should be instructed to touch the chair with the back of his unaffected leg before sitting down, so that he knows the chair is directly behind him. Figure 13-4 shows a patient getting from bed to chair with assistance and alone.

To teach the patient to return to his bed from a chair, the chair in which he sits should be placed so that his unaffected side is next to the bed. The patient moves forward to the edge of the chair with his feet touching the floor and the unaffected foot slightly back. Then he pushes down on the armrest with his unaffected arm to bring himself to a standing position, placing most of the weight on his unaffected leg. The nurse should support his involved knee with hers and can assist him to come

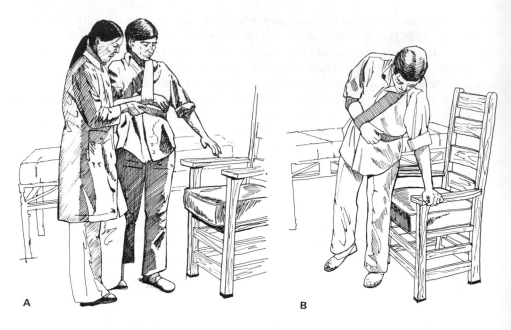

Figure 13-4
A. Transferring from bed to chair with assistance. B. Transferring from bed to chair without assistance.

to a standing position by grasping his waist belt and giving him a slight boost. The patient transfers his unaffected hand to the bed for support and pivots on his feet, so that he is standing with his buttocks against the mattress (Fig. 13-5), then gently lowers himself onto the bed in a sitting position. The patient then hooks his unaffected foot under the involved ankle and lifts his legs onto the bed, lies down on his unaffected side, and completes the transfer by rolling onto his back.

TRANSFERRING FROM WHEELCHAIR TO TOILET

When the patient has developed the ability to transfer safely from bed to chair either independently or with assistance, he is usually ready to attempt transfer from a wheelchair to the toilet. The patient who has difficulty coming to a standing position when transferring from bed to chair or chair to bed will have even more difficulty with toilet transfer. Providing a raised toilet seat and hand rails on either side of the toilet can make transfers easier and safer for the patient as well as for the person helping him. Handrails, or grab bars as they are frequently called, are usually mounted on the walls on either side of the toilet at a 45-degree angle with the high point of the rail installed away from the toilet.

In hospitals, rehabilitation centers, and nursing homes, toilet facilities are usually designed so that wall-mounted handrails can be installed on both sides of the toilet to accommodate patients with either right- or left-sided paralysis. This is rarely the case in the patient's home. If the bathroom layout allows, the bars should be

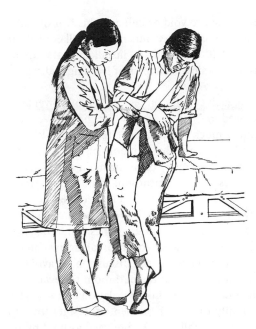

Figure 13-5
Chair to bed transfer.

mounted on the wall that will be next to the patient's unaffected side when he is seated on the toilet. If this is not feasible, right-angle handrails are available. One end is bolted to the wall behind the toilet and the other is bolted to the floor in front of the toilet [21]. These handrails should be installed at a proper height from the floor and distance from the toilet to accommodate the patient's size and provide maximum leverage for him as he raises himself to a standing position. As with the wall-mounted grab bars, they should be installed so that they are on the patient's unaffected side when he is seated on the toilet. Consideration must be given to placement of toilet tissue, so that the patient can reach it with his unaffected arm without undue stretching that might cause him to lose his balance. Families should be discouraged from making expensive structural alterations or purchasing costly equipment until a home visit is made. Often the therapist can make many valuable suggestions for self-help devices that can be devised from materials already in the home. No matter how skillfully the patient can transfer independently from bed to wheelchair and back to bed again, he should never be allowed to attempt toilet transfers unassisted until he has demonstrated that he can manage his clothing independently as well.

Because of the beneficial psychological effect and physical comfort of using the toilet in place of a bedpan, the patient may be transferred to the toilet with maximum assistance from the nursing staff as soon as he is able to maintain sitting balance. It is important that proper transfer techniques be used and that the nurses begin to reinforce learning patterns by repeating the steps in the transfer sequence.

Unfortunately the urgency of the patient's need to void or defecate, his fear of soiling or wetting himself, and the level of activity on a busy nursing unit will contribute too often to his being whisked down the hall at top speed and installed on the toilet with little regard for techniques of body mechanics, principles of learning and teaching, or a sense of modesty.

The deleterious physiological effects of such activity on restoration of bowel and bladder function have already been discussed in Chapter 10. In this chapter we are concerned with helping the patient regain as much independence as possible. We are especially concerned with that form of independence that can only be achieved with ease of mobility. In spite of the frenetic pace that many of us maintain in our active professional lives, the necessity to closet oneself in the bathroom from time to time is accepted as an undeniable right. The "bathroom" in our society is looked upon as not simply an efficient and sanitary convenience for disposal of our metabolic wastes but as a haven of retreat from cares, woes, and responsibilities. It has come to symbolize the one spot to which one can withdraw unassailed to weep, rail against an unfortunate turn of events, terminate an emotionally charged discussion, or avoid a potentially embarrassing encounter. One takes refuge in the bathroom to regain composure and put on a new face for the public, to rethink in isolation a new strategy when the original resulted in failure, or simply to enjoy a momentary respite from the bombardment of demands made by one's responsibilities. The privacy assured by the bathroom door is ordinarily inviolable. When one complains of not even having had two minutes of peace to use the bathroom it is fairly universally accepted that one has endured an exceedingly trying day.

Achieving independence in using the toilet then has a significance far more profound than simply relieving nurses and family members of the drudgery of dealing with bedpans and urinals or protecting the patient from the embarrassment of soiling his bed linen or clothing. It enables the patient to carry out very personal functions that he may well have managed unassisted and in privacy for well over one-half to three-quarters of a century. What is more, he will have regained the freedom to see to these functions at his convenience. The victim of stroke is too often left in isolation, due to either the nature of his neurological deficits or the absence of loved ones. However, an unmet need for companionship and affection does not necessarily negate the need for privacy and occasional moments of solitude. Knowledge that he is still able to retreat to the bathroom "under his own steam" can do much to foster a patient's sense of self-esteem.

For transfer to the toilet from a wheelchair, the patient angles the wheelchair so as to approach the toilet with his unaffected side closest to the seat and locks the wheelchair brakes with his unaffected hand. Next he removes his feet from the footrests and swings both footrests out to the side with his unaffected foot. He then adjusts clothing as necessary. Grasping the handrail with the unaffected hand, he leans forward, placing most of his weight on his unaffected leg, and rises from the wheelchair. It should be stressed that most of the lifting power should come from his uninvolved leg muscles and not from pulling on the handrail with his arm muscles. Once he is in an upright position, he uses the handrail to maintain balance and pivots on his feet until he is standing with his back to the toilet and directly in front of it.

He lowers his clothing and sits on the toilet while steadying himself with the handrail. These procedures are reversed for transfer from the toilet back to the wheelchair [17]. It should be noted that many men find it difficult to void in a sitting position. This may be particularly troublesome for older patients with prostatic hypertrophy. The nurse and therapist should establish a procedure that will give the patient adequate balance and support to allow him to urinate while standing. Providing right-angle bars on both sides of the toilet will certainly help.

USING THE TUB AND SHOWER
Most hospitals and nursing care facilities have shower stalls designed specifically for patients in wheelchairs. Tub and shower rooms are designed with ample space to maneuver and are usually fully equipped with safety features. Water temperature regulators, mechanical lifts, waterproof wheelchairs, and ancillary personnel are available to assist the patient with bathing and protect him from injury. This will not be the case in his own home. Assessment of the home will be discussed in more detail in the section on discharge planning. It is important to note here, however, that patient teaching should start early on and should take into account his previous pattern for activities of daily living and his current disabilities as well as the structural layout and limitations of his home.

During the more acute stages of illness, bathing will be directed primarily at keeping the skin clean and intact. The nurse will give bed baths. While in the hospital, the patient will probably be too ill and bewildered by his condition to understand, remember, or care about instructions for getting in and out of bathtubs. The nurse must impress upon the family, and the patient when he is ready to learn, that his day of a "quick shower" or "long, luxurious, hot soak in the tub" are over. It can be extremely frustrating to the patient who has been devastated by the loss of so many functions to learn that he will be deprived of still another of his "creature comforts." Certain structural changes in the bathroom may be necessary to guard against the risk of injury from falls and burns from hot water, and in any case the family will have to adapt its schedule to provide ample time and assistance to the patient in bathing. The patient should not be left unattended in the bath until he is completely independent. Even then, someone should be available to help immediately, and the patient must have a bell or other means of calling at hand.

TRANSFERRING IN AND OUT OF THE TUB
Transferring into and out of a bathtub are potentially quite hazardous. The patient may have difficulty raising his feet above the rim of the tub. His ability to reach and grasp with his upper extremities may be impaired, making it difficult for him to support himself or regulate the flow and temperature of the water. A slippery wet tub bottom or floor is a further danger, as is the possibility of hot water burns, particularly for patients with poor circulation and impaired sensation. Since the patient can lose his balance and fall while trying to step into the tub, or because his affected leg may be too weak to support his full weight while he raises his unaffected leg over the tub edge, this transfer should always be accomplished from a sitting position. The patient should be taught the procedure in a dry tub before trying to do it when he is actually taking a bath.

First, safety tread tape should be placed on the bottom of the tub and handrails should be installed on the wall alongside the tub. Horizontal tub seats that can be attached to the rim of the tub for use in bathing are available commercially. As an alternative the following technique can be used for transferring into the tub. Two firm wooden chairs may be placed side by side, both facing in the same direction, one adjacent to the edge of the tub and the other in the tub. The chair legs should be shortened so that both seats are even with the tub rim, and rubber tips should be placed over the ends to prevent the chairs from sliding and to protect the porcelain tub finish. The direction in which the chairs face is important and depends on which side is weak or paralyzed and the placement of the faucets. Since it is more difficult to get out of the tub than to get in, the patient should transfer into the tub toward his affected side so that he will be moving toward his unaffected side for the more difficult transfer out of the tub. If the tub does not also have an extensible hand-held shower head, a shampoo hose can be attached to the faucet. When the tub has separate faucets for hot and cold water, adapters can be used. In some cases consideration should be given to installing a device for controlling water temperature.

Whether the patient gets to the bathtub with a wheelchair, walker, or cane, the transfer is started by having him sit on the chair next to the tub. He is instructed to push down on the chair seat with his unaffected hand, push down on the floor with his unaffected leg, and slide his buttocks first to the side edge of the chair seat and then onto the edge of the tub. Using his unaffected hand he must then lift his affected leg and place it in the tub. Once again he is instructed to push down with his unaffected arm and leg while sliding his buttocks onto the chair that has been placed in the tub. When he is seated firmly, he can lift his unaffected leg into the tub. To transfer from the tub, the patient reverses the sequence, moving toward his unaffected side. He is instructed to dry the unaffected arm and hand as well as the adjacent tub edge first, to lessen the danger of losing his grip, then he is instructed to lean forward from his waist, push down on the side of the tub with his unaffected hand and on the bottom of the tub with his unaffected leg, and slide his buttocks onto the edge of the tub, then onto the chair. Once the patient is firmly seated on the chair outside the tub, he raises his unaffected leg out of the tub, then lifts the affected leg out with his unaffected hand. When the patient needs assistance to carry out any of these movements, it may be advisable to put a belt around his waist to provide a firm support but allow him complete freedom of movement of the unaffected limbs [17, 21]. The person assisting the patient should take care not to leave such items as wet washcloths, towels, soap, and lotions on the edge of the tub, chair, or the adjacent floor area, where they can interfere with the patient's transfer.

TRANSFERS FOR QUADRIPLEGICS

The patient with quadriplegia resulting from a brainstem stroke should be out of bed as much as possible for all the same reasons that the patient with hemiplegia is out of bed. However, he will have to have all transfers done for him. The transfer techniques used will depend upon his weight and height and the strength and agility of those who help him with the transfers.

The most frequently used technique is to have two people lift the patient from the bed into a chair placed at the side of the bed. The quadriplegic patient should have a wheelchair with removable arms. Bed and wheelchair heights should be adjusted so that the seat of the chair is even with the mattress surface. Footplates should be removed from the chair to prevent injury to the patient's feet and allow free movement of the nurses and attendants who are to transfer the patient. The chair is placed at a thirty-degree angle to the side of the bed with the seat adjacent to the patient's buttocks and the brakes locked. One person stands at the head of the bed behind the wheelchair with one foot on either side of the rear wheel that is closest to the bed. The second person stands in front of the wheelchair, facing the bed. The patient is brought to a semi-sitting position at the edge of the bed with his head and trunk flexed and his arms folded across his lower chest. The person behind the wheelchair is now also in back of the patient and places both arms around the patient's thorax from behind, grasping both the patient's folded arms and gripping the lower thorax to prevent the upper spine from elongating as the patient is lifted [2]. The person at the foot of the bed places his right arm under the patient's thighs and his left arm under the patient's lower legs. The heavier the patient, the higher up on the thighs this support should be provided. The two lift the patient in unison. Then the person supporting the patient's upper body takes one step sideways, the person supporting the legs takes one step backward, and the patient is lowered into the wheelchair.

Another method of transfer is often referred to as a "three man lift." This is required for heavy patients. Three people stand facing the side of the patient's bed. One places both arms under the patient's upper back, the second puts his arms under the patient's buttocks, and the third under his legs. The three lift the patient and step away from the bed in unison, then carry the patient to his chair. It is most important that the route to the chair be decided upon before the patient is in mid-air, so that he can be transferred safely and smoothly without unnecessary tugging and pulling in opposite directions and risk of being dropped.

Positioning of the patient with quadriplegia is most important. He has no voluntary movement and therefore is unable to adjust his position once he has been placed in the chair. He must be positioned to maintain balance and give maximum comfort, and this position must be checked often for safety and stability. If he has spasticity, the nurse must ensure that there are no factors present that are likely to initiate it. He should be sitting straight against the back of the chair and without pillows, since these encourage slouching. The chair should be equipped with an elevated backrest to support the head. The lower part of the patient's legs should be at right angles to the floor, and a safety belt should be placed across the lower legs to prevent extension, although this should be done carefully so as not to impair circulation. The arms must be supported to minimize strain on the shoulder joints. It is usually difficult to support the arms on the wheelchair armrests. Even though they are positioned carefully and properly, they tend to slide off the narrow armrests. An over-bed table or lap tray is useful for support; the hands and forearms can also be positioned on a cushion on the patient's lap. In Chapter 12 the proper sitting position for patients with impaired neuromuscular function was described.

The quadriplegic patient should be put into the same position. To provide mobility for the patient who has quadriplegia, a power-driven wheelchair can be obtained for long-term use. The control of the chair will depend on what remaining motor function the patient has. Often he will need to control it by pushing a sensitive lever in the appropriate direction with his chin. There are also electronic devices available — called puff-and-suck tubes — which are placed in the patient's mouth and allow him to control chair movement [2] .

Ambulation

For normal ambulation, coordination and balance of the head, trunk, pelvis, and lower extremities, muscle strength, joint mobility, and normal sensation are all required. Successful ambulation means that the patient can transfer from sitting to standing, is able to handle mechanical aids, is able to get to and from various types of chairs, the bed, toilet, and bath, and can negotiate over curbs and stairs. Factors that interfere with ambulation are (1) spasticity, which may cause sudden loss of balance and result in falls and injuries; (2) weak musculature of the trunk, which can result in poor sitting and standing balance; (3) weakness of the upper extremities that will prevent the patient from supporting himself while coming to a standing position; and (4) limited strength of the legs, which may prevent weight bearing necessary for standing and sitting transfers.

The characteristic gait of hemiplegia is primarily the result of the abnormal posture of the affected side — the leg in external rotation, slight flexion of the knee, and plantar flexion of the ankle, accompanied by loss of rhythmic motions of the trunk and alternating arm swing. The reasons for development of this posture have already been described. These patients generally have poor balance, with a tendency to fall to the paralyzed side. Often there is sensory impairment, loss of appreciation of spatial relationships, visual disturbances, and apraxia, all of which hamper progress with the goal of safe and independent ambulation. It is important to realize that voluntary muscle control of the leg is not the decisive factor in determining whether the patient will be able to walk. Patients with no voluntary quadriceps muscle function can stand without the knee giving way. It is thought that the proprioceptive reflex mechanism, which keeps the paralyzed leg in extension when the patient is in an upright position, allows the patient to support himself on that leg. It is for this reason that a long leg brace is rarely necessary for a patient with hemiplegia [11] , and that the patient should always be brought to a standing position to evaluate fully any potential for ambulation.

If the patient's arm is flaccid, an arm sling is recommended during ambulation, to prevent the weight of the arm from causing subluxation of the shoulder joint. Otherwise, unless the arm is painful or unduly heavy, he should be allowed to walk with the paralyzed arm hanging at his side [11] .

Initial balance practice is carried out in the parallel bars. The patient is wheeled between the bars. If he is unable to come to a standing position independently, the therapist will lift him up to it. Sometimes he may have to grasp one of the bars to pull himself up, but this is discouraged, because he must learn eventually to stand without the bars.

The patient is instructed to move close to the edge of his chair, place his unaffected foot on the floor as far under the chair as possible, then bend his trunk forward and stand, placing most of his weight on the affected leg while pushing downward on the armrest or seat of the chair with his unaffected arm. Once he is standing, he practices balance by releasing his grip of the bars for increasingly longer periods of time while shifting his weight onto his weaker leg [11, 21]. After he has demonstrated ability to shift weight and has a fair standing posture, the patient can progress to walking between the bars. Friedland states that the patient should be encouraged to take steps with either leg in as normal a fashion as possible and be instructed to keep his feet parallel and lean slightly to his unaffected side to keep himself from falling [11].

It is most important that the patient's physical condition be observed closely for any changes as he begins to ambulate and as he progresses to more difficult tasks. Ambulation training requires a great deal of physical effort, and patients with cardiovascular insufficiency, in particular, should be observed for any signs of paleness, sweating, tachycardia, or dyspnea. Patients with hemianopsia may bump into objects left in their path or walk directly into walls, furniture, or the path of others outside their range of vision. These patients should be taught to scan their surroundings as they proceed ahead to prevent collisions and injury to themselves and others.

The patient progresses from walking assisted by the therapist to walking unassisted but holding onto the parallel bars, and eventually to walking outside the bars [17]. At this time he may be measured for a cane that he can use with his unaffected arm. The length of the cane should be such as to allow it to touch the floor with minimum flexion of the elbow when the patient holds it by his side a few inches from his body. It should have a flat bottom and a large rubber tip to prevent slipping. When the patient's gait is unsteady and he needs a broader base of support, he may use a four-pronged cane. He should use a straight cane whenever possible, however, because a four-pronged cane is clumsy, can hook onto other objects, and is absolutely useless on the stairs [11]. To walk with the cane, the patient should hold it in his uninvolved hand, move it forward about 6–8 inches, then take a step with his paralyzed leg, bringing it just up to the cane, not beyond it. He then leans on the cane to keep himself from falling to the paralyzed side, while he swings the unaffected leg beyond the position of the cane. He shifts his weight back to the unaffected leg and begins the sequence over. As he gains confidence and becomes more skillful, the patient will be able to move the cane and paralyzed leg at the same time [11].

BRACING

A footdrop brace may improve the hemiplegic gait considerably, since even a mild degree of spastic plantar flexion of the ankle will lead to a steppage gait and interfere with ambulation. The conventional brace consists of double upright bars connecting a shoe plate and calf band. The brace is attached to the heel of the shoe by means of caliper tubing or a stirrup plate. The *caliper brace* controls footdrop by means of a posterior stop. It can be used to restrict ankle motion in both directions by means of anterior or posterior stops. The *stirrup type brace* has an ankle joint that is aligned to correspond with the physiological joint. It keeps the brace in an undisturbed relationship with the patient's leg, regardless of the flexion and extension of the knee and ankle. The cuff of the brace, regardless of the type, must be well padded to prevent undue pressure on the fibular head and peroneal nerve. Other types of footdrop braces have been developed mainly to improve their appearance. Plastic braces have become quite popular, because they are light in weight, and the clear plastic is thought to look better [11].

A *long leg brace* may be indicated, on occasion, when there are complications such as flexion contractures or an unstable knee due to an old injury or arthritic changes. This type of brace is rarely necessary for stabilizing the knee of a patient with hemiplegia. Friedland states that the use of a long leg brace should be avoided for the following reasons: (1) it makes the gait more awkward, (2) it increases the difficulty of clearing the floor during the leg's swing phase, (3) it adds to the risk of falling, (4) it is heavy and uncomfortable to wear all day, and (5) it limits independence because help is required to apply and remove it [11].

ADVANCED FUNCTIONAL ACTIVITIES

As ambulation progresses, more advanced functional activities are introduced, such as ascending and descending curbs and stairs and transferring in and out of automobiles. The patient cannot walk independently until he is able to negotiate stairs and curbs. *Stair climbing* is much easier with a handrail. Handrails are installed preferably on both sides of the stairs, so that the patient will have use of the rails when descending the stairs as well. On approaching the stairs, the patient is instructed to hang the cane over his arm or hook it onto a pocket, grasp the railing with his unaffected hand, and step up with his unaffected leg while simultaneously pulling on the rail with his hand. When his weight is firmly planted on the unaffected leg, the paralyzed leg is brought up to the same step, and the sequence is repeated until he reaches the top of the stairway. To descend, he is instructed to hold the railing firmly with his good hand and lead down with his paralyzed leg. With his full weight supported by the unaffected arm and the paralyzed leg, he proceeds to follow with his unaffected leg. This sequence is repeated for each step until he reaches the bottom of the stairs. When there is no handrail or bannister on his unaffected side, the patient must learn to use his cane for stability. To ascend the stair, he is instructed to lead with his good foot and follow with his cane and hemiplegic leg. To descend, he is instructed to lead with his hemiplegic leg, placing his full weight on the leg and cane, then to follow with his good leg [11, 21].

Curb climbing is performed in a manner similar to stair climbing. To ascend the curb the patient steps up, leading with his unaffected foot, shifts his weight onto his leg, then brings up his cane and paralyzed leg simultaneously. To step down from a curb, he leads with the paralyzed leg, placing his foot and cane down at the bottom of the curb, then steps down with his good leg [11, 21].

Automobile transfers do not pose any great problem for the patient who can ambulate well with or without a cane, particularly if he is slender. For purposes of safety, however, he should be taught to enter and leave the car on the passenger side rather than the driver's side. It is recommended that he sit in the front seat, since this usually offers more space in which to maneuver and greater leg room. He is taught to approach the front car door, open it, walk close to the seat, pivot so that his back is against the seat, and sit down. He can then move his legs into the automobile by supporting the paralyzed foot with his good foot and guiding the leg with his good hand. He may have some difficulty in closing the door if his paralyzed arm is on that side. A strip of plastic or cord can be attached to the door to permit him to close it by himself. He is instructed to get out of the car in reverse order.

Since most car seats are considerably lower than those of conventional chairs, it takes a good deal of effort to lower the trunk of the body down to the level of the car seat and an even greater effort to raise the body up to a standing position. This can be quite difficult for a heavy patient. Every effort should be made to have the patient enter and leave the car in a driveway or flat area away from the curb to give him additional leverage for this transfer. The patient may need to use his cane or grasp the car roof or the door to gain leverage and maintain his balance. If he comes to the automobile in a wheelchair, the front door on the passenger side should be opened diagonally for him and the window rolled down. He is instructed to approach the open door, set the wheelchair brakes, move foot and leg rests out of the way, and stand up by pushing down on the armrest with his unaffected arm and on the pavement with his good leg. Then he grasps the window frame with his unaffected hand, pivots to face the door with his back to the car seat, and sits down. He then brings his legs into the car as described above. The procedure is reversed in transferring from the automobile to the wheelchair [11].

Federal regulations stemming from the Rehabilitation Act of 1973 have set forth guidelines for structural changes in public buildings, walkways, parking lots, and public conveyances to accommodate the special needs of the handicapped. Specially equipped lavatories, enlarged doorways and corridors, ramps, and handrails are evident in many large community structures. Assigned parking areas and seating for the handicapped are found in more and more public places. Families should be encouraged to check for such facilities within their community and make use of them, so that trips away from the home can be accomplished as smoothly as possible.

Propelling the wheelchair

Generally the patient with hemiplegia can be taught to propel his wheelchair without assistance by using his unaffected arm and leg. The footrest on his unaffected side should be removed so that he will have freedom of movement of that leg to control the chair. If a hinged footrest is provided on the affected side, he can turn it away with his good foot when necessary to prevent interference with transfers. A heel loop attached to the back of the foot on the affected side can be used to prevent the paralyzed foot from slipping backward off the footrest.

The patient is instructed to propel the wheelchair by reaching back with his good arm to grasp the rim of the wheel and forward with his good foot to touch the floor with his heel, then to push the wheel forward and push his heel against the floor, flexing his knee to move the chair toward his foot. It is important for him to understand that it is his foot that controls the direction of the chair, not his hand. Initially he may have difficulty coordinating his hand and foot movements to guide the chair properly [21]. The importance of locking the brakes must be stressed often, so that it becomes second nature to him. Whenever he is not actually propelling the chair, he should apply the brakes to prevent accidents. He should also be taught not to lean too far forward while sitting in the chair and not to bear weight on the footrest, since the chair might tip over.

Self-care

Most self-care activities such as bathing, grooming, using the toilet, dressing, and eating are referred to as bilateral activities, because they normally involve the use of two hands. One of the greatest losses for the patient who has suffered a stroke can be the loss of a functional hand and arm. A functional hand requires motor control, intact sensory discrimination, and exquisite coordination to perform intricate movements with skill and speed. Following stroke the upper extremity frequently remains useless, because those qualities that make the difference between a functional and a nonfunctional hand are either totally lost or severely impaired. The occupational therapist can teach the patient various techniques for using his involved arm to assist his functional arm in carrying out self-care activities when no further return is possible. The most important motor ability of the body is that of opposition of the thumb and fingers to pinch, grasp, or clasp. When this function has been lost, the therapist will explore with the patient alternative methods that may be available to him for gripping and holding objects. Occasionally adaptive equipment for the hand may be used to improve function and assist in self-care. When the dominant side has been paralyzed, the therapist will initiate a restraining program for the good arm in which the patient is taught to write and use various implements such as keys, pins, and flatware. This is necessary because the patient will have had less dexterity of his nondominant hand even before he was paralyzed by the stroke. Once the patient begins to progress with use of the unaffected nondominant hand, he can be taught to use the affected hand for holding and stabilizing objects to be manipulated with the good hand [11, 15].

When the patient is able to participate in his own care, he should be encouraged to do so. Some of the major obstacles to independent performance in self-care activities are (1) paralysis or paresis of a hand and/or arm; (2) decreased sensation of a hand and/or arm; (3) incoordination of the upper extremities; (4) perceptual deficits, such as body image disturbances, spatial disorientation, and apraxias; (5) hemianopsia; (6) limited range of motion; and (7) poor or weak hand grasp. The following principles should be adhered to in assisting the patient to learn self-care activities:

1. Give simple directions, one step at a time, while the patient is being shown how to perform an activity.
2. Repeat directions many times, if necessary, and repeat them in the same words.
3. Let the patient know when he is doing something correctly, and do not push him if he doesn't.
4. Follow the same steps each time. If different methods are used each time, the patient will be confused and may have difficulty in learning.

5. Encourage use of the paralyzed arm as much as possible, even if it can only serve as a weight.

Feeding

Learning to feed himself is often the first self-care activity that the hemiplegic patient attempts. This may be the only area in which some achieve any independence. The feeding and nutritional problems of patients with stroke and the psychological aspects of these difficulties have already been discussed in Chapter 9. In this chapter the mechanics of manipulating food, beverages, utensils, and containers will be addressed. The patient with hemiplegia will have the greatest difficulty cutting up his food, buttering bread or rolls, and opening containers. He will always need some help with these activities, and this should be anticipated so as to reduce his sense of frustration. Before he starts to feed himself, he should have adequate sitting balance. It is most important that he be in a comfortable position for meals and that he be able to remain sitting up until he has finished eating.

Mealtimes are usually hectic in general hospitals. There are always too many patients to be fed, and staff are anxious to take their own meals. Invariably the emergency admission arrives in the midst of tray time. Rarely, if ever, is serving a meal looked upon as a therapeutic measure by the nursing staff. All too often meal trays are hastily served and distributed in assembly line fashion by ancillary personnel who have little if any knowledge of the patient's difficulties, then collected with little attention to what or how the patient has eaten or whether he has enjoyed it. At this point in his illness food is one of the few sources of pleasure available to the stroke victim. What is more, adequate nutrition is vital if he is to regain his strength. Special care must be taken that he is positioned properly and adequate assistance and time are provided. Initially the patient will be very slow, and approximately one hour should be allowed for meals. Meat should be cut, bread buttered, and all containers opened. Gradually he can be taught to manage most of these activities with one hand. Conventional eating utensils should be used as much as possible.

The major feeding difficulty will be cutting food, especially meat. The patient must be taught a new technique. If he is to cut a cooked vegetable, fish, or other soft food, he is instructed to grasp the fork with his good hand, insert the tines of the fork into the portion of food to be cut, then rock the fork back and forth. He then lifts the fork out and continues the process until he has severed a bite-sized piece. If he has a fairly tender portion of meat or other food of firm consistency, he can cut it with his knife in the following manner. Grasping the knife handle, blade down, with his index finger extended along the upper edge of the blade, he presses the knife tip into the food and rocks the knife handle up and down until there is a separation. He lifts the knife out and repeats the procedure to separate the food into bite-sized pieces. If the food is tough, this technique will not work, and someone will have to cut the food for him.

Every attempt should be made to teach the patient to use conventional eating utensils. However, special utensils are available for those patients who have particular difficulty manipulating a standard knife and fork. These include a knife—fork combination and a rocker knife. The combination knife—fork utensil enables the patient to use one piece of equipment rather than two and is available for both right- and left-handed use. The upper edge of the fork is sharp, and this section is inserted into the food to be cut. The same rocking motion as described for the conventional knife and fork is used to divide the food. The patient must be careful not to insert the fork so far into the mouth that he injures himself on the cutting edge. This drawback poses a significant risk for some patients. The rocker knife is simply a knife with a rounded blade that facilitates cutting with one hand. A plate guard is another device. This is a rim of metal that can be attached to the edge of a plate to prevent the food from sliding off the plate when the patient attempts to cut it. It also facilitates picking up portions of food with the fork or spoon [21].

It is not easy to butter bread with one hand, but it is possible to learn this technique with real determination, practice, and soft butter. The patient is instructed to place the bread on a flat surface and to hold the knife handle so that the flat side of the blade is in contact with the bread, between his thumb and his ring and fifth fingers, with his index finger slightly flexed and resting on top of the knife blade. With his middle finger he applies pressure to the bread to keep it from moving and rotates the knife blade to spread the butter [21].

At home it is easiest to serve beverages in the conventional cups or glasses, with cream or milk for tea and coffee in a small pitcher and sugar and condiments in the usual containers. The family should be reminded to consider the weight of containers, cups, and glasses as well as their base of support and their overall configuration to assure that they can be easily manipulated by the patient with one hand. When beverages and condiments are served in sealed containers, as is usually the case in hospitals and nursing homes, the patient should be assisted with these. With practice, those patients who have some return of arm flexion may be taught to stabilize the container with the affected arm and to open it with the unaffected hand.

It is extremely important for the patient's morale that his meals be served as attractively as possible and that he learn to eat in as customary a manner as possible. It is also important that thought be given to serving his food in a form that is easy for him to handle without spills and accidents but without undue emphasis on his handicap. Suction cups to stabilize dishes or placemats with cork backs may be helpful. Older patients seem to have more difficulty seeing objects against a white background and often will eat more when meals are served on brightly colored plates that contrast with the colors of the foods served. The specific feeding problems created by hemianopsia and perceptual deficits must be given particular attention when teaching the patient to feed himself and assisting his family to plan for his continuing care.

Bathing

Instructions for self-care in bathing, grooming, and oral hygiene should begin in the hospital as soon as the patient becomes alert and his medical condition begins to stabilize. While bathing the patient, the nurse has him first wash his own face, then gradually progress to completing a major portion of his bath. While he is confined to bed, the patient with hemiplegia will need help in applying soap to the washcloth and may have difficulty handling the washcloth and towel. When he is able to be up and transfer to the bathtub for bathing, he should be instructed to use a long-handled bath brush. This can be manipulated to wash the axillary region and upper portion of his unaffected arm. Some patients can also learn to place a bathmitt over the paralyzed hand and guide it with the unaffected hand to wash this area. Bath soaps that come attached to a rope are particularly helpful, because they can be suspended from a faucet or hook and thus reduce both the risk of slipping and frustration of trying to retrieve a bar that has slipped from the hand or soap dish. Those patients who have perceptual disorders with denial of parts of the body must be reminded with each bath to care for these areas.

To promote frequent, thorough hand washing, the task can be simplified by securing a small handbrush to the inside of the washbasin or sink with suction cups. The patient can turn on this tap, adjust the water temperature, and soap the brush with one hand. He is able then to cleanse both hands by rubbing his unaffected hand over the brush, then soaping and washing the paralyzed hand with the unaffected hand. A towel rack should be placed next to the sink at about waist height. The patient is taught to place one end of the towel under the affected arm or secure the edge of the towel in a belt or a pocket to hold it taut. Then the unaffected hand can be rubbed over the towel to dry it.

Oral hygiene

The various techniques for providing oral hygiene have already been presented in Chapter 11. It is emphasized here that loss of muscle function on one side of the face or mouth may interfere with easy access to the oral cavity. It is therefore necessary that special attention be given to the involved side of the mouth, because food will tend to collect between the cheek and the teeth. The patient should be instructed to check for food on the paralyzed side after eating. If he is unable to do this while in the hospital, it is the nurse's responsibility to do so and to teach those who will be caring for him after discharge to do so. Wall-hung plastic toothpaste dispensers are available in local drugstores and should be installed to allow the patient to brush his teeth independently. If the patient wears dentures, a denture brush should be attached to the washbasin with suction cups so that he can clean his own dentures [15]. It is recommended that the sink be filled with water when he washes the dentures, so that if he accidentally drops them, the water will cushion the impact.

Grooming

Use of an electric razor for shaving will eliminate the need for handling blades, shaving brush, and shaving cream. However, two hands may be needed to set the shaver up, insert the electrical cords, clean the shaver after use, and replace it. Even portable or battery-operated models may require an electrical cord for recharging. Much of the patient's frustration in trying to achieve independence in his personal care can be reduced by setting up a routine whereby the shaver is regularly set up for his use without undue manipulation on his part. Since he will be unable to hold the facial skin taut while he is shaving, he should be instructed to puff out his cheeks, which will accomplish the same thing.

Most men use a preshave preparation, which facilitates action of the electric razor, as well as an aftershave lotion. Many preparations are available in squeeze-type containers. The patient can be taught to secure the container between his affected elbow and chest while he removes the cap with his unaffected hand. He can then invert the bottle and allow the liquid to flow into the palm of his unaffected hand. Plastic squeeze-type bottles are also available in most drug stores, and various lotions can be transferred to them.

The patient is usually able to *manicure* his affected hand provided that he has no visual difficulties. To care for the normal hand, it may be helpful to have a nail file or emory board taped to the side of a table or counter to stabilize it. The patient then shapes the nails by running them against the file. The use of the handbrush for regular hand washing will pretty much eliminate the need for using the nail file to clean under the nails. If it is necessary that the nails be clipped, an ordinary nail clipper can be used for the affected hand. However, the patient will need help to trim the nails of the unaffected hand. While it is theoretically possible for the patient to trim his own toenails, his ability to accomplish this safely will depend on his size, agility, visual acuity, and the competence of his peripheral vascular system. He will usually need help in this area. If the circulation to his feet is in any way compromised, he must take great care not to injure the tissue.

An unkempt or unflattering hairdo can be very demoralizing. If the patient has a simple hair style, combing and brushing it can be accomplished with one hand. Patients should be encouraged to do this as soon as they are strong enough to begin their own bathing. Women who have long hair or a style that requires setting may have significant problems managing their hair and will need help. Some patients will be fortunate enough to be able to afford the luxury of regular trips to the hairdresser. Others may solve the problem with a wig. It may be necessary to have the patient's own hair cut or restyled to facilitate care and enhance grooming.

If the patient is able to transfer to the bathtub he can have a shampoo at that time. It is not advised that the patient attempt this on his own, because of the danger of falling. When the patient is not able to transfer to the bathtub, he can sit with his back to the sink for a shampoo. A shampoo hose can be attached to the faucet, if necessary. If the patient is unable to tilt his head back far enough, special protective trays can be used that fit snugly to the nape of the neck and slope down to the sink to direct the water and suds into the sink rather than down the patient's neck. Dry shampoo preparations are also available to help keep the hair clean between shampoos.

The use of cosmetics will vary among patients, depending upon age, life-style, and personal taste. Most women wear some form of makeup every day even if it is only a touch of lipstick. It is rare indeed to find a human being unaffected by personal vanity, and most of us will go to some lengths to improve upon nature's gifts. Unless the patient is severely depressed, she will usually take an interest in her appearance once her condition begins to stabilize. As soon as the patient begins to learn self-care techniques for bathing and grooming, she should be encouraged and assisted to apply her own makeup.

Unfortunately many cosmetics are packaged in containers that are almost impossible to open with one hand. If the patient has good strength in the unaffected hand, she can usually manage to open a bottle, if it is light in weight and small enough to grasp in the palm of the hand with the last three fingers, leaving the index finger and thumb free to unscrew the cap. Once the cap is loosened sufficiently, she can set the container down and remove the cap. Plastic containers are lighter in weight and present less risk of injury if dropped than glass. Lipstick tubes can be held in the same manner for lifting off the cap and unscrewing the lipstick.

Although pump-type dispensers for lotions are convenient for the person with two functioning hands, they can prove hazardous to the patient with hemiplegia, since she (or he) may be unable to pump and cup her hand to catch the lotion at the same time. Lotion spilled on the floor can cause a fall. Preparations that come in large unwieldy containers can be transferred to small plastic bottles of the type used for travel, which can be purchased at most drug or notion counters. Substances that will not evaporate or decompose when left unsealed can be transferred to containers with lift-off lids. Such things as perfumes and toilet waters can be purchased in spray form in small size or transferred to plastic spray containers. Needless to say, assistance will be required to accomplish this.

Depending upon the availability and sensitivity of family members, many of these niceties may have been thoughtfully provided. In many cases, however, little if any thought is given to this aspect of the patient's care. The nurse should encourage the family to look upon the patient's renewed interest in improving her appearance as a therapeutic goal. The family should be persuaded to consider that helping the patient use cosmetics is an important step in recovery of self-esteem and independence rather than catering to a frivolous whim.

Dressing

Training in dressing techniques can be started early on in the course of illness. When the patient begins to wash himself, he should also be taught to change his hospital gown or pajamas. As he progresses to sitting in a chair and ambulation, he should be taught to put on his bathrobe and slippers and eventually to put on street clothes. If the patient has poor balance, he can be taught to dress in bed. If he has good balance while sitting, he can learn to dress himself while sitting on the edge of the bed, with his feet either supported by a stool or flat on the floor. The patient should always start dressing by clothing the disabled limb first and undressing by removing clothing from the disabled limb last. In order to facilitate dressing as well as movement for transfers and practice in ambulation, clothing should not be constricting and should fasten easily, preferably at the front or side. Velcro closures can be sewn into clothing, since most patients with hemiplegia will have particular difficulty fastening garments with zippers, buttons, hooks and eyes, grippers, or snaps and even greater difficulty with tying bows or knots. Figures 13-6 through 13-10 illustrate dressing techniques that can be used for various items of clothing.

PULLOVER GARMENT

Figure 13-6 shows the sequence in which the patient with hemiplegia is taught to put on a pullover garment. This same technique can be used for sweaters, tee shirts,

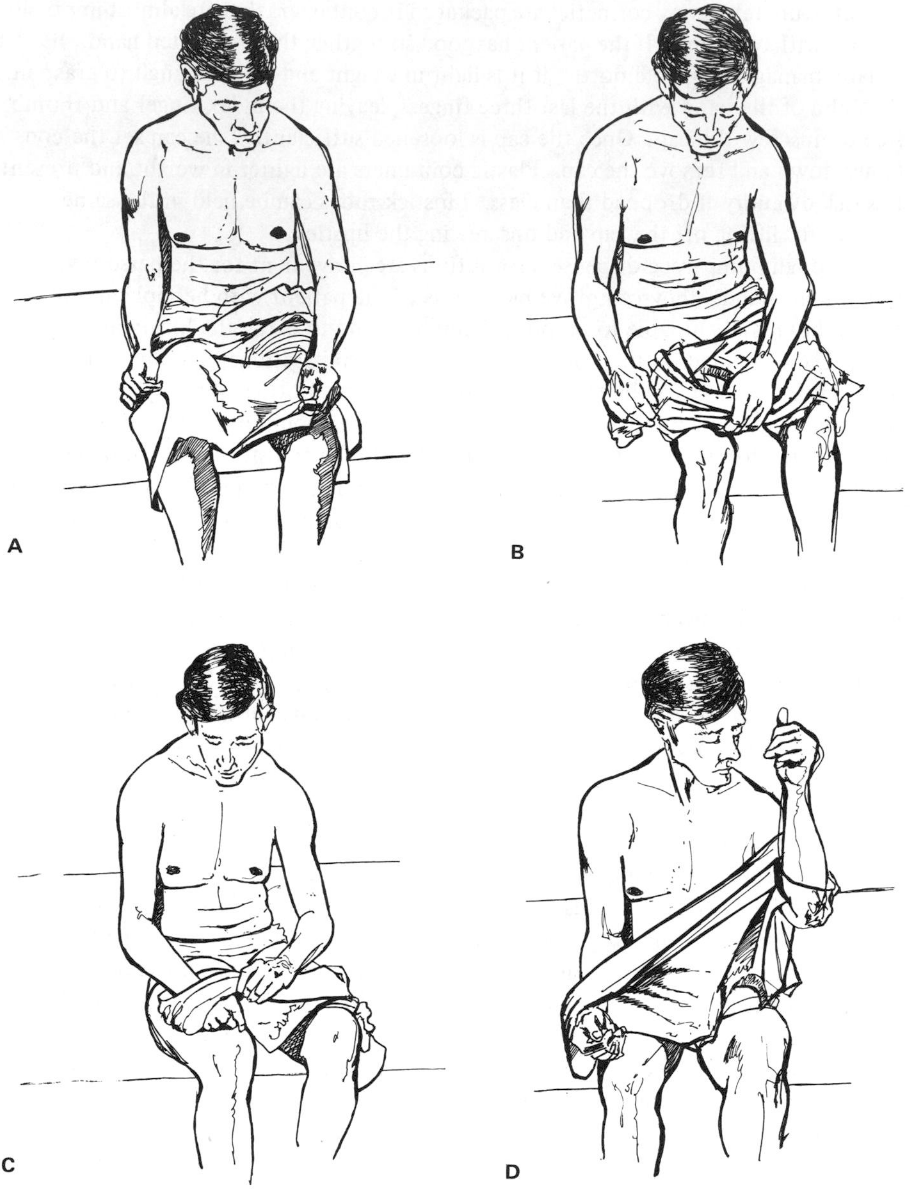

A

B

C

D

Figure 13-6
Sequence for putting on a pullover garment. (From Sister Kenny Institute. Self-Care
for the Hemiplegic *(Rehabilitation Publication #704). Minneapolis: Sister Kenny
Institute, 1970. Published by permission of the Institute. Further information on
rehabilitation may be obtained by writing Sister Kenny Institute, Publications Dept.,
Chicago Ave. at 27th St., Minneapolis, MN 55407.)*

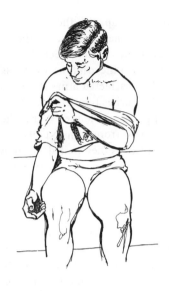

E

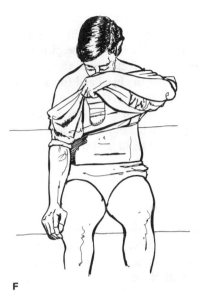

F

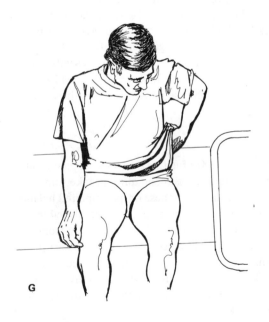

G

dresses, and slips. The garment is placed on the patient's lap with the neck away from him and the front of the garment down. With the unaffected hand, the patient gathers up the back of the garment to expose the armhole for the affected arm. He uses his unaffected hand to place the paralyzed hand into the armhole and pulls the sleeve over the hand and forearm. He then places the unaffected arm into its armhole and through the sleeve up to his elbow. Then he pushes the sleeve of the involved arm over the elbow and higher onto the upper arm. He then works the shirt up to his shoulders, gathers the back of the garment from hem to collar in his unaffected hand, and pulls it over his head. The garment is then pulled down over the body and adjusted. For undressing, this procedure is reversed, the affected arm being removed from the sleeve last.

OPEN-FRONT GARMENT

Figure 13-7 illustrates the steps suggested for putting on a garment that is opened down the front. This technique can be used for bathrobes, shirts, jackets, coats, blouses, vests, and front-opening dresses. The patient places the garment on his lap with the neck away from him, the inside of the garment up, and the armhole that corresponds to the affected arm resting on the opposite thigh. He slides his affected arm into the armhole and grasps the collar edge with the unaffected hand to pull the sleeve up onto the shoulder of the paralyzed arm. He then reaches up and grasps the back of the collar or neck band and brings the garment across his back, inserts his unaffected arm into the sleeve, and fastens the garment in front. It is important to remember that, while it is possible to learn to button clothes with one hand, the patient will not be able to fasten buttons or cufflinks on dress or shirt cuffs on the unaffected side. To remove the garment the patient reverses these steps, removing the sleeve from the paralyzed arm last.

TROUSERS

Figure 13-8 shows the technique that can be used for putting on trousers, pants and underpants, pajama bottoms, and shorts. Mastering this technique can take some practice, especially for the patient who is debilitated or obese or has impaired balance or visual difficulties. The patient uses his unaffected arm to cross his paralyzed leg over his unaffected leg. He places the garment on his lap with the legs away from him and the front side up. He grasps the garment by the center front of the waistband and tosses it downward to cover the paralyzed foot, then draws the garment up over the paralyzed limb to about the knee. He then uncrosses the paralyzed leg and places the foot on the floor. Then he can insert the unaffected leg into the other leg opening and pull the garment up over his knees.

    If his standing balance is adequate, he will stand up, while maintaining a firm grasp on the waistband, to pull the garment up to his waist (Fig. 13-8D). For pants or trousers that have a front or side opening rather than an elasticized waistband, he should arrange the unaffected side first and then the affected side, using his good elbow to keep the garment from sliding down. He then sits back down on the edge of the bed to fasten trousers and belt, if necessary. If his balance is not adequate to

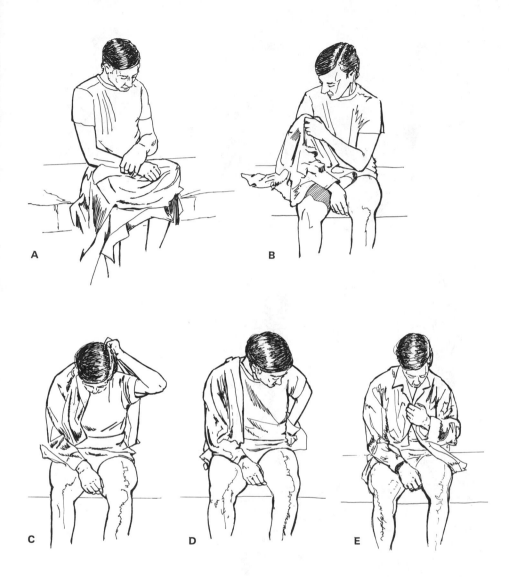

Figure 13-7
Sequence for putting on an open-front garment. (From Sister Kenny Institute. Self-
Care for the Hemiplegic *(Rehabilitation Publication #704). Minneapolis: Sister
Kenny Institute, 1970. Published by permission of the Institute. Further informa-
tion on rehabilitation may be obtained by writing Sister Kenny Institute, Publications
Dept., Chicago Ave. at 27th St., Minneapolis, MN 55407.)*

allow him to stand safely, he will lie back on the bed, after he has brought the garment
up over his knees, to complete the last two steps (Fig. 13-8F). If he cannot raise his
hips to pull the garment up to his waist, he can roll from side to side to accomplish
this. The patient must be cautioned not to lean too far forward when attempting to

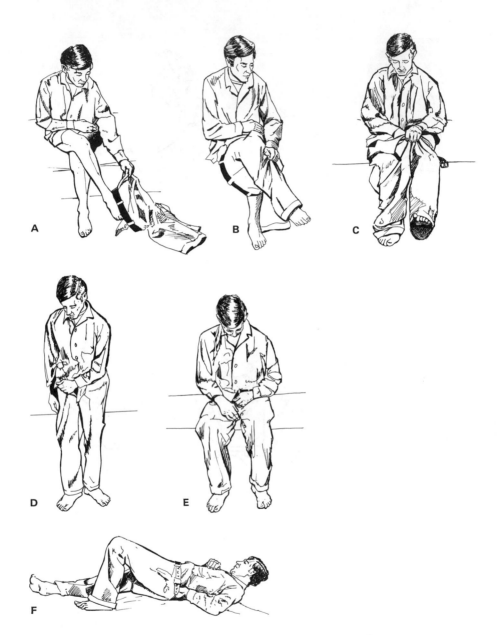

Figure 13-8
Sequence for putting on trousers. (From Sister Kenny Institute. Self-Care for the
Hemiplegic *(Rehabilitation Publication #704). Minneapolis: Sister Kenny Institute,*
1970. Published by permission of the Institute. Further information on rehabilita-
tion may be obtained by writing Sister Kenny Institute, Publications Dept., Chicago
Ave. at 27th St., Minneapolis, MN 55407.)

get the pant leg over the paralyzed foot, since he runs a danger of losing balance and falling. It may be necessary to have him rest his foot on an adjacent chair seat to bring his foot close enough for him to get the garment over it. There is also the potential problem of dropping the garment on the floor and being unable to retrieve it. A number of long-handled devices are available for picking up objects, and it may save the patient considerable exasperation and embarrassment and add to his independence if such a device is left handy for him while he is dressing. To remove the pants or trousers, the procedure is reversed, the uninvolved leg being removed from the pant leg first.

HOSE

Putting on hose is more difficult than donning pants or trousers, and the fragility of women's sheer hose adds to the challenge. The technique for applying short socks, illustrated in Figure 13-9, can be adapted for full-length stockings and pantyhose. The patient is instructed to cross the paralyzed limb over the unaffected limb, spread the opening of the sock with the thumb and fingers, then reach down and slip the sock over the toes. The sock is then pulled up to its full length. The patient can place his or her foot on a stool or adjacent chair seat to make it easier for him to reach. The same procedure is carried out for the opposite leg. For long hose, he inserts his hand into the top and gathers up the length of the stocking before slipping it over the toes. In both cases he must be careful that the heel is in the proper position and that there are no creases or wrinkles that may cause pressure or constriction of circulation and lead to tissue breakdown.

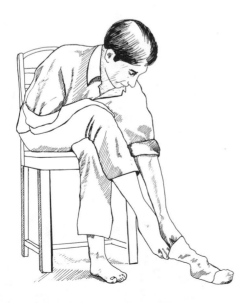

Figure 13-9
Technique for putting on hose.

SHOES

Figure 13-10 shows a technique for putting a shoe with a brace on the paralyzed foot. A long-handled shoehorn is a must for the patient with hemiplegia, and a footstool will make it easier for him to reach his foot and also provide him with something to push against when fitting his foot into the shoe. The patient is instructed to cross his paralyzed leg over his unaffected leg, grasp the shoe by the top of the brace, and fit the shoe over his toes. While maintaining the shoe in place, he uncrosses his leg and rests his foot on the footstool. He inserts the long-handled shoe horn between his heel and the back of the shoe, then pushes against his knee with his unaffected arm until his foot slides into the shoe. Then he removes the shoe horn and buckles the strap of the brace around the calf of the leg. Elastic shoe laces can be bought to fasten the shoes. Once they are inserted, there is no necessity to tie or untie them.

BRA

To put on a bra, the patient is instructed to grasp the end of the bra with her unaffected hand and slide it around her waist so that the inside is against her body, the straps are uppermost, and the front part is along her back. She can then tuck the end of the bra under the elbow of her paralyzed arm or into the elasticized waistband of her underpants to secure it while drawing the opposite end around her waist to fasten the hooks. If the patient has difficulty manipulating the hooks and eyes, Velcro fasteners can be sewn in their place. However, since the Velcro fasteners can come apart with stretching, the patient should be encouraged to learn to fasten the hooks

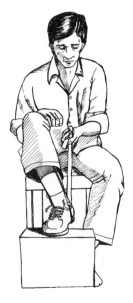

Figure 13-10
Technique for putting on a shoe with a brace.

with one hand. This can be accomplished with a bit of practice. The patient then slides the bra around so that the cups are in the front of the body, places her affected arm through the strap, and pulls the strap up over her shoulder. Then she places the unaffected arm through the other shoulder strap and adjusts the bra for comfort. This procedure is greatly facilitated when an elasticized bra is used. If the straps are not elasticized. a strip of elastic can be inserted between the strap and the bra itself. Although bras that fasten in the front are available, these are usually more difficult to fasten with one hand than the conventional back-closing type, because there is no way to stabilize the end of the bra while attaching the closure.

The occupational therapist is specially prepared to evaluate the patient's difficulties and set up a treatment program to help him with his self-care activities. The nurse should be familiar with the treatment program set up by the therapist and should supervise the patient's activities on the nursing division to assure that he is practising self-care activities properly. The patient must be allowed to practice the techniques that he has been taught, even if he is slow in carrying them out. If the nurse does these activities for the patient in the interest of time, she will only confuse the patient and hinder his progress in gaining independence with self-care.

DISCHARGE PLANNING

As plans for the patient's long-term care begin to be formulated, the nurse should keep in mind the patient's ability for self-care and begin to evaluate the kind of support that will be available to him in his home setting and whether it will allow him to function safely. A devoted family with strong bonds of affection greatly improves the patient's potential for adjusting to his disability and progressing in independent self-care. When family relationships are disturbed, the patient's illness can place an even greater strain on family ties, with deleterious effects on the patient's self-esteem and on his will to persevere in self-help training. For those patients with no family members available to care for them, discharge from the hospital almost invariably means placement in a nursing home or long-term care facility. This prospect will usually come as a terrible blow to the patient and often leads to a significant depression, the patient viewing himself as cast off with little hope of ever regaining his former state of independence. No two patients will ever face their illnesses in quite the same fashion. There are patients with profound deficits who will attain a remarkable degree of independence in spite of seemingly insurmountable obstacles, while others with apparently mild dysfunction will languish in an invalid state and never regain the slightest independence.

Whether the patient is in a hospital, nursing home, or rehabilitation facility, by the time he reaches the last phase of rehabilitation, discharge planning for continuing care should be well under way. The following elements should be included in discharge planning:

1. Establish early contact with the family to observe therapy.
2. Involve family in group sessions for education about stroke.

3. Provide counseling to patient and family.
4. Familiarize the family with self-care technique and assistive devices.
5. Set up a family meeting to learn about the patient's previous role in the family, his occupation, hobbies, and interests, and begin to establish goals for discharge.
6. Consider the type and amount of supervision that will be required at home and that which is currently available.
7. Teach the family the procedures the patient should perform regularly, such as range of motion exercises and techniques for activities of daily living.
8. Arrange weekend passes to assess the patient's ability to function at home and determine whether his rehabilitation program needs to be altered.
9. Schedule follow-up clinic visits to assess the patient's function and adaptation to his home and society and to evaluate the effectiveness of the program designed for him.

Assessment of neuromuscular abilities and disabilities prior to discharge

When the patient with stroke has a neuromuscular disability, it is recommended that, prior to discharge, a full assessment of the patient's disability be carried out and a home visit be made to determine how he can function with his disability in that setting. The evaluation should be geared to identification of limitations and deciding whether the patient can compensate for his functional disability and whether adjustments can be made in the home to facilitate this.

In assessing the patient's physical capabilities and limitations, the head, neck, and upper extremities should be evaluated for range of movement, strength, muscle tone, coordination, and presence of abnormal movements. The manner in which a particular deficit interferes with functional performance, particularly hand dexterity, should be looked at. It should be determined whether the patient has voluntary motor control or only motion in synergy. If there is no motion, he will be unable to perform bilateral hand activities. The trunk and lower extremity function should also be evaluated for movement, strength, muscle tone, coordination, and abnormal movements. The way in which deficits interfere with mobility and the need for aids such as a brace, wheelchair, or cane should be identified. Adjustments in the existing approach should be considered at this time. Perhaps the patient could become more mobile if he used a transfer board, cane, or wheelchair, for instance. Adaptive hand equipment might allow more independent self-care and recreational activities. Once the overall patient performance has been assessed adequately, the home should be looked at in terms of whether it contributes to or inhibits independent functioning.

Assessment of physical layout of home

In many cases information that can be obtained from the patient and family concerning the home setting will be adequate to plan self-care procedures. For instance, if the layout of the bathroom is provided, hospital personnel can review special techniques for transferring to the toilet and tub and use of the sink with the patient and his family while he is still in the hospital and can make suggestions for adjustments in either the transfer techniques or the layout itself. In some cases, however, it is more appropriate to have a visiting nurse or therapist visit the home and review the techniques there. This is especially important when it appears that there are architectural barriers to the patient's independent functioning. In general, the areas to be looked at in the home are the entrance to the house, the main rooms, the bedroom, the bathroom, and the kitchen. Within each of these rooms the doors, doorways, thresholds, carpeting, and hallways and stairs leading to the area should be looked at specifically. Particular attention should be given to the layout of furniture. This should be evaluated specifically for safety, ease of mobility, transfers, and maneuverability. The placement of appliances and the location of fixtures such as the telephone, thermostats, and light switches contribute to overall functioning and are important to consider from the standpoint of safety.

Following are the various areas of the home to be evaluated, with examples of those disabilities that present limiting factors, suggestions for improvement of patient performance with self-care, and recommendations for adjustments to the physical setting that might be considered.

ENTRANCES
Entrances should be evaluated in terms of accessibility from an outside walk and from a garage. If stairs lead to the entrance, it should be noted how many steps there are and whether or not there are handrails. Some patients will not have sufficient endurance to climb stairs, others will not be able to climb without the use of handrails. A high incline leading to the entrance is an obstacle to the use of a wheelchair.

Recommendations
    Install handrails.
    Purchase a wheelchair ramp.

DOORWAYS
Doorways should be wide enough to allow passage with walking aids such as canes and walkers and enough clearance for a wheelchair. A width of 36 inches is recommended. It should be noted whether doors open in or out and whether there is enough space for the patient to manipulate opening and closing. Evaluation of the patient's ability to manipulate doorknobs, latches, handles, and keys is essential. The presence of thresholds should be noted, since they may pose a hazard to the patient with hemiplegia and will present an obstacle to the patient in a wheelchair.

Recommendations
    Widen doorways, when necessary, for clearance.
    Replace existing doors with swing-through doors or folding doors.
    Obtain a wheelchair narrower.
    Install special knobs designed specifically for patients with poor hand function.
    Remove thresholds for patients who use walking aids or wheelchairs.

STAIRS

A flight of stairs may be a major obstacle to a patient with limited range of motion, decreased strength, or incoordination, and it will of course pose an absolute barrier to a patient confined to a wheelchair. The patient's ability to climb as well as descend stairs should be evaluated carefully. This is especially important for those patients who use walking aids. The presence or absence of handrails on both sides of the stariwell should be noted.

Recommendations
    Install a built-in stair lift or elevator.
    Construct a ramp in areas where there are four steps or less and sufficient space
        to provide an incline gradual enough for the patient to negotiate.
    Install handrails.

HALLWAYS

Hallways should be wide enough to permit a wheelchair to be turned around in them.

Recommendations
    If the hallway is only a few inches too narrow, change to a narrower wheelchair
        or obtain a device for reducing the width of the wheelchair temporarily.

CARPETING

All carpeting should be secured to the floor. Scatter rugs are a hazard, since the patient can trip or slide on them and fall. The pile of the carpet should allow for ease of mobility with a cane, walker, or wheelchair. Deep pile or shag rugs make ambulation and propelling a wheelchair very difficult. Any loose edges of carpeting or linoleum should be noted, and shag rugs should be avoided.

Recommendations
    Remove scatter rugs.
    Nail down borders of all rugs, carpeting, and other floor coverings, or secure edges
        with carpet tape.
    Although it may not be economically feasible to replace existing carpeting, before
        any new carpets are purchased, test the walking aids or wheelchair on them.
    Limit the patient's access to rooms carpeted with a deep shag, if it is a hazard.

SEATING

Seating should be evaluated for height and width of all chairs and sofas. Patients with limited range of motion or poor muscle strength may have difficulty getting up from a low seat. The ability to transfer from one seat to another has implications for the patient's mobility within a room, and transfer is greatly facilitated when the two points of transfer are the same height. It should be noted whether the chairs prevent the patient from getting close enough to the table or work areas to function. Some patients need the support of armrests.

Recommendations
> Elevate seats by padding with pillows so that the person has less distance from which to rise.
>
> Provide transfer boards for a transfer from wheelchair to another chair.

BATHROOM

The layout of the bathroom may be a major obstacle to independent self-care for the patient with stroke. The special techniques taught the patient for getting into and out of a bathtub or shower and transferring to and from the toilet must be evaluated in light of any structural constraints to be certain that he will be able to function safety in the bathroom. A patient with limited range of motion, poor strength, or incoordination may not be able to raise his legs over a tub rim or step over a shower threshold. A shower door may further hamper a transfer. The patient with hemiplegia may not be able to rise from a tub, or he may not be able to reach and/or manipulate the faucets. If the patient has poor balance, he will not be able to stand unassisted in a shower without the use of special grab bars. For any patient with impaired neuromuscular function there is always the danger of falling, especially with bathtub transfers. With poor strength in the lower extremities he may not be able to rise from a toilet seat. He may be further hampered by limitations of the upper extremities, which may prevent him from using grab bars to help pull himself up. The width of conventional bathroom doors — approximately 24–26 inches in apartments and 28 inches in houses — is the major obstacle to wheelchair entry.

Recommendations
> Install a raised toilet seat.
>
> Place grab bars adjacent to the toilet, tub, or shower.
>
> Install safety treads or provide nonslip mats for use in the bathtub and shower.
>
> Provide a shower seat in the bathtub.
>
> Provide a chair outside the tub or shower, so that the patient can transfer in and out of the tub from a sitting position.
>
> Provide detachable bathtub rails that can be clamped onto a tub rim to assist the patient in a transfer.

KITCHEN

A kitchen can be a particularly hazardous place for a patient with upper extremity impairment, such as hemiplegia, incoordination, limited range of motion, and/or decreased strength. When the patient has only one functional hand, he will have difficulty in operating a stove, handling pots and dishes, and removing or placing food in the refrigerator. With incoordination, items frequently may be dropped or spilled. Some dishes, pots, and pans may be too heavy to carry for patients with poor strength. Because of paralysis or weakness of the leg, the patients may be unable to get close enough to counters or cupboards. The patient who requires a wheelchair may not be able to reach the stove, counter, or refrigerator. Many utensils, staple foodstuffs, and other items used for cooking may be placed too far back on shelves or counters for the patient to reach safely.

Recommendations
A few very basic suggestions are listed below. A homemaker who is handicapped
should consult an occupational therapist for a complete homemaking evaluation.

Provide a tea cart or utility tray on wheels that may be used to wheel items that
cannot be carried from area to area.
Lower counters to accommodate the patient who is confined to a wheelchair.
Obtain a high chair so that the patient who cannot stand for a long period can
work at a high counter.
Remove cabinets (or cabinet doors) under sinks or counters to allow the patient
in a wheelchair to approach the counter.
Place kitchen items on lower shelves and on a readily accessible table to eliminate
opening and closing doors, unsafe reaching, etc.

UTILITIES
It is important that patients with limited mobility due to stroke be able to use and
control utilities such as electric lighting, heat, and hot water as well as communication devices such as the telephone, radio, and television. In reviewing the layout of
the home, the location of lighting switches, thermostats, and controls for heating
and electrical units should be noted. The placement of lamps and telephone exten-
sions should also be considered and the patient's ability to manipulate switches,
controls, and windows and to use the telephone be assessed. Patients confined to
wheelchairs may not be able to reach switches, lamps, windows, thermostats, or
telephones. The patient with a nonfunctional hand may have difficulty in turning
a regular dial to a given position or pushing a switch. He may also be unable to open
or close a window or use the dial on a telephone. These activities may be complicated further if he has visual problems.

Recommendations
If possible, have the patient move to housing specially designed to allow the handi-
capped person to live alone.
Provide pull-down lamps for people with limited reach.
Install casement windows.
Purchase a push button remote control to operate a TV.
Contact the phone company to install a special telephone designed for the handi-
capped, or simply dial "O."
Procure specifically devised rods for individual switches, knobs, or dials.

Homemaking

The need to perform household tasks will depend upon the patient's previous living
arrangements and family role and the amount of assistance that will be available upon
his return home. The patient who lives alone should be able to prepare simple meals
and carry out limited homemaking chores safely, unless arrangements can be made
for live-in help. Most women will want to resume some of their former household

responsibilities. Often men who are unable to return to work following stroke will be able to assist with household chores and preparation of meals.

Just what the patient will be capable of doing will depend on his physical limitations and ability to learn new activities and problem-solving techniques. The major obstacle to performing homemaking activities safely in hemiplegia is a nonfunctioning hand and inability to stand or ambulate without assistance. If the patient is confined to a wheelchair, the traditional household layout may pose innumerable architectural barriers. Most patients who are able to perform self-care activities, ambulate with the aid of a brace or cane, or propel a wheelchair independently can learn to prepare light meals.

In assessing the patient's ability to function safely in the kitchen, where potentially dangerous equipment must be used, memory, judgment, integrity of sensation, and visual and auditory acuity must be considered in addition to motor skills. It may be that the patient should not be allowed to perform any more complex kitchen activity than simply removing from the refrigerator a lunch that has been set up for him. Patients with impaired memory, judgment, or attention span may be able to perform certain household tasks but should never be left unattended while assisting with meal preparation. Patients with aphasia should not be left alone in the kitchen, because they will be unable to call for help in the event of an accident involving the stove, sharp knives, broken glass, or burns from hot water. Some patients who display good cognitive abilities and sound judgment will be physically unable to perform the tasks themselves but will be able to maintain responsibility for planning and supervising cooking, laundry, cleaning and shopping. Others may be able to assume responsibility for all duties involved in maintaining a household, with assistance for particularly heavy chores such as transporting laundry and carrying shopping bags full of groceries.

For the patient with only one functional hand, household chores can be simplified through the use of simple inexpensive gadgets and special techniques developed for this purpose. A cutting board with two long nails hammered into it can stabilize potatoes and other firm vegetables while they are being peeled. Mixing bowls can be held in place by means of suction cups. Quite often, even with two functional hands and a very firm grip, it is nearly impossible to remove lids from new screwtop jars. There are gadgets available to increase leverage and facilitate removal. If the cap is not sealed, usually it can be released with one hand. One method is to stabilize the jar by placing it inside a drawer that is not as deep as the jar and then to lean against the drawer to exert pressure on the jar and keep it from moving. Tongs can be substituted for forks in turning or transferring foods during preparation [15].

Quite often the affected hand is used for stabilizing food or dishes. A second hand is indispensable in meal preparation to hold food containers and utensils and keep them from sliding about while being cut, opened, or stirred. In most cases the paralyzed hand can be used to assist in holding utensils in place so that they are convenient for a one-handed approach [16]. A utility cart can be used to transport objects for meals, laundry, and other tasks that would ordinarily require two hands. The stability of the cart can be increased by placing heavy objects such as a sandbag or books on the bottom shelf. The occupational therapist can teach the patient who will be assuming full responsibility for household chores special techniques for handling cleaning implements, making beds and changing linens, and using the stove and oven as well as a variety of procedures for preparation of meals [15].

Vocational rehabilitation

Stryker has described work as central to the meaning of life for most individuals and as being as important to mental well-being as it is for economic security [26]. Vocational programs are essential for the disabled patient, who may need new techniques to continue in his present position, help in changing his job, or education or training to secure employment. Unfortunately the employment potential for patients who have suffered a stroke is quite limited.

Such disorders as aphasia, agnosia, and apraxia will pose significant problems in finding a work situation in which the patient can function safely and effectively. Severe perceptual disorders and visual disturbances may preclude employment. While the majority of patients with hemiplegia will be unable to work because of their physical limitations, some studies have indicated that as many as 30–40 percent of all hemiplegics are employable. According to Mossman, however, such statistics can be misleading, since the methods of selecting patients for rehabilitation programs preclude applying these study findings to all patients. These study results reflect the achievement of selected subjects [21]. The Community Rehabilitation Industries, Inc. of Long Beach, California, studied hemiplegia and employability and found that the most common barriers to employment were physical limitations and a reduced learning capacity due to brain damage. The potential employers cited "second injury insurance risks," "possibility of a second stroke," and "danger on the job" as their most common objections to hiring stroke victims who were left with hemiplegia [21]. The Rehabilitation Act of 1973 addressed the issue of discrimination against handicapped persons in hiring practices. However, even though a hemiplegic may have employment potential, those with the least marketable skills within the labor force will suffer when the labor market is unable to absorb all the unemployed.

Because stroke occurs more frequently in the older population, early retirement is the most frequent solution to the problem. There are, however, many patients, young and old, who might benefit from vocational counseling and placement. In the early phases of rehabilitation, the occupational therapist may begin prevocational testing to determine competence in previous skills and consider the introduction of new skills. Some hospitals and rehabilitation facilities have vocational counselors available to provide vocational evaluation. Many also have sheltered workshops, where the patient is assigned to a work area with supervision and where his performance is evaluated by a rehabilitation team to determine the feasibility of employment. Even if the patient's disability precludes his resumption of the role of a major wage earner, learning to master an avocational skill is an important part of his rehabilitation in terms of self-esteem.

Community resources

Upon completion of the rehabilitation program, the patient may still need assistance in one or more areas. The following resources are available in most communities:

(1) visiting nurse associations, which provide nursing care and supervision, physical, occupational, and speech therapy, dietary consultation, and home health aides; (2) homemaker services; (3) meals-on-wheels programs; (4) neighborhood day-care centers; (5) housing for the elderly and the handicapped; (6) outpatient rehabilitation centers and clinics; (7) counseling agencies; (8) transportation services; (9) nursing homes; and (10) state social and rehabilitative services, which provide financial assistance [26].

The nurse should be aware of the social service and health care resources available in the community and work closely with the patient's physician, social worker, therapist, dietitian, vocational counselor, and family in planning for his long-term care needs. To be truly effective this planning must begin as soon as the patient is admitted and continue on through discharge. It involves teaching and counseling as well as listening and providing emotional support to the patient and his family. Often it involves placement of a patient in a long-term care facility. Assessment of the patient's assets and liabilities at discharge and establishment of a plan for continuing care are as important as his initial neurological assessment, for they hold the key to the success or failure of the entire rehabilitative effort [21].

CONCLUSION

All the techniques for self-care described in the previous section require a great deal of effort. They may entail considerable discomfort and even pain as the patient learns to adapt to his disability. What is more, these techniques presuppose the presence of a concerned and knowledgeable individual who can provide supervision, support, both physical and emotional; and the necessary structural changes in the environment to allow the patient to function safely. Patients who have strong, supportive families and who have previously functioned well in response to stress will have less difficulty adapting to their functional losses than will patients who do not have these assets. Patients and families who have traditionally adjusted to change in only a marginal fashion may be completely incapable of dealing with the drastic alterations in body image, aspirations, interpersonal relationships, and lifestyle that will occur with stroke.

Often the nurse will be looked to for support and guidance by the family as well as by the patient. Both patient and family will be adjusting to a loss. The nurse must be aware that both may go through the stages of psychological shock, denial depression, and anxiety before coming to grips with the reality of the situation and accepting the disability. She must also be able to recognize these various stages. Unfortunately there is no simple technique for getting the patient or his family from one stage to the next. The nurse must be flexible enough to vary her approach as each stage arises. She must also understand that no real progress in rehabilitation can be achieved until the patient accepts his disability. The degree to which the family is able to accept the patient's disability will determine to what extent his disability becomes a handicap.

It is important that the nurse be able to interpret to the family the significance of any disorders the patient has, such as hemiplegia, agnosia, apraxia, or aphasia, in relation to his ability to learn new techniques and progress in self-care. She must however, be attentive to their questions and concerns, recognizing that they also may be dealing with the stages of denial, depression, and anxiety. She may have to repeat explanations and instructions. She will have to be alert for clues that indicate they are ready to learn more about the patient's disability and their role in helping him deal with it. Often she will have to help them to deal with unrealistic expectations for the patient's recovery.

Primary nursing clearly provides the ideal organizational setting for care of the patient with stroke. The primary nurse is in the best position to assess the patient's needs and structure his care so that there will be a consistent pattern with some latitude for flexibility. Her continuing relationship with the patient and his family will be most helpful in establishing realistic goals, anticipating failures, reinforcing learning, and modifying approach. By interacting with the therapists assigned to the patient in the hospital and the professional staff of the VNA, nursing home, or rehabilitation center who will be responsible for his care after discharge, she can determine that he will be prepared to function outside the hospital setting. This coordination can ease the transition process and promote continuity of care.

How close to his full potential the patient is able to come in gaining independence will rely to a great extent on his courage and determination to overcome his handicaps. The two most important sources of strength and inspiration for this are the patient's family and his primary nurse. In the end the patient's achievement of his potential, no matter how limited that may be, comes down to caring: the *patient* caring enough about himself as a person and his place in the world to fight against all odds to function independently; the *family members* caring enough to alter the structure and tempo of their lives, rearrange their homes, and call upon all their resourcefulness and ingenuity to anticipate the needs of the patient during a period when he can contribute little to the family unit; and finally the *nurse* caring enough to look beyond the ugly and annoying aspects of the stroke to the person and his particular needs.

REFERENCES

1. Bobath, B. *Adult Hemiplegia Evaluation and Treatment.* London: W. Heinemann, 1970. Pp. 1–29.
2. Bromley, I. *Tetraplegia and Paraplegia.* London: Churchill/Livingstone, 1975. Pp. 122–146.
3. Brunnstrom, S. *Movement Therapy in Hemiplegia.* New York: Harper & Row, 1970. Pp. 1–128.
4. Carroll, D. Hand function in hemiplegia. *J. Chronic Dis.* 18:493–500, 1965.
5. Clipper, M. Nursing Care of the Stroke Patient. In S. Licht (Ed.), *Stroke and Its Rehabilitation.* Baltimore: Williams & Wilkins, 1975. Pp. 171–205.
6. Covalt, N. Preventive techniques of rehabilitation for hemiplegia patients. *G. P.* 17:131–143, 1958.
7. Dervitz, H. A medical perspective of physical therapy and stroke rehabilitation. *Geriatrics* 25:123–132, 1970.

8. Feldman, D. J., Lee, P. R., et al. A comparison of functionally oriented medical care and formal rehabilitation in the management of patients with hemiplegia due to cerebrovascular disease. *J. Chronic Dis.* 15:297, 1962.

9. Feldman, L. J., and Schultz, M. E. Rehabilitation after stroke. *Cardiovasc. Nurs.* 11:29–34, 1975.

10. Flanagan, E. M. Methods of facilitation and inhibition of motor activity. *Am. J. Phys. Med.* 46:1006–1011, 1967.

11. Friedland, F. Physical Therapy. In S. Licht (Ed.), *Stroke and Its Rehabilitation.* Baltimore: Williams & Wilkins, 1975. Pp. 221–255.

12. Gersten, J. Rehabilitation Potential. In S. Licht (Ed.), *Stroke and Its Rehabilitation.* Baltimore: Williams & Wilkins, 1975. Pp. 435–471.

13. Gordan, E. E., and Kohn, K. H. Evaluation of rehabilitation methods on the hemiplegic patient. *J. Chronic Dis.* 19:3–16, 1966.

14. Hurd, G. Teaching the hemiplegic self-care. *Am. J. Nurs.* 62:64–68, 1962.

15. Kamenetz, H. Occupational Therapy for the Stroke Patient. In S. Licht (Ed.), *Stroke and Its Rehabilitation.* Baltimore: Williams & Wilkins, 1975. Pp. 347–379.

16. Klinger, J. L., Frieden, F. H., and Sullivan, R. *Mealtime Manual for the Aged and Handicapped.* New York: Institution of Rehabilitation Medicine, 1970. Pp. 2–7.

17. Krusen, F., Kottke, F., and Ellwood, P. *Handbook of Physical Medicine and Rehabilitation.* Philadelphia: Saunders, 1971. Pp. 452–472; 521–565.

18. Lawton, E. *Activities of Daily Living for Physical Rehabilitation.* New York: McGraw-Hill, 1963. Pp. 1–7.

19. Licht, S. Stroke Rehabilitation Program. In S. Licht (Ed.), *Stroke and Its Rehabilitation.* Baltimore: Williams & Wilkins, 1975. Pp. 206–220.

20. Lowman, E., and Klinger, J. *Aids to Independent Living.* New York: McGraw-Hill, 1969. Pp. 234–266.

21. Mossman, P. *A Problem Oriented Approach to Stroke Rehabilitation.* Springfield, Ill.: Thomas, 1976. Pp. 154–169; 171–185; 250–360.

22. Peszczynski, M. Rehabilitation of the Hemiplegic. *Annual Volume of Physiology and Experimental Sciences,* Vol. 4, 1962–1963.

23. Peszczynski, M. Rehabilitation in Hemiplegia. In S. Licht (Ed.), *Rehabilitation and Medicine.* Baltimore: Williams & Wilkins, 1968. Pp. 390–410.

24. Report of the Joint Commission for Stroke Facilities. Stroke rehabilitation. *Stroke* 3:373–407, 1972.

25. Reynolds, G. G. Problems of sensorimotor learning in the evaluation and treatment of the adult hemiplegic patient. *Rehabil. Lit.* 20:163–174, 1959.

26. Stryker, R. *Rehabilitative Aspects of Acute and Chronic Nursing Care.* Philadelphia: Saunders, 1972. Pp. 146–215.

27. Twitchell, T. The restoration of motor function following hemiplegia in man. *Brain* 74:443–480, 1951.

Index

Acalculia, 117, 125, 128
Acid-base balance, 163, 164, 228, 235, 239–245
 buffer systems, 240
Acidosis, 164, 206, 236, 238, 242–243
Activities of daily living, (ADL), 72, 147, 151, 325–339
Agnosia, 2, 31, 129, 135, 140–143, 147, 151–152, 362
 auditory, 125, 141–142, 152
 verbal, 125, 127, 129, 141–142
 tactile, 142–143
Agraphia, 117, 120, 125, 147
Airway obstruction, 160, 162, 164–166, 182, 242
 airway patency maintenance, 166–170, 173–174, 178, 250, 285, 295
 communication with patient, 168, 169, 172–173
 complications of, 164
 infection prevention, 169–170, 171, 173
 secretion control and suctioning, 166–172, 178, 180, 181
 by tube, 166–173, 177–178, 291
  tracheostomy, 166, 168, 170, 172, 173, 177, 178, 181, 295
Alertness, 38, 42, 52, 76–77, 104
Alexia, 117, 120, 125, 127
Alkalosis, 164, 237, 239, 240, 241–245
Ambulation, 286, 320, 321, 324, 328, 338–341, 361. See also Walking (gait) impairment
Amygdala, 45, 46, 63
Anemia, 4, 165, 185, 192
Aneurysm. See Saccular aneurysm, ruptured
Angina pectoris, 189, 191, 212, 213, 219
Angiography (arteriography), 3, 6, 11, 108–109, 191
Angular gyrus, 116, 117, 120
Ankle impairment, 93–94, 100, 296, 298, 299, 311, 321–323
Anomia, 116, 120, 125, 127, 241–242
Anoxia, 170, 191, 211, 282
Antiarrhythmic agents, 208–211
Anticoagulant therapy, 4, 7, 185, 196, 197, 202, 209, 212

Antidiuretic hormone (ADH; vasopressin) secretion, 43, 44, 229, 234, 235
 inappropriate (IADH syndrome), 234
Antifibrolysin (Amicar), 11
Antihypertensive agents, 214–224
Aorta, 53, 59, 187–189
Aphasia, 24, 32, 78, 114–134, 141–142
 communication problems, 172, 248, 253, 320
 and feeding difficulties, 252
 psychological aspects, 130–133
 and rehabilitation, 361, 362
 sign of stroke, 1, 2, 3, 6, 8, 10, 11, 13
Apraxia, 13, 14, 31, 127, 143–145, 147, 150–151, 253, 321, 338, 342, 362
 constructional, 144
 dressing, 145
Archicerebellar syndrome, 49
Arm impairment and care, 99, 105–106, 297–301, 306, 322–325, 328, 338, 342. See also Hand, wrist, and finger impairment and care
 exercises, 314–315
 flaccidity, 294
 muscle stretch reflexes, 103
 screening procedure, 93–96
 and Wallenberg syndrome, 90
Arm sling, 301, 328, 331, 338
Arrhythmias, 5–6, 76, 191–192, 194, 202, 203, 205, 208–212, 236
Arteries, 2, 12–16, 188, 199. See also Cerebral arteries and specific arteries
Arteriosclerosis, 187, 189
Astereognosia. See Body image and self-awareness disturbances
Asynergy, 15, 49, 97, 98
Ataxia, 1, 13, 15, 16, 49, 88, 95, 97–99, 106, 223, 324
 cerebellar, 3, 16, 97
Atelectasis, 71, 160, 164, 171, 174–175, 181, 198
Atherosclerosis, 2, 4, 5, 16, 76, 185, 189–191, 192
Auditory area, 26
Auditory pathway, 41